Free Video  **Free Video**

Essential Test Tips Video from Trivium Test Prep

Dear Customer,

Thank you for purchasing from Trivium Test Prep! We're honored to help you prepare for your EMT exam.

To show our appreciation, we're offering a **FREE** *EMT Essential Test Tips* **Video by Trivium Test Prep.*** Our video includes 35 test preparation strategies that will make you successful on the EMT. All we ask is that you email us your feedback and describe your experience with our product. Amazing, awful, or just so-so: we want to hear what you have to say!

To receive your **FREE** *EMT Essential Test Tips* **Video**, please email us at 5star@triviumtestprep.com. Include "Free 5 Star" in the subject line and the following information in your email:

1. The title of the product you purchased.

2. Your rating from 1 – 5 (with 5 being the best).

3. Your feedback about the product, including how our materials helped you meet your goals and ways in which we can improve our products.

4. Your full name and shipping address so we can send your **FREE** *EMT Essential Test Tips* **Video.**

If you have any questions or concerns please feel free to contact us directly at 5star@triviumtestprep.com.

Thank you!

– Trivium Test Prep Team

*To get access to the free video please email us at 5star@triviumtestprep.com, and please follow the instructions above.

EMT STUDY GUIDE:

Comprehensive Review Materials
with Practice Test Questions for
the NREMT Exam

E. M. Falgout

TABLE OF CONTENTS

ONLINE RESOURCES

To help you fully prepare for your EMT exam, Ascencia includes online resources with the purchase of this study guide.

Practice Test

In addition to the practice test included in this book, we also offer an online exam. Since many exams today are computer based, getting to practice your test-taking skills on the computer is a great way to prepare.

From Stress to Success

Watch "From Stress to Success," a brief but insightful YouTube video that offers the tips, tricks, and secrets experts use to score higher on the exam.

Reviews

Leave a review, send us helpful feedback, or sign up for Ascencia promotions—including free books!

Access these materials at **ascenciatestprep.com/emt-online-resources.**

INTRODUCTION

Congratulations on choosing to take the National Registry of Emergency Medical Technicians (NREMT) exam! Passing the EMT exam is an important step forward in your health care career. In the following pages, you will find information about the exam, what to expect on test day, how to use this book, and the content covered on the exam.

The Certification Process

The **National Registry of Emergency Medical Technicians (NREMT)** provides certifications for prehospital emergency providers. To become certified, the **Emergency Medical Technician (EMT)** candidate must:

- complete a state-approved EMT course within the two years prior to certification

- possess a current Basic Life Support (BLS) for health care provider card (or equivalent)

- pass the NREMT cognitive exam (a written multiple-choice test)

- pass the NREMT psychomotor exams (a practical skills test)

Candidates must have completed or be currently enrolled in an EMT course before they are approved to take the NREMT exams. If the candidate does not pass both exams within two years of completing the course, they must repeat the EMT course.

To apply for the exams, the EMT candidate should create an account at www.NREMT.org and submit an application. Approved candidates will receive an **Authorization to Test (ATT)** that is valid for 90 days. Candidates who successfully complete their EMT certification will then need to obtain the necessary state licensure to practice as an EMT.

Most states do not require the EMT to maintain their NREMT certification after receiving a state license. However, some EMTs may need to go through the recertification every two years to maintain their NREMT certification. These EMTs can recertify in one of two ways:

1. Complete 40 hours of continuing education.

2. Take the written exam (only one attempt is allowed).

The Cognitive Exam
QUESTIONS AND TIMING

The NREMT **cognitive exam** includes 70 to 120 multiple-choice questions. Ten of these questions are not scored and are instead used by NREMT to test new questions. Candidates have two hours to complete the exam.

The exam covers five content areas (see table below). In all content areas except EMS Operations, 85 percent of the questions are related to adults and 15 percent are related to pediatrics.

EMT Cognitive Exam Content Outline	
Content Area	**Percentage of Exam**
Airway, Respiration, and Ventilation	18 – 22%
Cardiology and Resuscitation	20 – 24%
Trauma	14 – 18%
Medical; Obstetrics and Gynecology	27 – 31%
EMS Operations	10 – 14%

The cognitive exam is a computer-adaptive test (CAT). In a CAT, the computer adapts to the examinee's abilities, selecting questions based on the examinee's responses. When the examinee answers a question correctly, the next question the computer presents is more difficult than the last. If the examinee answers a question incorrectly, the computer offers a question of lesser difficulty.

Remember: because CAT adapts to your abilities, once you submit an answer, you CANNOT go back to change your answer to a previous question.

ADMINISTRATION

The EMT cognitive exam is administered by Pearson VUE at testing centers around the nation. Arrive at least 30 minutes before the exam. Bring proper ID and a printed copy of your ATT (found in your online NREMT account). Expect the testing center to use biometric scanning (a fingerprint or palm print) and to take your picture.

You must bring two forms of ID to the testing center. The primary ID must be government issued and include a recent photograph and signature. The secondary ID must have your name and signature. The names on both IDs must match the name on your ATT. If you do not have proper ID, you will not be allowed to take the test.

You will not be allowed to bring any personal items, such as calculators or phones, into the testing room. You may not bring pens, pencils, or scratch paper. Prohibited items also include hats, scarves, and coats. You may wear religious garments, however. Most testing centers provide lockers for valuables.

An untimed tutorial will be provided before the exam. You will also have time to read and sign a nondisclosure agreement before the exam begins.

RESULTS

Cognitive exam results are posted within five business day to the candidate's NREMT account. The results for each test category will be denoted as follows:

- Above Passing: The candidate displayed enough knowledge to pass.

- Near Passing: The candidate may or may not have displayed enough knowledge to pass.

- Below Passing: The candidate has not displayed enough knowledge to pass.

Candidates who pass each category can apply to a state for an EMT license. Candidates who do not pass the exam can apply to take the exam again after 15 days. If the candidate fails three times, they must complete remedial training before they can take the test again. If the candidate fails the test six times, they must retake an initial EMT course.

The Psychomotor Exam
SKILLS

The **psychomotor exam** is a standardized, hands-on test in which the EMT candidate must perform specific emergency medical skills. Skills are demonstrated on simulated patients using real equipment. The EMT candidate is graded using standard NREMT performance checklists. Each skill has **critical criteria**, which is a list of items that if performed incorrectly will lead to automatic failure.

The psychomotor exam consists of seven skills:

- Patient Assessment/Management – Trauma

- Patient Assessment/Management – Medical

- Bag-Valve Mask (BVM) Ventilation of an Apneic Adult Patient

- Oxygen Administration by Non-Rebreather Mask

- Cardiac Arrest Management/AED

- Spinal Immobilization (Supine Patient)

- Random EMT Skill (one)
    - Spinal Immobilization (Seated Patient)
    - Bleeding Control/Shock Management
    - Long Bone Immobilization
    - Joint Immobilization

ADMINISTRATION

The psychomotor exam is administered by state EMS officials or other agents approved by the state EMS. Candidates should schedule the exam either through their EMT training course or through the state EMS office.

On the day of the exam, candidates will gather at the testing site. You should bring a government-issued ID and plan to leave your phone or other communication devices locked in a secure location. When it is your turn to test, you will be called into the testing room where a skill examiner will guide you through the scenarios and grade your performance. (See chapter twelve, "The Psychomotor Exam," for more details on how the exam is conducted.)

RESULTS

Availability of exam results will vary depending on state EMS guidelines. They may be communicated to candidates on testing day, or candidates may have to wait longer. All results will be available in the candidate's NREMT account.

Candidates must pass all seven skills to earn their certification.

- If a candidate fails three or fewer skills, they are eligible to retake those skills twice. If the candidate fails those skills twice, they must take remedial education courses before retaking the full exam.

- If a candidate fails four or more skills, they must take remedial education courses before retaking the full exam.

- Candidates who fail the exam twice must take another complete EMT training course before retesting.

Using This Book

This book is divided into two sections. In the content area review, you will find a summary of the knowledge and skills included in the exam content outline. Throughout the chapter you'll also see practice questions that will reinforce important concepts and skills.

The book also includes two full-length practice tests (one in the book and one online) with answer rationales. You can use these tests to gauge your readiness for the test and determine which content areas you may need to review more thoroughly.

Ascencia Test Prep

With health care fields such as nursing, pharmacy, emergency care, and physical therapy becoming the fastest-growing industries in the United States, individuals looking to enter the health care industry or rise in their field need high-quality, reliable resources. Ascencia Test Prep's study guides and test preparation materials are developed by credentialed industry professionals with years of experience in their respective fields. Ascencia recognizes that health care professionals nurture bodies and spirits, and save lives. Ascencia Test Prep's mission is to help health care workers grow.

ONE: HUMAN ANATOMY and PHYSIOLOGY

The Biological Hierarchy

- The biological hierarchy is a systematic breakdown of the structures of the human body organized from smallest to largest (or largest to smallest).

- The smallest unit of the human body is the **cell**, a microscopic, self-replicating structure that performs many different jobs.

- **Tissues** comprise the next largest group of structures in the body; they are a collection of cells that all perform a similar function. The human body has four basic types of tissue:

  - **Connective** tissues—which include bones, ligaments, and cartilage—support, separate, or connect the body's various organs and tissues.

  - **Epithelial** tissues are found in the skin, blood vessels, and many organs.

  - **Muscular** tissues contain contractile units that pull on connective tissues to create movement.

  - **Nervous** tissue makes up the peripheral nervous systems that transmit impulses throughout the body.

- **Organs** are a collection of tissues within the body that share a similar function (e.g., the esophagus or heart).

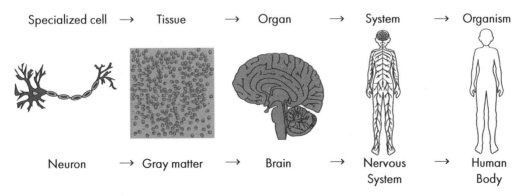

Figure 1.1. Biological Hierarchy and Levels of Organization

- **Organ systems** are a group of organs that work together to perform a similar function (e.g., the digestive system).

- Finally, an **organism** is the total collection of all the parts of the biological hierarchy working together to form a living being; it is the largest structure in the biological hierarchy.

PRACTICE QUESTION

1. The meninges are membranes that surround and protect the brain and spinal cord. What type of tissue would the meninges be classified as?

HELPFUL HINT

In anatomy, the terms *right* and *left* are used with respect to the subject, not the observer.

Directional Terminology and Planes

- When discussing anatomy and physiology, specific terms are used to refer to directions.

- Directional terms include the following:
  - **inferior**: away from the head
  - **superior**: closer to the head
  - **anterior**: toward the front
  - **posterior**: toward the back
  - **dorsal**: toward the back
  - **ventral**: toward the front
  - **medial**: toward the midline of the body
  - **lateral**: farther from the midline of the body
  - **proximal**: closer to the trunk
  - **distal**: away from the trunk

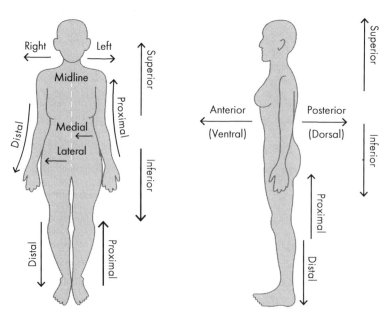

Figure 1.2. Directional Terminology

- The human body is divided by three imaginary planes.
  - The transverse plane divides the body into a top and bottom half.
  - The coronal (frontal) plane divides the body into a front and back half.
  - The sagittal plane divides the body into a right and left half.

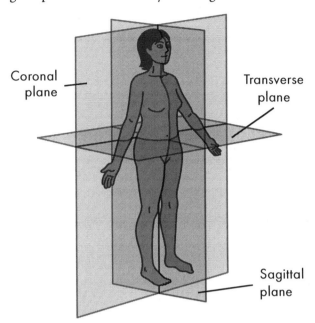

Figure 1.3. Planes of the Human Body

PRACTICE QUESTION

2.   Which directional term describes the neck relative to the head?

The Cardiovascular System
STRUCTURE AND FUNCTION OF THE CARDIOVASCULAR SYSTEM

- The cardiovascular system circulates **blood**, which carries nutrients, waste products, hormones, and other important substances dissolved or suspended in liquid **plasma**.
  - **Red blood cells (RBCs)** transport oxygen throughout the body. RBCs contain **hemoglobin**, a large molecule with iron atoms that bind to oxygen.
  - **White blood cells (WBCs)** fight infection.
- The circulatory system is a closed double loop.
  - In the **pulmonary loop**, deoxygenated blood leaves the heart and travels to the lungs, where it loses carbon dioxide and becomes rich in oxygen. The oxygenated blood then returns to the heart.
  - The heart then pumps blood through the **systemic loop**, which delivers oxygenated blood to the rest of the body and returns deoxygenated blood to the heart.

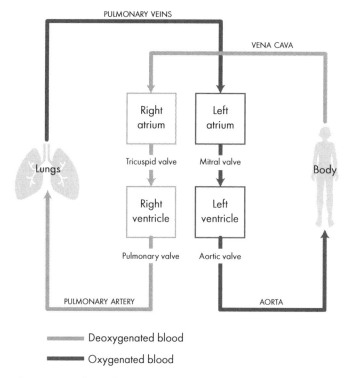

Figure 1.4. The Pulmonary and Systemic Loops

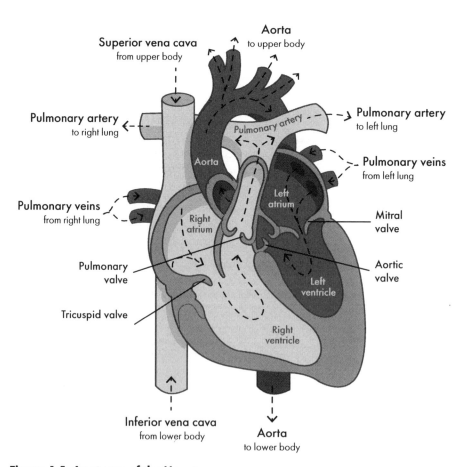

Figure 1.5. Anatomy of the Heart

- The heart has four chambers: the left atrium, right atrium, left ventricle, and right ventricle.
  - The **right atrium** collects blood from the body.
  - The **right ventricle** pumps blood to the lungs.
  - The **left atrium** collects blood from the lungs.
  - The **left ventricle** pumps blood to the body.
  - The atria are separated by the **atrial septum**, and the ventricles by the **ventricular septum**.
- The **atrioventricular valves** are located between the atria and ventricles and cause the first heart sounds (S1) when they close.
  - The **tricuspid valve** separates the right atrium and right ventricle.
  - The **mitral valve** separates the left atrium and left ventricle.
- The two **semilunar valves** are located between the ventricles and great vessels and cause the second heart sound (S2) when they close.
  - The **pulmonic valve** separates the right ventricle and pulmonary artery.
  - The **aortic valve** separates the left ventricle and aorta.
- The heart includes several layers of tissue:
  - **pericardium**: the outermost protective layer of the heart, which contains a lubricative liquid
  - **epicardium**: the deepest layer of the pericardium, which envelops the heart muscle
  - **myocardium**: the heart muscle
  - **endocardium**: the innermost, smooth layer of the heart walls

HELPFUL HINT
The movement of blood to tissues through the capillaries is called **perfusion**.

- Blood leaves the heart and travels throughout the body in **blood vessels**, which decrease in diameter as they move away from the heart and toward the tissues and organs.
- Blood exits the heart through **arteries**.
- The arteries branch into **arterioles** and then **capillaries**, where gas exchange between blood and tissue takes place.
- Deoxygenated blood travels back to the heart through **veins**.
- Some veins have valves that prevent deoxygenated blood from flowing back to the extremities.
- Blood is supplied to the heart by coronary arteries: the **right coronary artery (RCA)**, **left anterior descending (LAD) artery**, and **left circumflex artery**.

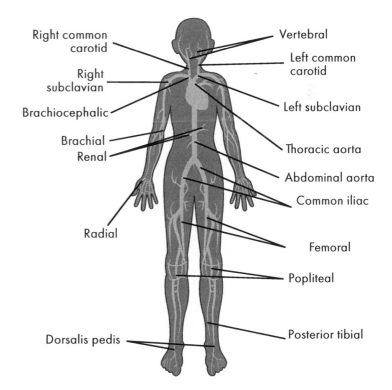

Figure 1.6. Major Arteries

- The heart's pumping action is regulated by the **cardiac conduction system**, which produces and conducts electrical signals in the heart.
  - The **sinoatrial (SA) node** sets the heart's pace by sending out electrical signals that cause the atria to contract. It is located in the anterior wall of the right atrium.
  - The **atrioventricular (AV) node** relays the electrical impulse of the sinoatrial node to the ventricles. The impulse is delayed to allow the atria to fully contract and fill the ventricles. The node is located at the base of the right atrial wall.
- **Stroke volume (SV)**, the volume of blood pumped from the left ventricle during one contraction, depends on several conditions:
  - **preload**: how much the ventricles stretch at the end of diastole
  - **afterload**: the amount of resistance needed for the heart to open the aortic valve and force blood into circulation
  - **contractility**: the force of the heart, independent of preload and afterload
- Normal SV is 60 – 130 mL per contraction.
- **Heart rate (HR)** is how many times the ventricles contract each minute.

Table 1.1. Normal Heart Rates		
Age	**Normal Heart Rate: Awake (bpm)**	**Normal Heart Rate: Sleeping (bpm)**
Newborn to 3 months	85 – 205	80 – 160
3 months to 2 years	100 – 180	75 – 160
2 – 10 years	60 – 140	60 – 90
10 years	60 – 100	50 – 90

- **Cardiac output (CO)** is the volume of blood that the heart pumps every minute.
  - To calculate CO, multiply SV by HR.
  - Normal CO is 4 – 8 L per minute.

PRACTICE QUESTION

3. Left-sided heart failure can cause pulmonary edema, while right-sided heart failure is more likely to cause edema in the abdomen and extremities. How does the anatomy of the heart produce this difference?

CARDIAC MONITORING

- An **electrocardiogram (ECG)** is a noninvasive diagnostic tool that records the heart's cardiac rhythm and rate.
- An ECG can help diagnose myocardial infarctions (MI), electrolyte imbalances, and other damage to the heart.

- The readout from the ECG, often called an **ECG strip**, is a continuous waveform whose shape corresponds to each stage in the cardiac cycle.

  - **P wave**: right and left atrial contraction

  - **QRS complex**: contraction of the ventricles

  - **T wave**: relaxation of the ventricles

- A normal heart rhythm and rate is called **normal sinus rhythm.**

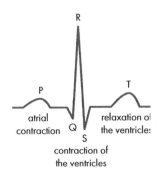

Figure 1.7. Waveforms and Intervals on an ECG

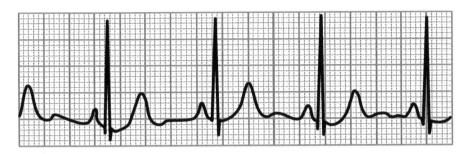

Figure 1.8. ECG: Normal Sinus Rhythm

- A **12-Lead ECG** is performed by placing 10 electrodes in specific locations on the patient's chest, arms, and legs.

  - In order for the leads to stick to the skin, the patient's skin has to be clean and dry.

  - If there is excess chest hair, it is sometimes necessary to shave the area to keep the lead on the skin.

  - Patients, especially those with breasts, should be offered a cover for the chest once electrode lead placement is done.

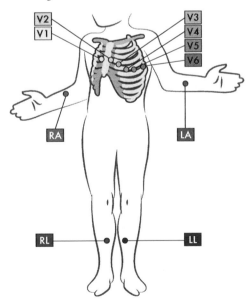

Figure 1.9. 12-Lead ECG Electrode Placement Diagram

Table 1.2. 12-Lead ECG Electrode Placement

Electrode	Placement
V1	fourth intercostal space to the right of the sternum
V2	fourth intercostal space to the left of the sternum
V3	midway between V2 and V4
V4	fifth intercostal space at the midclavicular line
V5	anterior axillary line at the same level as V4
V6	midaxillary line at the same level as V4 and V5
RA	between right shoulder and right wrist
LA	between left shoulder and left wrist
RL	above right ankle and below the torso
LL	above left ankle and below the torso

PRACTICE QUESTION

4. If a rhythm is missing P waves or has an excessive number of P waves, which area of the heart is having difficulty conducting?

CARDIAC DEVICES

- A **pacemaker** is a device that uses electrical stimulation to regulate the heart's electrical conduction system and maintain a normal heart rhythm.

  - **Permanent pacemakers** are implanted subcutaneously, and the leads are then run through the subclavian vein into the heart. The device is battery operated and allows the physician to continuously monitor the patient's rhythm.

  - **Temporary pacemakers** can include transvenous leads or transcutaneous adhesive pads attached to the chest. Temporary pacemakers are controlled by an external pulse generator and are used to maintain normal heart rhythm in critical care settings.

  - Signs of pacemaker malfunction include chest pain, palpitations, dizziness, syncope, and weakness.

  - If the patient has an implanted pacemaker, ensure that automated external defibrillator (AED) pads are placed at a distance from the pacemaker to avoid interference with the shock (about 1 inch is recommended).

DID YOU KNOW?
Strong magnets can reset the settings on pacemakers and ICDs, causing them to malfunction.

- An **implantable cardioverter defibrillator (ICD)** continuously monitors heart rhythms and emits an electric shock that terminates emergent dysrhythmias such as V-tach and V-fib, preventing cardiac arrest.

- **Left ventricular assist devices (LVADs)** provide support for weakened left ventricles in patients with end-stage heart failure.

- A mechanical pump is placed in the left ventricle. The pump moves blood from the left ventricle to the ascending aortic branch, from which it can be further circulated to the rest of the body.
- The LVAD is battery operated, and patients can remain on the device for months to years.
- EMTs should check with medical control before beginning CPR or administering nitroglycerin to patients with LVADs.

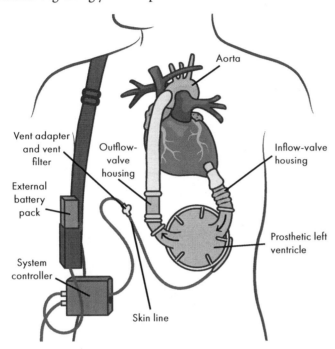

Figure 1.10. Left Ventricular Assist Device

PATHOLOGIES OF THE CARDIOVASCULAR SYSTEM

- **Ischemia** is reduced or restricted blood flow to tissues caused by:
  - occlusion of blood vessels by an **embolus** (a mass made of fat, bacteria, or other materials) or **thrombus** (blood clot; also called a thromboembolism)
  - narrowed blood vessel (e.g., aneurysm or atherosclerosis)
  - trauma
- **Infarction** is the death of tissue caused by restricted blood flow and the subsequent lack of oxygen.
- **Atherosclerosis**, also called atherosclerotic cardiovascular disease (ASCVD), is a progressive condition in which **plaque** (composed of fat, white blood cells, and other waste) builds up in the arteries.
  - Atherosclerosis can occur in any artery and is categorized according to the location of the plaque buildup.
    - **coronary artery disease (CAD):** narrowing of the coronary arteries
    - **peripheral artery disease (PAD):** narrowing of the peripheral arteries

- The presence of advanced atherosclerosis places patients at a high risk for several cardiovascular conditions.
  - Arteries may become **stenotic**, or narrowed, limiting blood flow to specific areas of the body (e.g., carotid stenosis).
  - When a plaque **ruptures**, the plaque and the clot that forms around it (superimposed thrombus) can quickly lead to complete occlusion of the artery (e.g., MI).
  - The clots or loosened plaque released by a rupture may also move through the bloodstream and occlude smaller vessels (e.g., ischemic stroke).
  - Atherosclerosis is also a cause of **aneurysms** (widened arteries), which weaken arterial walls, increasing the risk of arterial dissection or rupture (e.g., abdominal aortic aneurysm [AAA]).
- **Dysrhythmias** are abnormal heart rhythms.
  - **Bradycardia** is a heart rate < 60 bpm.
    - Bradycardia is normal in certain individuals and does not require an intervention if the patient is stable.
    - Symptomatic patients, however, need immediate treatment to address the cause of bradycardia and to correct the dysrhythmia.
  - **Atrial fibrillation (A-fib)** is a rapid, irregular contraction of the atria.
    - During A-fib, the heart cannot adequately empty, causing blood to pool and clots to form. These clots can break off and travel to the heart or brain, causing a heart attack or stroke.
    - The irregular atrial contractions also decrease cardiac output.
  - **Atrioventricular (AV) block** is the disruption of electrical signals between the atria and ventricles. The electrical impulse may be delayed (first degree), intermittent (second degree), or completely blocked (third degree).
  - During **ventricular fibrillation (V-fib)** the ventricles contract rapidly (300 – 400 bpm) with no organized rhythm. There is no cardiac output.

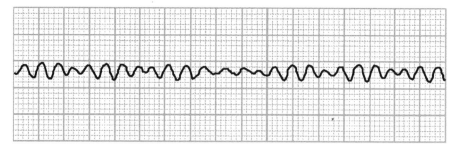

Figure 1.11. Ventricular Fibrillation

- **Ventricular tachycardia (V-tach)** is tachycardia originating in the ventricles with > 3 consecutive ventricular beats occurring at a rate > 100 bpm.
  - Because the ventricles cannot refill before contracting, patients in this rhythm may have reduced cardiac output, resulting in hypotension.

- V-tach may be short and asymptomatic, or it may precede V-fib and cardiac arrest.

- ○ **Pulseless electrical activity (PEA)** is an organized rhythm in which the heart does not contract with enough force to create a pulse. PEA is a nonshockable rhythm with a poor survival rate.

- ○ **Asystole**, also called a "flat line," occurs when there is no electrical or mechanical activity within the heart. Like PEA, asystole is a nonshockable rhythm with a poor survival rate.

DID YOU KNOW?
V-fib and V-tach are the two *shockable rhythms*, meaning they can be corrected using an automatic external defibrillator.

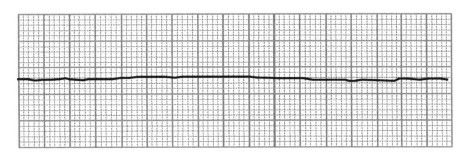

Figure 1.12. Asystole

- **Heart failure** occurs when either one or both of the ventricles in the heart cannot efficiently pump blood.

  - ○ The condition is typically due to another disease or illness, most commonly CAD.

  - ○ Because the heart is unable to pump effectively, blood and fluid back up into the lungs (causing pulmonary congestion), or the fluid builds up peripherally (causing edema of the lower extremities).

  - ○ Heart failure is most commonly categorized into **left-sided heart failure** or **right-sided heart failure**, although both sides of the heart can fail at the same time.

- **Hemophilia** is a recessive, X-chromosome-linked bleeding disorder characterized by the lack of coagulation factors.

  - ○ Generally, the condition is seen in males. Females usually only act as carriers, but female carriers can develop symptoms.

  - ○ The deficiency in coagulation factors causes abnormal bleeding after an injury or medical procedure, and spontaneous bleeding can occur in patients with severe hemophilia.

- **Sickle cell disease** is an inherited form of hemolytic anemia that causes deformities in the shape of the RBCs.

  - ○ When oxygen levels in the venous circulation are low, the RBCs dehydrate and form a sickle shape. This process can be exacerbated by exposure to cold temperatures or high altitudes.

  - ○ Sickle cell disease is a chronic disease that can lead to complications that require emergency care:

HELPFUL HINT

See chapter 4, "Cardiovascular Emergencies," for a more detailed discussion of cardiac conditions commonly seen by EMTs.

- **Vaso-occlusive pain** (previously called sickle cell crisis): sickle-shaped cells clump together and restrict blood flow, causing localized ischemia, inflammation, and severe pain.
- **Acute chest syndrome (ACS)**: vaso-occlusion in the lungs (often after an infection) that exacerbates the sickle formation of RBCs.
- Infection: the leading cause of death for children with sickle cell disease; common infections include bacteremia, pneumonia, and osteomyelitis.
- Priapism: a common complication for men with sickle cell disease.

PRACTICE QUESTION

5. An EMT has attached an AED to a patient, and the AED advised a shock is necessary. What possible cardiac rhythms has the AED identified in the patient?

The Respiratory System
STRUCTURE AND FUNCTION OF THE RESPIRATORY SYSTEM

- The **respiratory system** is responsible for the exchange of gases between the human body and the environment.

- **Oxygen** is brought into the body for use in glucose metabolism, and the **carbon dioxide** created by glucose metabolism is expelled.

- Gas exchange takes place in the **lungs.**
  - Humans have a **right lung** and **left lung**. The right lung is slightly larger than the left.
  - The right lung has three **lobes**, and the left has two.
  - The lungs are surrounded by a thick membrane called the **pleura.**

- Respiration begins with pulmonary ventilation, or **breathing.**

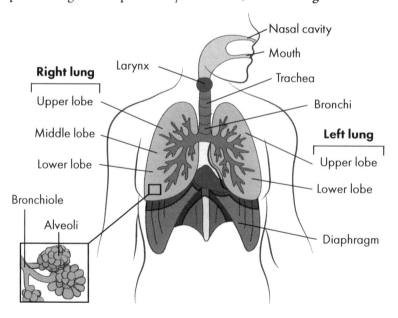

Figure 1.13. The Respiratory System

- The first stage of breathing is **inhalation**. During this process, the thoracic cavity expands and the diaphragm muscle contracts, which decreases the pressure in the lungs, pulling in air from the atmosphere.

- Air is drawn in through the **nose** and **mouth**, then into the throat, where cilia and mucus filter out particles before the air enters the **trachea**.

- The **epiglottis** prevents food or other materials from entering the trachea.

- Once it passes through the trachea, the air passes through either the left or right **bronchi**, which are divisions of the trachea that direct air into the left or right lung.

- These bronchi are further divided into smaller **bronchioles**, which branch throughout the lungs and become increasingly smaller.

- Eventually, air enters the **alveoli**—tiny air sacs located at the ends of the smallest bronchioles. The alveoli have very thin membranes, only one cell thick, and are the location of gas exchange with the blood.

- Carbon dioxide is then expelled from the lungs during **exhalation**, the second stage of breathing. During exhalation, the diaphragm relaxes and the thoracic cavity contracts, causing air to leave the body because the lung pressure is now greater than the atmospheric pressure.

- Lung function can be gauged by measuring the volume of air moved by the lungs. Important values include:
  - **total lung capacity**: amount of air in the lungs when full
  - **tidal volume**: amount of air inhaled or exhaled during normal breathing
  - **residual volume**: amount of air left in the lungs after a large exhalation

PRACTICE QUESTION

6. Describe the pathway air follows once it has been inhaled through the nostrils.

PATHOLOGIES OF THE RESPIRATORY SYSTEM

- Disruptions to the respiratory system can result in abnormal breathing patterns.
  - **eupnea**: normal breathing
  - **tachypnea**: rapid breathing
  - **bradypnea**: slow breathing
  - **dyspnea**: difficulty breathing
  - **apnea**: not breathing
  - **hyperventilation**: increase in rate or volume of breaths, which causes excessive elimination of CO_2
  - **agonal breathing**: irregular gasping breaths accompanied by involuntary twitching or jerking. Agonal breathing is associated with severe hypoxia and is a sign the patient requires immediate medical treatment.

- **Biot's breathing**: alternating rapid respirations and apnea. Causes include stroke, trauma, and opioid use.
- **Cheyne-Stokes breathing**: deep breathing alternating with apnea or a faster rate of breathing; associated with left heart failure or sleep apnea
- **Kussmaul breathing**: type of hyperventilation characterized by deep, labored breathing that is associated with metabolic acidosis

HELPFUL HINT

See chapter 3, "Respiratory Emergencies," for a more detailed discussion of respiratory conditions EMTs commonly see.

- The lungs and kidneys work together to maintain a blood pH between 7.35 and 7.45.
  - **Acidosis** is abnormally low (acidic) blood pH.
  - **Alkalosis** is abnormally high (alkaline or basic) blood pH.
  - Disruption in blood pH can be caused by respiratory or metabolic factors (see Table 1.3).

Table 1.3. Causes and Symptoms of Acidosis and Alkalosis

Abnormality	pH	Common Causes	Symptoms
Respiratory acidosis	decreased	asthma, COPD	anxiety, dyspnea, lethargy, confusion, delirium
Respiratory alkalosis	increased	hyperventilation	dyspnea, dizziness, numbness or tingling in extremities, spasms of hands and feet
Metabolic acidosis	decreased	diabetic disorders, diarrhea or vomiting, kidney dysfunction	Kussmaul breathing; non-specific symptoms such as chest pain, altered mental status, and nausea
Metabolic alkalosis	increased	kidney dysfunction or diabetic disorders	usually asymptomatic; patient may have symptoms related to underlying condition

PRACTICE QUESTION

7. Kussmaul breathing is a symptom associated with what disorder?

The Skeletal System
STRUCTURE AND FUNCTION OF THE SKELETAL SYSTEM

- The skeletal system is made up of over 200 different **bones**, a stiff connective tissue in the human body.
- The bones have many functions, including:
  - protecting internal organs
  - synthesizing blood cells
  - storing necessary minerals
  - providing the muscular system with leverage to create movement

- Bones are covered with a thin layer of vascular connective tissue called the periosteum, which serves as a point of muscle attachment, supplies blood to the bone, and contains nerve endings.

- **Osseous tissue** is the primary tissue that makes up bone. There are two types of osseous tissue: cortical (compact) bone and cancellous (spongy) bone.

  o **Cortical bone** is the dense, solid material that surrounds the bone and gives it hardness and strength. It is usually concentrated in the middle part of the bone.

  o **Cancellous bone** is less dense, more porous, and softer. It is located at the ends of long bones, where it does not bear a structural load.

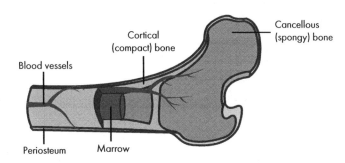

Figure 1.14. Structure of Bone

HELPFUL HINT

Long bones are longer than they are wide. The term is usually used to refer to the long bones of the arm and leg, such as the femur and humerus.

- Bone marrow is stored in cancellous bone.

  o **Red bone marrow** is responsible for producing red blood cells, platelets, and white blood cells.

  o **Yellow bone marrow** is composed mostly of fat tissue and can be converted to red bone marrow in response to extreme blood loss in the body.

- The hundreds of bones in the body make up the human **skeleton.**

- The **axial skeleton** contains 80 bones that support and protect many of the body's vital organs. It has 3 major subdivisions:

  o the skull, which contains the cranium and facial bones

  o the thorax, which includes the sternum and 12 pairs of ribs

  o the vertebral column, which contains the body's vertebrae

- The **vertebral column,** or the **spine,** is made up of 24 vertebrae, plus the sacrum and the coccyx (the tailbone). These 24 vertebrae are divided into three groups:

  o the cervical, or the neck vertebrae (7 bones)

  o the thoracic, or the chest vertebrae (12 bones)

  o the lumbar, or the lower back vertebrae (5 bones)

- The **appendicular skeleton's** 126 bones make up the body's appendages. The main function of the appendicular skeleton is locomotion.

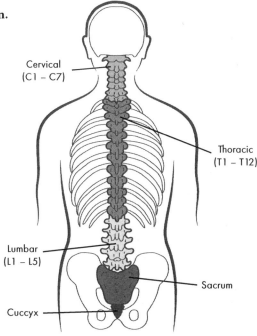

Figure 1.15. The Vertebral Column

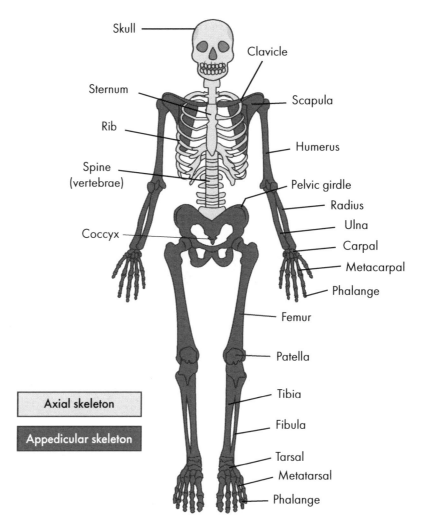

Skull
Clavicle
Sternum
Scapula
Rib
Humerus
Spine (vertebrae)
Pelvic girdle
Radius
Ulna
Coccyx
Carpal
Metacarpal
Phalange
Femur
Patella
Tibia

Axial skeleton

Appedicular skeleton

Fibula
Tarsal
Metatarsal
Phalange

Figure 1.16. The Axial and Appendicular Skeletons

- Various connective tissues join the parts of the skeleton together to other systems.

  ○ **Ligaments** join bone to bone.

  ○ **Tendons** join bones to muscles.

  ○ **Cartilage** cushions the bones in joints, provides structural integrity for many body parts (e.g., the ear and nose), and maintains open pathways (e.g., the trachea and bronchi).

- The point at which a bone is attached to another bone is called a joint. There are three basic types of joints:

  ○ **Fibrous joints** connect bones that do not move.

  ○ **Cartilaginous joints** connect bones with cartilage and allow limited movement.

  ○ **Synovial joints** allow for a range of motion and are covered by articular cartilage that protects the bones.

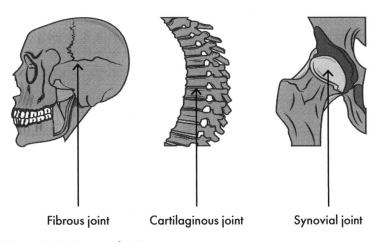

| Fibrous joint | Cartilaginous joint | Synovial joint |

Figure 1.17. Types of Joints

PRACTICE QUESTION

8. A patient is complaining of severe lower back pain after a fall. Which vertebrae has the patient possibly injured?

PATHOLOGIES OF THE SKELETAL SYSTEM

- **Rheumatoid arthritis** is a type of inflammation at the joint caused by chronic autoimmune disorder, which can lead to excessive joint degradation. The immune system attacks healthy joint tissue, making the joints stiff and causing the cartilage and bone to deteriorate.

- **Osteoporosis** is poor bone mineral density due to the loss or lack of the production of calcium content and bone cells, which makes bones more likely to fracture.

- **Osteomyelitis** is an infection in the bone that can occur directly (after a traumatic bone injury) or indirectly (via the vascular system or other infected tissues).

PRACTICE QUESTION

9. An EMT is doing a head-to-toe assessment of a 75-year-old patient who fell in the bathtub. The patient states she has severe pain in both hands. She states the pain has increased recently, and she is progressively losing function of her hands. The EMT notes that the joints in both hands are reddened, swollen, and disfigured. What condition should the EMT suspect is causing her pain?

The Muscular System

STRUCTURE AND FUNCTION OF THE MUSCULAR SYSTEM

- The primary function of the muscular system is movement: muscles contract and relax, resulting in motion.

- The muscular system consists of three types of muscle: cardiac, visceral, and skeletal.

  ○ **Cardiac muscle** is only found in the heart. It is a **striated** muscle, with alternating segments of thick and thin filaments, that contracts involuntarily, creating the heartbeat and pumping blood.

  ○ **Visceral**, or **smooth**, **muscle** tissue is found in many of the body's essential organs, including the stomach and intestines. It slowly contracts and relaxes to move nutrients, blood, and other substances throughout the body. Visceral muscle movement is involuntary.

  ○ **Skeletal muscle** is responsible for voluntary movement and, as the name suggests, is linked to the skeletal system.

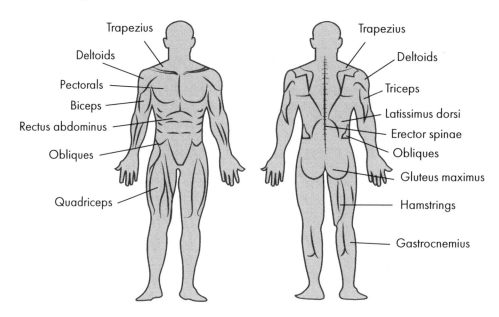

Figure 1.18. Major Muscles of the Body

PRACTICE QUESTION

10. During assessment of a patient with possible heat cramps, the patient complains of severe pain in his lower right leg. What muscle is most likely causing the patient's pain?

PATHOLOGIES OF THE MUSCULAR SYSTEM

- **Muscular dystrophy (MD)** is a genetically inherited condition that results in progressive muscle wasting, which limits movement and can cause respiratory and cardiovascular difficulties.

- **Rhabdomyolysis** is the rapid breakdown of dead muscle tissue.

  ○ Common symptoms of rhabdomyolysis include dark urine, muscle pain, and muscle weakness.

- Rhabdomyolysis can be caused by crush injuries, overexertion (particularly in extreme heat), and a variety of drugs and toxins (particularly statins, which are prescribed to lower cholesterol levels).

- Muscle cramps are involuntary muscle contractions (or **spasms**) that cause intense pain.

PRACTICE QUESTION

11. What symptoms should an EMT expect to see in an adult patient with muscular dystrophy?

The Nervous System
STRUCTURE AND FORM OF THE NERVOUS SYSTEM

- The **nervous system** coordinates the processes and action of the human body.

- **Nerve cells,** or **neurons,** communicate through electrical impulses and allow the body to process and respond to stimuli.

  - Neurons have a nucleus and transmit electrical impulses through their axons and dendrites.

  - The **axon** is the stem-like structure, often covered in a fatty insulating substance called **myelin,** that carries information to other neurons throughout the body.

  - **Dendrites** receive information from other neurons.

- The nervous system is broken down into two parts: the **central nervous system (CNS)** and the **peripheral nervous system (PNS).**

  - The CNS is made up of the brain and spinal cord.

    - The **brain** acts as the control center for the body and is responsible for nearly all the body's processes and actions.

    - The **spinal cord** relays information between the brain and the peripheral nervous system; it also coordinates many reflexes.

    - The spinal cord is protected by the vertebral column, a structure of bones that enclose the delicate nervous tissue.

  - The PNS is the collection of nerves that connect the central nervous system to the rest of the body.

- The brain is composed of myelinated **white matter** and unmyelinated **gray matter.**

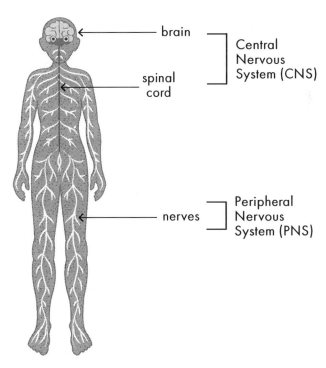

Figure 1.19. The Nervous System

- The **meninges** form a protective coating over the brain and spinal cord. They consist of three layers:
  - The outermost layer is the **dura mater.** The epidural space (above the dura) and the subdural space (below the dura) contain vasculature that can bleed following injury to the brain.

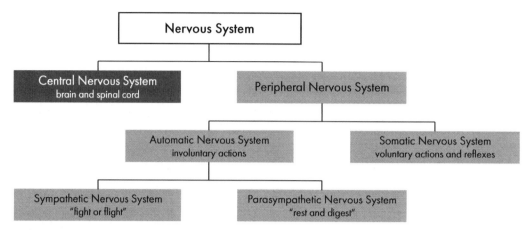

Figure 1.20. Divisions of the Nervous System

- The **arachnoid mater** is below the dura mater.
- The **pia mater** is the innermost layer that is attached to the CNS.
- The functions of the nervous system are broken down into the somatic nervous system and the autonomic nervous system.
  - The **somatic nervous system** is responsible for the body's ability to control skeletal muscles and voluntary movement as well as the involuntary reflexes associated with skeletal muscles.
  - The **autonomic nervous system** controls involuntary actions that occur in the body, such as respiration, heartbeat, digestive processes, and more.
- The autonomic nervous system is further broken down into the sympathetic nervous system and parasympathetic nervous system.
  - The **sympathetic nervous system** is responsible for the body's reaction to stress and induces a "fight or flight" response to stimuli. The "fight or flight" reaction includes accelerated breathing and heart rate, dilation of blood vessels in muscles, release of energy molecules for use by muscles, relaxation of the bladder, and slowed or stopped movement in the upper digestive tract.
  - The **parasympathetic nervous system** is stimulated by the body's need for rest or recovery. The parasympathetic nervous system responds by decreasing the heart rate, blood pressure, and muscular activation when a person is getting ready for activities such as sleeping or digesting food.

PRACTICE QUESTION

12. Many neurological disorders are the result of demyelination, the loss of myelin from neurons. Why would the lack of a myelin sheath impact the functions of the nervous system?

PATHOLOGIES OF THE NERVOUS SYSTEM

- **Syncope** (fainting) is the temporary loss of consciousness caused by the brief decrease of blood flow to the brain brought on by hypotension.
  - Syncope typically causes muscle weakness and collapse, which may lead to fall injuries.
  - The causes of syncope are generally grouped into three categories:
    - Syncope can also be caused by underlying cardiac conditions, such as dysrhythmias or coronary artery disease.
    - **Reflex syncope** is neurologically mediated and occurs as a result of stress, pain, or specific triggers such as coughing.
    - **Orthostatic syncope** is caused by a drop in blood pressure after standing.

- **Alzheimer's disease** is characterized by the loss of memory and deteriorating cognitive function, usually later in life, due to the degeneration of neurons in the brain.
  - The disease is a form of dementia that progresses gradually and has no known cure.
  - Onset usually occurs past age 60 but can also occur as early as age 40.

- **Multiple sclerosis (MS)** involves the gradual breakdown and scarring of the myelin sheaths on axons, causing disruption of nervous transmission of impulses.
  - The nerve damage associated with MS causes vision trouble, difficulty walking, fatigue, pain, involuntary spasms, and numerous other symptoms.
  - This disease is thought to be genetic, and there is no known cure. However, treatments are available to slow the disease's progression.

- **Amyotrophic lateral sclerosis (ALS)**, sometimes called Lou Gehrig's disease, is a neurodegenerative disorder that affects the neurons in the brain stem and spinal cord.
  - ALS presents with progressive, asymmetrical weakness.
  - Symptoms progressively worsen until the respiratory system is affected; ALS is ultimately fatal.

- **Peripheral neuropathy** is impairment of the peripheral nerves.
  - Common causes include diabetes (diabetic neuropathy), autoimmune conditions, and infections.
  - Peripheral neuropathy can cause pain and impair motor or sensory function.

PRACTICE QUESTION

13. An EMT responds to a call for an unconscious 56-year-old male. When she arrives at the scene, the EMT finds the patient alert and oriented. What details in the patient's history should lead an EMT to suspect orthostatic syncope?

The Gastrointestinal System
STRUCTURE AND FORM OF THE GASTROINTESTINAL SYSTEM

- The gastrointestinal system is responsible for the breakdown and absorption of food necessary to power the body.

- The gastrointestinal system starts at the **mouth**, which allows for the consumption and mastication of nutrients via an opening in the face.
  - The mouth contains the muscular **tongue** to move food and uses the liquid **saliva** to assist in the breakdown of food.

- The chewed and lubricated food travels from the mouth through the **esophagus** via **peristalsis**, the contraction of smooth muscles.

- The esophagus leads to the **stomach**, the organ of the digestive tract found in the abdominal cavity that mixes food with powerful acidic liquid for further digestion.
  - The stomach creates an acidic bolus of digested food known as **chyme**.

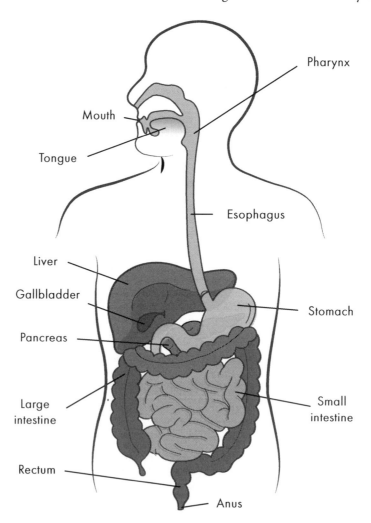

Figure 1.21. The Gastrointestinal System

- Chyme travels to the **small intestine,** where a significant amount of nutrient absorption takes place.
  - The tube-like small intestine contains millions of finger-like projections known as **villi** and microvilli to increase the surface area available for the absorption of nutrients found in food.
- The small intestine then transports food to the **large intestine.**
  - The large intestine is similarly tube-like but larger in diameter than the small intestine.
  - The large intestine assists in water absorption, further nutrient absorption, waste collection, and the production of feces for excretion.
- At the end of the large intestine is the **rectum,** which stores feces.
- Feces are expelled through the **anus.**
- Along the digestive tract are several muscular rings, known as **sphincters,** which regulate the movement of food through the tract and prevent reflux of material into the previous cavity.
- The digestive system also includes accessory organs that aid in digestion:
  - **salivary glands:** produce saliva, which begins the process of breaking down starches and fats
  - **liver:** produces bile, which helps break down fat in the small intestine
  - **gallbladder:** stores bile
  - **pancreas:** produces pancreatic juice, which neutralizes the acidity of chyme, and digestive enzymes

PRACTICE QUESTION

14. What role does the liver play in digestion?

PATHOLOGIES OF THE DIGESTIVE SYSTEM

- **Food poisoning** occurs when an acute infection (bacterial or viral) affects the lining of the digestive system and the resulting immune response triggers the body to void the contents of the digestive system.
- **Irritable bowel syndrome (IBS)** refers to recurrent abdominal pain, bloating, diarrhea, or constipation.
- **Crohn's disease** is an inflammatory bowel disorder that occurs when the immune system attacks the digestive system.
- **Cirrhosis** is a chronic disease in which the liver has permanent scarring and loses cells, impairing normal functioning.
  - Symptoms of cirrhosis include jaundice, bruising easily, ascites, and asterixis.
  - Cirrhosis can also decrease blood flow to the liver; the resulting hypertension in the portal vein can lead to related conditions, including an enlarged spleen and esophageal varices.

- Common causes of liver cirrhosis include hepatitis, chronic alcohol abuse, and hemochromatosis (excess iron).
- **Heartburn** occurs when the lower esophageal sphincter does not close completely, allowing stomach acid to move into the esophagus.
- **Peritonitis** is inflammation of the peritoneum (the lining of the abdominal cavity). It can cause **ileus**, paralysis of the digestive tract, resulting in severe pain, nausea, and vomiting.

PRACTICE QUESTION

15. Why do patients with cirrhosis often experience bleeding in their esophagus?

The Immune System
STRUCTURE AND FUNCTION OF THE IMMUNE SYSTEM

- The human **immune system** protects the body against bacteria and viruses that cause disease.
  - The **innate immune system** includes nonspecific defenses (physical barriers and immune cells) that work against a wide range of infectious agents.
  - The **adaptive immune system** "learns" to respond only to specific invaders.
- The body has a number of innate defense systems against pathogens that enter the body.
  - **Barriers to entry** (e.g., skin, mucus) prevent pathogens from entering the body.
  - **Inflammation** increases blood flow to the infected area, bringing large numbers of **white blood cells** (WBCs, also called **leukocytes**) to fight the infection.
- The adaptive immune system relies on molecules called antigens that appear on the surface of pathogens to which the system has previously been exposed.
  - In the cell-mediated response, **T cells** destroy any cell that displays an antigen.
  - In the antibody-mediated response, **B cells** are activated by antigens and release antibodies that destroy the targeted cells.
- During an infection, **memory B cells** specific to an antigen are created, allowing the immune system to respond more quickly if the infection appears again.

PRACTICE QUESTION

16. Breastmilk contains antibodies from the mother's immune system. How do these antibodies protect breastfeeding infants from infection?

PATHOLOGIES OF THE IMMUNE SYSTEM

- The immune system of individuals with an **autoimmune disease** will attack healthy tissues. Autoimmune diseases (and the tissues they attack) include:
    - psoriasis (skin)
    - rheumatoid arthritis (joints)
    - multiple sclerosis (nerve cells)
    - lupus (kidneys, lungs, and skin)

- **Leukemia** is cancer of the WBCs. It occurs in the bone marrow, disrupting the production of WBCs and platelets.

- **Human immunodeficiency virus (HIV)** attacks T cells, eventually causing **acquired immunodeficiency syndrome (AIDS)**, which allows opportunistic infections to overrun the body.

PRACTICE QUESTION

17. What signs and symptoms should an EMT expect to see in a patient diagnosed with leukemia?

The Endocrine System
STRUCTURE AND FORM OF THE ENDOCRINE SYSTEM

- The endocrine system is made up of **glands** that regulate numerous processes throughout the body by secreting chemical messengers called **hormones.**

- Hormones regulate a wide variety of bodily processes, including metabolism, growth and development, sexual reproduction, the sleep-wake cycle, and hunger.

Table 1.4. Endocrine Glands and Their Functions

Gland	Regulates	Hormones Produced
Adrenal glands	"fight or flight" response and regulation of salt and blood volume	epinephrine, norepinephrine, cortisol, androgens
Hypothalamus	pituitary function and metabolic processes including body temperature, hunger, thirst, and circadian rhythms	thyrotropin-releasing hormone (TRH), dopamine, growth-hormone-releasing hormone (GHRH), gonadotropin-releasing hormone (GnRH), oxytocin, vasopressin
Ovaries	maturation of sex organs, secondary sex characteristics, pregnancy, childbirth, and lactation	progesterone, estrogens
Pancreas	blood glucose levels and metabolism	insulin, glucagon, somatostatin

Table 1.4. Endocrine Glands and Their Functions (continued)

Gland	Regulates	Hormones Produced
Parathyroid	calcium and phosphate levels	parathyroid hormone (PTH)
Pineal gland	circadian rhythms (the sleep-wake cycle)	melatonin
Pituitary gland	growth, blood pressure, reabsorption of water by the kidneys, temperature, pain relief, and some reproductive functions related to pregnancy and childbirth	human growth hormone (HGH), thyroid-stimulating hormone (TSH), prolactin (PRL), luteinizing hormone (LH), follicle-stimulating hormone (FSH), oxytocin, antidiuretic hormone (ADH)
Placenta	gestation and childbirth	progesterone, estrogens, human chorionic gonadotropin, human placental lactogen (hPL)
Testes	maturation of sex organs and secondary sex characteristics	androgens (e.g., testosterone)
Thyroid gland	energy use and protein synthesis	thyroxine (T_4), triiodothyronine (T_3), calcitonin

PRACTICE QUESTION

18. Which endocrine gland regulates blood glucose levels?

PATHOLOGIES OF THE ENDOCRINE SYSTEM

- Hormone production in endocrine glands can be disrupted by disease, tumors, or congenital conditions.

- **Diabetes mellitus** is a metabolic disorder that affects the body's ability to produce and use **insulin**, a hormone that regulates cellular uptake of glucose (sugar).
  - Uncontrolled diabetes can lead to high blood glucose levels (**hyperglycemia**) or low blood glucose levels (**hypoglycemia**).
  - Diabetes mellitus is classified as type 1 or type 2.
    - **Type 1 diabetes** is an acute-onset autoimmune disease predominant in children, teens, and adults < 30 years. Beta cells in the pancreas are destroyed and are unable to produce sufficient amounts of insulin, causing blood glucose to rise.
    - **Type 2 diabetes** is a gradual-onset disease predominant in adults 40 years, but it can develop in individuals of all ages. The person develops insulin resistance, which prevents the cellular uptake of glucose and causes blood glucose to rise. Type 2 diabetes accounts for 90 percent of all diabetes diagnoses in the United States.
  - Diabetes requires long-term management with insulin or oral hypoglycemic drugs.

DID YOU KNOW?
Over 30 million Americans have been diagnosed with diabetes. In the US, more money is spent on health care related to diabetes than on any other single medical condition.

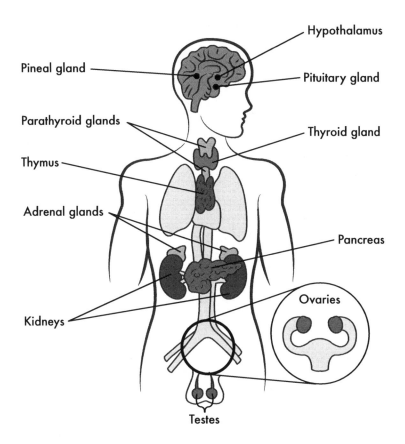

Figure 1.22. The Location of Endocrine Glands

- **Hypothyroidism** occurs when insufficient thyroxine is produced and can result in fatigue, weight gain, and cold intolerance.

- **Hyperthyroidism** occurs when too much thyroxine is produced and can cause anxiety, mood swings, weight loss, and palpitations.

- **Adrenal insufficiency** (Addison's disease) is the chronic underproduction of steroids.

  o Signs and symptoms of adrenal insufficiency include fatigue, nausea, hypotension, and darkening of the skin.

  o Adrenal insufficiency can cause shock.

PRACTICE QUESTION

19. How is insulin production and use affected by type 1 and type 2 diabetes?

The Reproductive System
THE MALE REPRODUCTIVE SYSTEM

- The male reproductive system produces **sperm**, or male gametes, and passes them to the female reproductive system.

- Sperm are produced during **spermatogenesis** in the **testes** (also called testicles), which are housed in a sac-like external structure called the **scrotum**.

- Mature sperm are stored in the **epididymis**.

- During sexual stimulation, sperm travel from the epididymis through a long, thin tube called the **vas deferens**. Along the way, the sperm are joined by fluids from three glands:

  ○ The **seminal vesicles** secrete a fluid composed of various proteins, sugars, and enzymes.

  ○ The **prostate** contributes an alkaline fluid that counteracts the acidity of the vaginal tract.

  ○ The **Cowper's gland** secretes a protein-rich fluid that acts as a lubricant.

- The mix of fluids and sperm, called **semen**, travels through the **urethra** and exits the body through the **penis**, which becomes rigid during sexual arousal.

- The main hormone associated with the male reproductive system is **testosterone**, which is released mainly by the testes.

  ○ Testosterone is responsible for the development of the male reproductive system and male secondary sexual characteristics, including muscle development and facial hair growth.

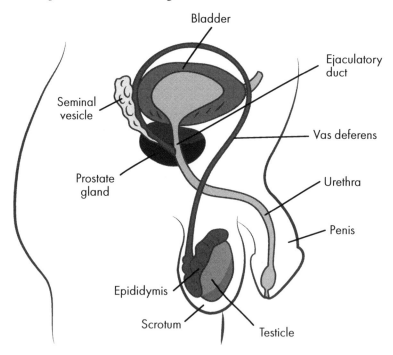

Figure 1.23. The Male Reproductive System

PRACTICE QUESTION

20. What role does the urethra play in the male reproductive system?

THE FEMALE REPRODUCTIVE SYSTEM

- The female reproductive system produces **eggs**, or female gametes, and gestates the fetus during pregnancy.

- Eggs are produced in the **ovaries** and travel through the **fallopian tubes** to the **uterus**, which is a muscular organ that houses the fetus during pregnancy.

- The uterine cavity is lined with a layer of blood-rich tissue called the **endometrium**.

  - If no pregnancy occurs, the endometrium is shed monthly during **menstruation**.

- An opening in the uterus called the **cervix** leads to the **vagina**.

- **Fertilization** occurs when the egg absorbs the sperm; it usually takes place in the fallopian tubes but may happen in the uterus itself. (See chapter 9, "Obstetrical Emergencies" for anatomy and physiology of pregnancy.)

- The female reproductive cycle is controlled by several different hormones, including **estrogen** and **progesterone**.

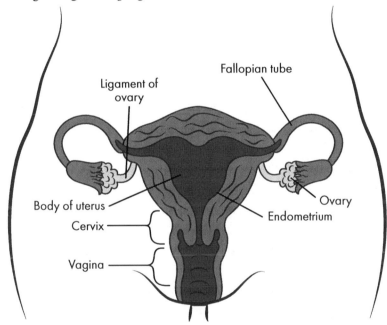

Figure 1.24. The Female Reproductive System

PRACTICE QUESTION

21. What is the role of the fallopian tubes in the female reproductive system?

PATHOLOGIES OF THE REPRODUCTIVE SYSTEM

- **Sexually transmitted infections (STIs)** occur in both males and females.

  - **Chlamydia** is caused by the bacteria *Chlamydia trachomatis*; it is the most commonly reported STI in the United States.

- The infection can be found in the cervix, urethra, rectum, or pharynx.
- Symptoms include vaginal, penile, or rectal discharge; vaginal bleeding; and lower abdominal pain.
- Chlamydia infections may be asymptomatic for long periods.
  - **Gonorrhea** is caused by the gram-negative diplococcus *Neisseria gonorrhoeae*; it is the second highest reported STI in the United States.
    - Common infection sites include the cervix, vagina, rectum, and pharynx.
    - Symptoms include painful urination; itching and burning; and vaginal, penile, or rectal discharge.
    - Gonorrhea infections may be asymptomatic, especially in women.
  - **Genital herpes** is an STI caused by the two strains of the herpes simplex virus (HSV-1 and HSV-2).
    - Both strains cause blisters on the mouth, anus, or genital area.
    - The first outbreak after the initial infection is the most severe; recurrent outbreaks, which vary in frequency and duration, will generally be less severe.
  - **Syphilis** is an STI caused by the bacteria *Treponema pallidum*.
    - The first sign of infection is **chancres** (sores) that appear 3 to 6 weeks after infection.
    - Syphilis is a progressive disease: severe cardiovascular and neurological symptoms may appear if the disease is left untreated for years.
- Inflammation of the epididymis (**epididymitis**), testes (**orchitis**), and prostate (**prostatitis**) can cause pain, swelling, and painful urination in males. The inflammation is usually caused by infection.
- **Pelvic inflammatory disease (PID)** is an infection of the upper organs of the female reproductive system, including the uterus, fallopian tubes, and ovaries.
  - The infection, usually chlamydia or gonorrhea, ascends from the cervix or vagina.
  - PID is often asymptomatic; left untreated, it can lead to infertility and increased risk of cancer.
- **Ovarian cysts** form in the ovaries and are usually asymptomatic. However, the cysts can burst, causing sudden, intense pelvic pain.
- **Priapism** is an unintentional, prolonged erection that is unrelated to sexual stimulation and is unrelieved by ejaculation.
  - **Ischemic (low-flow) priapism** occurs when blood becomes trapped in the erect penis.
  - Ischemic priapism is considered a medical emergency requiring immediate intervention to preserve function of the penis.
- **Penile fractures** occur when there is a rupture of the penis's internal membranes; they are medical emergencies that require immediate treatment.

- **Testicular torsion** occurs when the spermatic cord, which supplies blood to the testicles, becomes twisted, leading to an ischemic testicle. The condition is considered a medical emergency that requires immediate treatment to preserve the function of the testicle.

PRACTICE QUESTION

22. Why is it important for patients diagnosed with an STI to be treated even if they have no symptoms?

The Urinary System

STRUCTURE AND FUNCTION OF THE URINARY SYSTEM

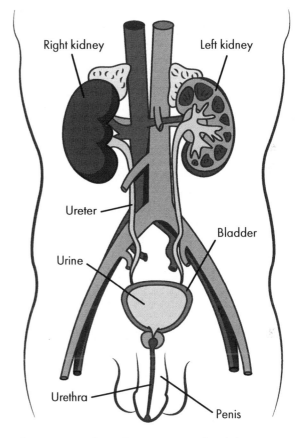

Figure 1.25. The Urinary System (Male)

- The **urinary system** excretes water and waste from the body and is crucial for maintaining the balance of water and salt in the blood (also called electrolyte balance).

- The main organs of the urinary system are the **kidneys**, which perform several important functions:
  - filter waste from the blood
  - maintain the electrolyte balance in the blood
  - regulate blood volume, pressure, and pH

- **Nephrons** in the kidneys filter the blood and excrete the waste products as **urine**.

- Urine passes out of the kidneys through the **renal pelvis** and then through two long tubes called **ureters**.

- The two ureters drain into the **urinary bladder**, which holds up to one liter of liquid.

- Urine exits the bladder through the **urethra**.
  - In males, the urethra goes through the penis and also carries semen.
  - In females, the much shorter urethra ends just above the vaginal opening.

PRACTICE QUESTION

23. What structure drains the urine into the bladder?

PATHOLOGIES OF THE URINARY SYSTEM

- **Renal calculi** (kidney stones) are hardened mineral deposits that form in the kidneys. They are usually asymptomatic but will cause debilitating pain and urinary symptoms once they pass into the urinary tract.

- **Urinary tract infections (UTIs)** can occur in the lower urinary tract (bladder and urethra) or in the upper urinary tract (kidneys and ureters). Symptoms include frequent, painful urination; cloudy, foul-smelling urine; and pelvic or lower abdominal pain.
- **Pyelonephritis**, infection of the kidneys, occurs when bacteria reach the kidney via the lower urinary tract or the bloodstream.
    - The clinical triad for kidney infections is fever, nausea or vomiting, and costovertebral pain.
    - Pyelonephritis can damage organs, can be a life-threatening infection, and will lead to renal scarring without prompt diagnosis and treatment.
- **Renal failure** is the loss of kidney function that leads to buildup of waste in the bloodstream. It can be acute or chronic.
    - **Acute renal failure** (also called acute kidney injury) occurs quickly as a result of hypovolemia, shock, infection, or obstruction of the urinary tract.
    - **Chronic kidney disease** is the progressive and irreversible loss of kidney function over months or years. The most common causes of chronic kidney disease are diabetes mellitus and hypertension.

PRACTICE QUESTION

24. An EMT is assessing a patient with complaints of bloody urine and severe side and back pain. The patient is alert and oriented with no abnormal vital signs. What condition should the EMT suspect?

The Integumentary System

- The **integumentary system** refers to the skin (the largest organ in the body) and related structures, including the hair and nails.
- **Skin** is composed of three layers.
    - The **epidermis** is the outermost layer of the skin. This waterproof layer contains no blood vessels and acts mainly to protect the body.
    - Under the epidermis lies the **dermis**, which consists of dense connective tissue that allows skin to stretch and flex. The dermis is home to blood vessels, glands, and **hair follicles**.
    - The **hypodermis** is a layer of fat below the dermis that stores energy (in the form of fat) and acts as a cushion for the body. The hypodermis is sometimes called the **subcutaneous layer**.
- The skin has several important roles.
    - It acts as a barrier to protect the body from injury, the intrusion of foreign particles, and the loss of water and nutrients.
    - Skin helps **thermoregulation**: blood vessels near the surface of the skin can dilate to release heat and contract to conserve heat.
    - The skin houses nerve endings that sense temperature, pressure, and pain.

- Skin produces vitamin D when exposed to sunlight.
- **Sweat glands** release the water and salt mixture (sodium chloride, NaCl) called **sweat.**
  - Sweat helps the body maintain the appropriate salt-water balance.
  - Sweat can also contain small amounts of other substances the body needs to expel, including alcohol, lactic acid, and urea.

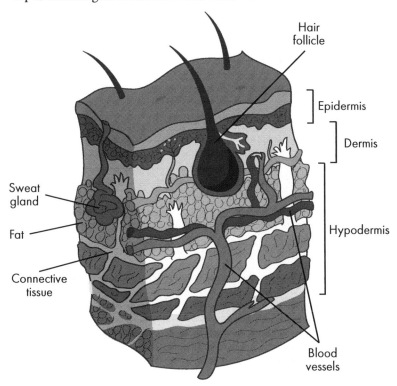

Figure 1.26. The Skin

PRACTICE QUESTION

25. What is the outermost layer of the skin called?

Pharmacology

- **Pharmacology** is the science of drugs and their effects on the human body.
  - Medications work by bonding to receptors on cells in the body and either amplifying or inhibiting the activity of those cells.
  - **Agonists** bond to receptors to amplify activity.
  - **Antagonists** (blockers) bond to receptors to block the receptor sites, inhibiting the cell's normal functioning.
- Drugs are grouped into classes based on their chemical structures and the conditions they treat. The major drug classes, their general purpose, and examples of each are given in Table 1.5.

Table 1.5. Common Medications

Drug Class	Purpose	Example(s) generic name (brand name)
Antibiotics	inhibit growth of or kill bacteria	penicillin; amoxicillin; ciprofloxacin
Anticoagulants (blood thinners)	prevent blood clots	rivaroxaban (Xarelto); warfarin (Coumadin)
Anticonvulsants	prevent seizures	carbamazepine (Tegretol); topiramate (Topamax)
Antidepressants	treat depression and mood disorders	fluoxetine (Prozac); sertraline (Zoloft); bupropion (Wellbutrin, Zyban)
Antihistamines	treat allergies	diphenhydramine (Benadryl)
Antipsychotics	manage psychosis	aripiprazole (Abilify); lithium carbonate
Antivirals	inhibit growth of or kill viruses	docosanol (Abreva); oseltamivir (Tamiflu)
Barbiturates	depress the central nervous system	amobarbital (Amytal Sodium); butabarbital (Butisol Sodium); phenobarbital (Nembutal)
Benzodiazepines	reduce anxiety and relax muscles	alprazolam (Xanax); clonazepam (Klonopin); diazepam (Valium); lorazepam (Ativan)
Beta blockers	reduce blood pressure and improve blood flow	acebutolol (Sectral); atenolol (Tenormin); metoprolol (Lopressor); propranolol (Inderal)
Calcium channel blockers	relax and widen blood vessels	amlodipine (Norvasc); diltiazem (Cardizem); felodipine (Plendil); nifedipine (Procardia)
Corticosteroids	reduce inflammation	dexamethasone (Decadron); prednisone (Sterapred)
Diuretics	increase the output of urine	furosemide (Lasix); valsartan (Diovan)
Histamine-2 blockers	reduce stomach acid	famotidine (Pepcid); ranitidine (Zantac)
Hypnotics	reduce anxiety and induce sleep	eszopiclone (Lunesta); zolpidem (Ambien)
Immunosuppressants	suppress the immune system	adalimumab (Humira); methotrexate (Trexall)
Local anesthetics	block sensation in a small area	benzocaine; lidocaine (Xylocaine, Lidoderm)
Neuromuscular blockers	paralyze skeletal muscles	pancuronium (Pavulon); rocuronium (Zemuron)

Drug Class	Purpose	Example(s) generic name (brand name)
Nonsteroidal anti-inflammatory drugs (NSAIDs)	reduce pain and inflammation	ibuprofen (Motrin, Advil); naproxen (Aleve, Naprosyn)
Opioid pain relievers	block pain signals in brain	morphine (Astramorph, Duramorph); oxycodone (Percocet, OxyContin)
Proton pump inhibitors	reduce stomach acid	esomeprazole (Nexium); lansoprazole (Prevacid); omeprazole (Prilosec)

- **Adverse drug reaction** is a broad term used to describe unwanted, uncomfortable, or dangerous effects resulting from taking a specific medication.
  - Most adverse drug reactions are dose related, but they can also be allergic or idiosyncratic (unexpected responses that are neither dose related nor allergic responses).
  - Adverse drug reactions are one of the leading causes of morbidity and mortality in health care.
  - They can be classified by severity as:
    - mild (e.g., drowsiness)
    - moderate (e.g., hypertension)
    - severe (e.g., abnormal heart rhythm)
    - lethal (e.g., liver failure)
  - Adverse drug reactions are classified into six types, which are described in Table 1.6.

Table 1.6. Adverse Drug Reactions

Type	Description	Example
A augmented	predictable reactions arising from the pharmacological effects of the drug; dependent on dose	diarrhea due to antibiotics; hypoglycemia due to insulin
B bizarre	unpredictable reactions; independent of dose	hypersensitivity (anaphylaxis) due to penicillin
C chronic	reactions caused by the cumulative dose (the dose taken over a long period of time)	osteoporosis with oral steroids
D delayed	reactions that occur after the drug is no longer being taken	teratogenic effects with anticonvulsants
E end of use	reactions caused by withdrawal from a drug	withdrawal syndrome with benzodiazepines
F failure	unexpected failure of the drug to work; often caused by dose or drug interactions	resistance to antimicrobials

- The following routes are used to administer medications:
  - buccal: placed between the cheek and gum via spray, gel, or tablet
  - inhalation: inhaled into the respiratory system via mist, spray, or mask
  - intradermal (ID): injected into the dermal skin layer at a 15-degree angle via a 25- to 27-gauge needle
  - intramuscular (IM): injected into the muscle at a 90-degree angle via an 18- to 23-gauge needle
  - intravenous (IV): injected into a vein via an 18- to 22-gauge needle
  - ophthalmic: placed in the eye via ointment or drops
  - oral: taken by mouth and swallowed via capsule, tablet, liquid, gel, or solution
  - otic: placed in the ear via drops
  - parenteral: any injected medication (SC, IM, ID, or IV)
  - rectal: placed in the rectum via applicator (cream or suppository)
  - subcutaneous (SC): injected into the subcutaneous tissue at a 45- to 90-degree angle via a 22- to 25-gauge needle
  - sublingual: placed under the tongue via gel or tablets
  - topical: placed on the skin via patch, ointment, cream, liquid, or spray
  - transdermal: placed on the skin via patch
  - urethral: placed in the urethra and bladder via catheter
  - vaginal: placed in the vagina via applicator (cream or suppository)
  - Z-track: a specific IM injection method used to prevent the medication from irritating the subcutaneous tissue.
- To prevent errors, the "six rights of medication administration" should be followed every time a patient is given any medication.
  - Right patient
  - Right drug
  - Right route
  - Right dose
  - Right time
  - Right documentation
- Medications can be packaged in a variety of ways depending on the medication form, intended use, shelf stability, and more.
  - **Tablets** and **capsules** are usually taken orally.
  - **Metered-dose inhalers (MDIs)** allow droplets of medication to be inhaled.
  - **Transcutaneous patches** deliver medication through the skin.

PRACTICE QUESTION

26. What physiological changes should an EMT expect to see in a patient who has taken clonazepam (Klonopin)?

ANSWER KEY

1. The meninges are connective tissue.

2. The neck is inferior, or below, the head.

3. Blood from the lungs is returned to the left side of the heart. When the left side cannot pump this blood back out to the body, fluid builds up in the lungs. Blood from the body is returned to the right side of the heart, so right-sided failure causes fluid to build up in the abdomen and extremities.

4. The P wave shows atrial contraction. If a rhythm shows abnormalities in the P waves, then the patient's atria are not functioning properly.

5. An AED will advise a shock is necessary when it recognizes V-tach or V-fib.

6. Air that has been inhaled through the nostrils enters the trachea and then passes through the bronchi and bronchioles. The pathway for the inhaled air ends in the alveoli, where gas exchange takes place.

7. Kussmaul breathing is deep, labored hyperventilation associated with metabolic acidosis. Patients with this type of breathing are likely experiencing diabetic or kidney disorders, with diabetic ketoacidosis being the most common cause.

8. The lumbar vertebrae are located in the lower back. The patient may have injured their lumbar vertebrae.

9. The patient likely has rheumatoid arthritis which has led to progressive, bilateral degeneration of the joints in her hands.

10. The patient most likely has a cramp is his gastrocnemius (calf) muscle, which is posterior on the lower leg.

11. The patient will likely have muscle weakness and limited range of motion that will limit his mobility. He may also have muscle spasms. If the MD is advanced, the patient may have difficulty breathing.

12. Myelin insulates nerve cells and increases the speed that signals travel through the nervous system. When the myelin sheath disintegrates, signals between nerve cells slow down or are not transmitted at all.

13. Orthostatic syncope is the temporary loss of consciousness caused by a sudden drop in blood pressure upon standing. If the patient reports fainting immediately after standing from a sitting or lying position, the EMT should suspect orthostatic syncope.

14. The liver produces bile, which helps break down fat in the small intestine.

15. The vasculature of the lower esophagus drains into the portal vein, which becomes hypertensive in patients with advanced cirrhosis. This hypertension prevents the blood from the capillaries in the esophagus from draining. As a result, they become dilated and may burst.

16. Antibodies attach to antigens and destroy pathogens that cause infection. Because the mother and child have likely been exposed to the same pathogens, the mother's antibodies can help protect the infant from pathogens to which he has been exposed.

17. Patients with leukemia have dysfunctional white blood cells, so they are prone to frequent infections. Leukemia also disrupts the production of platelets, so patients with leukemia may bruise easily or bleed excessively.

18. The pancreas controls blood glucose levels by producing and releasing insulin and glucagon.

19. Type 1 diabetes is an autoimmune disease in which the body destroys cells in the pancreas that produce insulin. People with type 1 diabetes do not produce enough

insulin. Type 2 diabetes is the result of developed insulin resistance: the body produces insulin, but cells do not respond appropriately.

20. Semen passes through the urethra as it exits the penis.

21. The fallopian tubes are the passages through which eggs travel from the ovaries to the uterus.

22. Untreated STIs can spread to other organs, including the uterus, ovaries, and testes. The resulting infections can create a range of serious health problems including severe pain and infertility.

23. Urine passes through the ureters from the kidneys into the urinary bladder.

24. Bloody urine and flank and back pain are symptoms of renal calculi (kidney stones).

25. The epidermis is the outermost layer of the skin.

26. Clonazepam (Klonopin) is a benzodiazepine that relaxes muscles and reduces anxiety. A patient who has taken clonazepam may appear drowsy and have slowed breathing and heart rate.

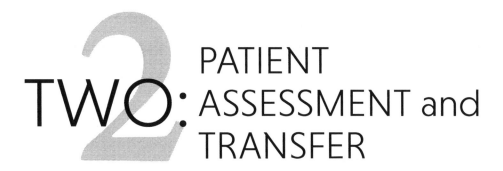

TWO: PATIENT ASSESSMENT and TRANSFER

Assessing the Scene

SCENE HAZARDS

- Provider safety is the most important aspect of patient care.

- The priority is to protect:

  1. yourself
  2. your partner
  3. the patient
  4. bystanders

- To ensure scene safety, a quick assessment, or **scene size-up**, should be conducted to determine:

  ○ scene hazards

  ○ number of patients

  ○ need for additional resources

  ○ mechanism of injury or nature of illness

- Scene hazards may include environment hazards, hazardous substances, violence, and rescue hazards.

  ○ **Environmental hazards** can include inclement weather, traffic, poor lighting, or loud noises.

  ○ **Hazardous substances** can include hazardous chemicals or biological agents, radioactive agents, or explosives.

  ○ **Violence hazards** can include violent patients or bystanders, active crime scenes, or animals.

  ○ **Rescue hazards** can include traffic, water, fire, or collapsed buildings.

- If the scene is safe, make patient contact and begin the patient assessment.

- When hazards are present, the EMT should remove the hazard or remove the patient from the hazard if this can be done safely.

HELPFUL HINT
Park upwind, uphill, and up-stream of hazardous materials incidents.

HELPFUL HINT
If the scene is not safe for bystanders, EMTs should request additional resources (e.g., police) to move bystand-ers to safety.

- If the scene hazards cannot be addressed, request additional resources.
  - Fires: Request the fire department.
  - Rescue operations: Request the fire department and a technical rescue team.
  - Hazardous chemicals and biological agents: Request the fire department and a hazardous materials (HazMat) response team.
  - Traffic hazards and violent or active crime scenes: Request the police.
- At hazardous scenes, EMTs may need to **stage**: wait off-scene in a safe location with the crew until responders on the scene request EMT presence.

PRACTICE QUESTION

1. The EMT has arrived on the scene of a car that struck a utility pole. What hazards should the EMT look for before entering the scene?

MASS CASUALTY INCIDENTS

- If there is more than one patient, immediately request additional ambulances or EMS personnel.
- A **mass casualty incident** is an event in which the number of patients overwhelms the capabilities of the initial EMS responders.
- In a mass casualty incident, the first EMS responders on scene should triage patients.
  - **Triage** is the sorting of patients by their injuries to determine in what order they will be treated and transported.
  - The goal of triage is to direct immediate resources to patients with life-threatening but treatable injuries (red).
  - Patients with less serious injuries (yellow and green) can receive delayed treatment and may be transported longer distances.
  - Patients with a very small chance of survival (black) are treated last.

Table 2.1. SALT Triage Classifications

Priority	Color	Description
Minor	green	minor injuries that require minimal treatment, including abrasions, sprains, and minor fractures
Delayed	yellow	serious injuries whose treatment can be delayed for a short period, including fractures and burns without airway compromise or major bleeding
Immediate	red	treatable life-threatening injuries, including respiratory compromise and uncontrolled bleeding
Expectant	gray	injuries incompatible with life
Dead	black	not breathing after life-saving measures have been attempted

- **Incident Command System (ICS)** is a system of control and command that emergency responders throughout the United States use.
  - The ICS provides recognizable command structure in emergencies and helps organizations work together effectively.
  - The **incident commander (IC)** is in charge of managing the emergency response across all agencies or organizations.
  - The IC will divide workers into sections, branches, and/or divisions, each of which has a designated supervisor.
  - When an EMT is dispatched to the scene of a mass casualty incident, they should know who their designated direct supervisor is on the scene.

PRACTICE QUESTION

2. An EMT arrives at the site of a motor vehicle crash (MVC). When assessing the scene, he notes that a school bus was involved in the accident, and multiple students appear to be injured. What should be the EMT's priority at this scene?

HAZARDOUS MATERIALS

- A **hazardous material** poses a threat to the safety of emergency responders, patients, bystanders, or the environment.
- A scene with hazardous materials present is referred to as a **HazMat incident**.
- HazMat protocols differ between regions and organizations. The EMT should be familiar with their local protocols.
- EMTs need specialized training to respond to most HazMat incidents.
- Commons sources of hazardous materials on a scene include:
  - fuel containers (e.g., car gas tank)
  - tanker trucks
  - leaks or fires at industrial facilities
  - sewage or natural gas infrastructure
- The EMT should assess the scene for signs of hazardous materials. These may include:
  - chemical storage containers
  - Department of Transportation (DOT) placards
  - multiple non-traumatic patients
  - shipping papers or **material safety data sheets (MSDS)** identifying chemicals on scene
- If the EMT suspects hazardous materials are present on a scene, they should immediately request the appropriate additional resources.
- Hazardous materials are categorized as Level 0 – 4 based on their level of toxicity, with Level 0 materials causing little damage and Level 4 materials causing death after minimal contact.

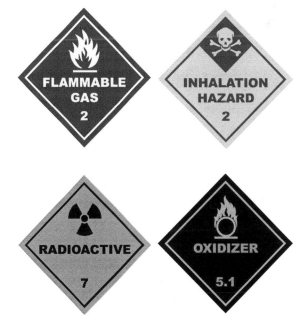

Figure 2.1. DOT Placards

- HazMat scenes are divided into three zones:
  - **hot zone**: area of contamination
  - **warm zone**: where decontamination occurs
  - **cold zone**: clear of contamination
- EMTs should wear the appropriate personal protective equipment (PPE) in each containment area.

PRACTICE QUESTION

3. An EMT is the first responder at the scene of an MVC. At the scene, the EMT sees a tanker truck leaking large amounts of fluid onto the road. What should the EMT do first?

PERSONAL PROTECTIVE EQUIPMENT (PPE)

DID YOU KNOW?

Universal precautions were introduced in the 1980s to protect health care workers from blood-borne pathogens. These were later replaced by *body isolation standards*, which in turn were replaced by *standard precautions* in 1996. The three terms are often used interchangeably.

- **Standard precautions** are a set of infection prevention measures crafted by the Centers for Disease Control and Prevention (CDC) to protect health care workers from infections in blood, feces, mucus, and other bodily substances.
- EMTs should use standard precautions any time they interact with a patient or scene.
- Standard precautions are based on the idea that health care workers should assume all patients are carrying a microorganism.
- Standard precautions relevant to the EMT include:
  - Use PPE, including gloves, masks, gowns, and protective eyewear.
  - Wear gloves during any contact with patients.
  - Change gloves after contact with patients and before touching equipment or other patients.
  - Practice good hand hygiene by washing with soap and water or using antimicrobial foam.
  - Wear appropriate PPE if at risk of body fluids splashing or spraying.
  - Clean and disinfect surfaces and equipment that come in contact with patients' bodily fluids.
  - Use an N-95 respirator mask when patients are suspected or known to be carrying an airborne infection (e.g., measles).
- PPE may also include gear to protect EMTs from scene hazards.
  - PPE may include firefighting turnout gear, reflective vests, helmets, or steel-toed boots.
  - The PPE needed will be determined by the hazards on an emergency scene. For example, wear firefighting turnout gear with goggles and helmet when extricating a patient from a car; wear reflective vests while working on roadways.
  - Specialized rescue PPE (e.g., self-contained breathing apparatus) should only be worn by rescuers who are trained to wear it.

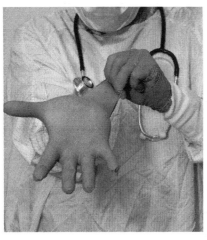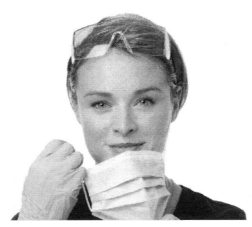

Figure 2.2. Personal Protective Equipment (PPE)

PRACTICE QUESTION

4. The EMT is caring for a patient who has been cut by a chainsaw. The patient has blood spurting from the leg wound. What PPE should the EMT wear during this patient encounter?

Assessing the Patient

- Providing a quality patient assessment will allow the EMT to form a **field impression**, the EMT's determination of the patient's likely condition.

- Patient assessment includes scene size-up, initial assessment, medical assessment or trauma assessment, and reassessment.

  - During the primary or **initial assessment**, the EMT looks for life-threatening conditions that need immediate attention.

  - A **medical assessment** is done on a patient with a medical ailment.

  - A **trauma assessment** is done on a patient with an injury.

  - **Reassessment** is done throughout the course of patient care to determine response to treatments or if any changes have occurred.

INITIAL ASSESSMENT

- The purpose of the initial assessment is to look for and address life-threatening issues.

- If life-threatening issues are found during the initial assessment, they should be promptly addressed, and the patient should be immediately transported to the ED.

- The initial assessment should always be completed in this order:

  1. general impression
  2. level of consciousness (LOC)

HELPFUL HINT

During the initial assessment, do not be distracted by injuries that are not immediately life threatening. Also, be aware that patients may be too distracted by their own injuries to accurately respond to questions about their condition.

3. airway

4. breathing

5. circulation

- After determining that the scene is safe, the EMT can approach the patient. As the EMT approaches the patient, they can begin to form their **general impression**, or first impression, of the patient.

  ○ The general impression is an initial indicator of whether the patient is stable or unstable. A patient is considered **unstable** if their injury or illness is immediately life threatening.

  ○ During the general impression, the EMT should note the patient's age, sex, race, and general condition.

  ○ Look for obvious signs of distress, such as respiratory difficulty or indicators that the patient is in pain.

- After the general impression, determine the patient's **level of consciousness (LOC)**, a measure of a person's responsiveness to stimuli.

  ○ LOC can be unaltered, altered, or unconscious.

    • **unaltered LOC**: alert and able to answer simple questions

    • **conscious with altered LOC**: alert but confused

    • **unconscious**: not responsive

  ○ LOC can also be described using the AVPU scale (Table 2.2).

HELPFUL HINT
Use your senses to form a general impression.
- Look at the patient's appearance.
- Listen for sounds such as wheezing or gasping.
- Note foul smells that may indicate gangrene or other medical issues.

Table 2.2. Assessing Level of Consciousness

Level of Consciousness	Designation	The patient will . . .
Alert	A	interact with EMTs without being prompted
Alert to Verbal Stimuli	V	respond only when they are spoken to
Alert to Painful Stimuli	P	respond only to painful stimuli
Unresponsive	U	not respond to any stimuli

HELPFUL HINT
Check for response to painful stimuli by applying pressure to the earlobe, supraorbital nerve, or trapezius muscle.

- The EMT may also determine the patient's Glasgow Coma Scale (from 3 to 15).

Table 2.3. Scoring on the Glasgow Coma Scale

Eye Opening (E)	Verbal Response (V)	Motor Response (M)
4 = spontaneous 3 = to sound 2 = to pressure 1 = none NT = not testable	5 = orientated 4 = confused 3 = to words 2 = to sounds 1 = none NT = not testable	6 = obeys command 5 = localizes 4 = normal flexion 3 = abnormal flexion 2 = extension 1 = none NT = not testable

- Next, check the **airway** and determine if it is open.
  - If the patient is alert, speak with the patient to determine if there is any obstruction to the airway.
  - If the patient cannot speak or is holding their hand on their throat in distress, they may have an airway obstruction.
  - If the patient is not alert, open the airway and check for good air exchange.
    - No spinal injury: use the head tilt–chin lift maneuver.
    - Possible spinal injury: use the jaw-thrust maneuver.
  - If the patient cannot maintain an open airway, use an airway adjunct to keep the airway open.
    - oropharyngeal airway if no gag reflex
    - nasopharyngeal airway if there is a gag reflex
- Once the airway has been opened, check for **breathing** to assure adequate ventilation.
  - Form a general impression of breathing (e.g., fast/slow, shallow/deep); do not obtain a specific rate in the initial assessment.
  - If breathing is not adequate, the EMT should provide the appropriate intervention. (See chapter 3, "Respiratory Emergencies," for a detailed discussion of artificial ventilation and oxygen delivery.)
  - Address injuries interfering with respirations (e.g., impaled object in the cheek or a flail rib).
- The final part of the initial assessment is **circulation**.
  - Look for major bleeding, and address it immediately if found.
  - Check for the presence of pulses. (Do not obtain a specific rate in the initial assessment.)
    - Unconscious patients: start with a carotid pulse in adults and children and a brachial pulse in infants.
    - Conscious patients: palpate a radial pulse. If no pulse is found, check the femoral or carotid pulse.
  - The EMT should compare central (carotid) and peripheral (radial) pulses. If the pressures differ, the patient could be suffering from shock.
  - Immediately begin CPR on unconscious patients with no pulse and prepare AED.
  - Check the patient's skin color, condition, and temperature.
    - skin color: pale, cyanotic, flushed, or jaundiced (yellow)
    - condition: diaphoretic, dry, or poor skin turgor
    - temperature: cold, warm, or hot

HELPFUL HINT

Do not palpate both carotid arteries at once, as it can reduce blood flow to the brain and cause syncope.

HELPFUL HINT

Pale skin that is cold and clammy is a potential sign of shock, which should be treated immediately.

PRACTICE QUESTION

5. An EMT is dispatched to a call for a 56-year-old male with chest pain. At the scene, the EMT finds the patient prone on the floor, and the patient does not respond to the EMT's questions. What should the EMT do next to further assess the man's LOC?

VITAL SIGNS

- EMTs must take a full set of vital signs to determine how to care for patients.

- A full set of vital signs includes:
  - alertness level
  - pulse
  - blood pressure
  - respirations
  - lung sounds
  - pulse oximetry (SpO_2)
  - pupillary response
  - blood glucose

- Vital signs do not have to be taken in order. The EMT should first choose vital signs relevant to the patient's chief complaint. For example, if a patient is complaining of difficulty breathing, evaluate the patient's respiratory rate, lung sounds, and pulse oximetry first.

- Determine **alertness level** by asking simple questions that everyone should know (e.g., What month is it? Where are you?).
  - The EMT should only ask questions they know the answers to.
  - The patient is described as "alert and oriented by" the number of questions answered correctly "of" the number of questions asked (e.g., A&O × 3 of 5).

- Check a patient's **pulse** (measured in beats per minute [bpm]) for rate, regularity, and strength.
  - Obtain a pulse rate with a pulse oximeter or by palpating the pulse.
  - Check carotid, femoral, brachial, radial, or pedal pulses (dorsalis pedis and posterior tibial).

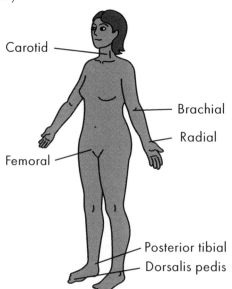

Figure 2.3. Location of Pulses

○ Heart rate is described as normal, **tachycardia** (fast), or **bradycardia** (slow).

Table 2.4. Normal Heart Rate

Age	Beats per Minute (bpm)
Adults and adolescents	60 – 100
Children (2 – 10 years)	60 – 140
Infants and toddlers	100 – 190
Newborns (< 3 months)	85 – 205

○ Pulse rhythm is described as **regular** (equal time between contractions) or **irregular** (missed beats or changes in time between beats).

○ Pulse strength is described as normal, **bounding** (stronger than normal), or **thready** (weaker than normal).

● **Blood pressure (BP)** is the measurement of the force of blood as it flows against the walls of the arteries, measured in mm Hg.

○ **Systolic pressure** is the pressure that occurs while the heart is contracting; **diastolic pressure** occurs while the heart is relaxed.

○ Blood pressure can be taken at the brachial artery by auscultation, palpation, or automated blood pressure cuff.

　• An automated blood pressure cuff is placed on the patient's bicep and provides a readout of their blood pressure.

　• During auscultation, the EMT places the blood pressure cuff on the patient's bicep and the stethoscope on the brachial artery. The EMT should inflate the cuff and listen for **Korotkoff sounds**. The first sound will be the systolic pressure, and the absence of sound is the diastolic pressure.

　• To palpate blood pressure, the EMT places the blood pressure cuff on the upper arm and palpates a radial pulse. The cuff is inflated. The systolic pressure is determined when the EMT feels the radial pulse return as the cuff is deflating. Palpating blood pressure is the least accurate method.

○ A healthy adult blood pressure is a systolic value of 100 to 139 mm Hg and a diastolic value of 60 to 79 mm Hg.

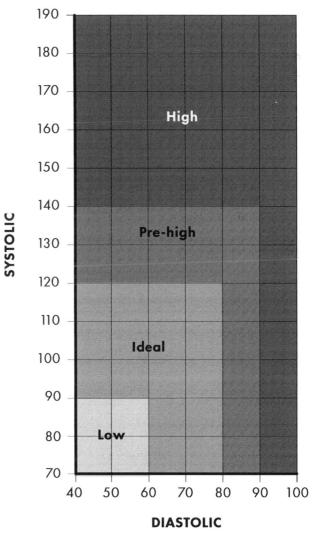

Figure 2.4. Classifying Blood Pressure

- For infants and children, the normal systolic blood pressure is 80 + 2 × patient's age in years; the diastolic pressure is about 2/3 the systolic.

- **Respirations** should be evaluated for rate, rhythm, depth, and quality.

  - Respiratory rate (measured in breaths per minute) can be described as normal, **tachypnea** (fast), or **bradypnea** (slow).

  - Respiratory rhythms can be normal, irregular, or **apneic** (no breathing).

  - Respiratory depth can be normal, **shallow**, or **deep**.

  - **Respiratory quality** can be normal or labored, with the patient working harder than normal to breathe. Evidence of labored breathing includes **tripod position**, using accessory muscles, bobbing the head, or flaring the nostrils.

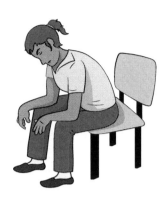

Figure 2.5. Tripod Position

Table 2.5. Normal Respiratory Rate	
Age	**Breaths per Minute**
Adult	12 to 20
Child 11 – 14 years	12 to 20
Child 6 – 10 years	15 to 30
Child 6 months – 5 years	20 to 30
Infant 0 – 6 months	25 to 40
Newborn	30 to 50

- **Lung sounds** should be taken by listening to the upper and lower lungs on the right and left side of the patient's back. Lung sounds may also be taken from the patient's front or side if the back is inaccessible.

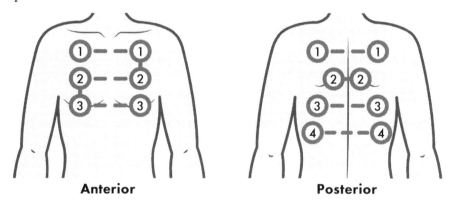

Anterior   Posterior

Figure 2.6. Respiratory Auscultation

Table 2.6. Lung Sounds		
Sound	**Description**	**Etiology**
Normal	air heard moving through the lungs with no obstructions	normal function of the lungs
Wheezes	continuous musical-like sound; can occur on inspiration or expiration	air being forced through narrowed passages in the airway (e.g., asthma, COPD)

Sound	Description	Etiology
Rhonchi	low-pitched, coarse rattling lung sounds	secretions in the airway (e.g., pneumonia, cystic fibrosis)
Stridor	high-pitched wheezing sound	air moving through narrowed or obstructed passages in the upper airway (e.g., aspiration, laryngospasm)
Rales (crackles)	crackling, rattling sound that can be coarse or fine	fluid in the small airways of the lung (e.g., pulmonary edema, pneumonia)
Pleural friction rub	grating, creaking sound	inflamed pleural tissue (e.g., pleuritis, pulmonary embolism)
Diminished or absent breath sounds	decreased intensity of breath sounds due to lack of air in lung tissues	air or fluid around the lungs (e.g., pleural effusion, pneumothorax) or blocked airway

- **Pulse oximetry** (SpO_2) measures the percentage of red blood cells that are carrying oxygen.

Table 2.7. Pulse Oximetry (SpO_2)

Reading	Assessment
96% – 100%	normal
91% – 95%	mild hypoxia
85% – 90%	moderate hypoxia
Less than 85%	severe hypoxia

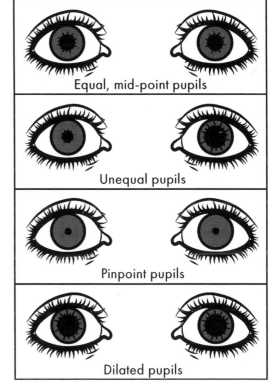

Figure 2.7. Pupil Assessment

- ○ Pulse oximetry can provide false readings in patients who have suffered carbon monoxide poisoning: the actual oxygenation saturation will be lower.

- ○ Pulse oximetry may not work well on patients with cold hands, anemia, or nail polish.

- **Pupils** should be assessed for size and reactivity.
  - ○ Pupils may be **equal** (the same size) or **unequal** (different sizes).
  - ○ Pupil size is described as **constricted**, **mid-point** (normal size), or **dilated**.
  - ○ The pupils' response to light is described as **reactive** or **non-reactive**.
  - ○ Unequal pupils may indicate a brain injury.
  - ○ Unreactive constricted pupils or pinpoint pupils may indicate opioid overdose.
  - ○ Unreactive dilated pupils may indicate alcohol or drug usage.

- **Blood glucose** can be used to identify hypoglycemia or hyperglycemia.
  - ○ Take the blood glucose of any patient who is unconscious or has altered LOC.

- The EMT should use a **glucometer** to take a blood glucose: clean the patient's finger with an alcohol wipe, prick the patient's skin with a lancet, and apply a drop of blood to the test strip.
- The normal blood glucose range is 60 – 110 mg/dL.
- After the finger stick, dispose of the lancet in a sharps container.

HELPFUL HINT

False low-glucose readings can occur if the EMT does not allow the alcohol to dry before performing the finger stick.

PRACTICE QUESTION

6. An EMT is dispatched on a call for an adult female complaining of headache and difficulty breathing. The EMT finds the patient alert with unaltered LOC. The EMT gathers the following vital signs: heart rate 110 bpm, respiratory rate 22 breaths per minute, BP 190/100 mm Hg, SpO$_2$ 92%. Which finding indicates a need for immediate medical treatment?

SECONDARY ASSESSMENT: MEDICAL PATIENTS

- **Nature of illness (NOI)** is the cause of the patient's current illness or **chief complaint** (the patient's main concern).

- If the medical patient is conscious, ask questions to determine a field impression and treatment strategy.

- Ask conscious patients about the history of the present illness. This can be done using the **OPQRST** mnemonic.
  - **O**nset: When did the symptoms start?
  - **P**rovocation: What causes the pain? What were you doing when the pain started?
  - **Q**uality: Please describe the pain.
  - **R**adiation: Where is the pain? Does it go anywhere?
  - **S**everity: On a scale of 1 to 10, with 10 being the worst pain you ever had, what is your pain level?
  - **T**ime: When did the pain start?

- Take a **SAMPLE** history.
  - **S**ymptoms
  - **A**llergies
  - **M**edications
  - **P**ertinent history
  - **L**ast oral intake
  - **E**vents leading to the incident

- Tailor the physical examination to the chief complaint, vital signs, history of present illness, and SAMPLE history. Examine the affected body system thoroughly.

- If the patient is unconscious, perform a rapid physical exam.

Table 2.8. Rapid Physical Exam of an Unconscious Patient

Area	What to Look For
Neck	jugular vein distension, medical alert tags
Chest	equal chest rise and fall, lung sounds
Abdomen	rigidity, distension
Pelvis	incontinence, symmetry
Extremities	symmetry, pulse, motor function, sensation, medical alert tags

- Attempt to obtain OPQRST and SAMPLE histories from bystanders or family.

- Complete a **reassessment** every 5 minutes for unstable patients and every 15 minutes for stable patients.

  o Look for trends in the vital signs to determine if the interventions are improving the patient's condition.

  o Reassess if there is any change in the patient's condition and after giving medications.

PRACTICE QUESTION

7. The EMT has completed the initial assessment and checked the vital signs on a conscious medical patient. What should the EMT do to complete the secondary assessment?

SECONDARY ASSESSMENT: TRAUMA PATIENTS

- **Mechanism of injury (MOI)** is how an injury occurred; use the mechanism of injury to obtain clues about possible injuries.

- A trauma patient could have multiple injuries; the patient should be systematically assessed so that injuries are not missed.

  o If the patient is alert and stable, obtain a SAMPLE history and perform a detailed assessment on scene.

  o If the patient is unstable, perform a **rapid head-to-toe assessment** looking for immediate life threats, and then immediately transport the patient to the hospital. The detailed assessment can be done en route.

- The detailed assessment should include checking the head, neck, chest, abdomen, pelvis, extremities, and posterior for **DCAP-BTLS**:

  o **D**eformity

  o **C**ontusions

  o **A**brasions

  o **P**unctures and penetrations

  o **B**urns

○ Tenderness

○ Lacerations

○ Swelling

Table 2.9. Revised Trauma Score

	Criterion	Revised Trauma Score Points
Glasgow Coma Scale	13 – 15	4
	9 – 12	3
	6 – 8	2
	4 – 5	1
	3	0
Systolic Blood Pressure	> 89 mm Hg	4
	76 – 89 mm Hg	3
	50 – 75 mm Hg	2
	1 – 49 mm Hg	1
	0 mm Hg	0
Respiratory Rate	10 – 29/min	4
	> 29/min	3
	6 – 9/min	2
	1 – 5/min	1
	0/min	0

- The EMT's goal is to get the trauma patient to the hospital within the **golden hour**: the first hour after a patient suffers a traumatic injury.

  ○ The concept of the golden hour is controversial. Multiple studies have suggested that time to initiation of definitive treatment has minimal impact on patient outcomes.

  ○ Patients with cardiac arrest, intracranial hemorrhage, and abdominal hemorrhage are most affected by delays in treatment.

- Assess the patient's **trauma score** (Table 2.9).

  ○ The trauma score will determine what level of trauma center the patient should be transported to.

  ○ A low revised trauma score indicates the need for a higher-level trauma facility.

Table 2.10. Trauma Center Levels

Level	Description
I	Provides complete care for any level of injury.
II	Able to initiate definitive care for all injured patients. Some procedures may require transfer to a Level I trauma center.

Level	Description
III	Able to assess, resuscitate, and stabilize injured patients. Patients requiring intensive care will be transferred to Level I or II trauma center.
IV	Provides advanced trauma life support (ATLS) before transferring patients to a higher level of care; common in remote areas with long transport times to higher-level trauma centers.
V	Provides ATLS before transferring patients to a higher level of care (designation used only in some states).

PRACTICE QUESTION

8. An EMT is assessing a construction worker who has fallen off a roof. During the initial assessment, the EMT determines that the patient is unconscious but breathing with a weak pulse. What type of assessment should the EMT perform next?

Moving the Patient
MOVING PATIENTS

- The EMT should choose the best device to move, lift, and transfer the patient.
    - When possible, use a **power stretcher** to avoid back injuries.
    - If the patient is in a bed, push the stretcher next to the bed. Then transfer the patient to the stretcher using a sheet.
    - Use a **stair chair** for conscious patients who need to be moved downstairs. When backing down the stairs, have a spotter to help maintain balance.
    - Use a **commercial sheet with handles** for patients who need to be moved through tight quarters.
    - Use a **backboard** to move unconscious or traumatic patients.
    - Use a **litter basket stretcher** to carry patients across rough terrain. There should be 4 to 6 EMTs carrying the litter basket stretcher.
- Use proper lifting techniques when moving patients.
    - When lifting, the EMT should keep their legs shoulder-width apart and lift with the legs.
    - The EMT should avoid lifting to the side or twisting.
    - The EMT should avoid reaching more than 15 to 20 inches from their body when lifting.
- The EMT should know their limitations and call for additional help if needed.
- Communicate with the patient and other EMTs when lifting and moving patients or heavy items.
- In all patient transfers and moves, EMT and patient safety must be a priority.

LOAD-AND-GO

- Any patient in a potentially life-threatening condition is considered a **load-and-go** patient.
  - The load-and-go patient should be immediately moved to the ambulance and transported to the hospital.
  - Patient care should be completed en route to the hospital.
- Load-and-go patients have an issue that has been discovered during the primary assessment, including:
  - shock
  - heart attack
  - stroke
  - cardiac arrest
  - respiratory arrest
  - anaphylaxis
  - significant trauma
- Upon recognition of a load-and-go patient, request an advanced life support (ALS) intercept.
  - An **ALS intercept** is a request for an ALS unit to be sent to meet the EMTs. The patient is transferred to the ALS unit for treatment.
  - The EMT should not wait on scene with a load-and-go patient if the ALS intercept has not arrived. Attempt to meet the ALS unit en route to the hospital. If the hospital is closer than the ALS unit, transport the patient to the hospital.

PATIENT TRANSFERS

- Transferring patients can be emergent, urgent, and non-urgent.
- **Emergent** moves are performed when there is an immediate threat to the safety of patients or EMTs.
  - Emergent moves may be used when:

- the patient needs to be removed from a hazard before treatment for a life-threatening condition
- there is a life-threatening condition that requires the patient to be repositioned before treatment
- the patient must be moved to get to other patients with life-threatening conditions
  - No spinal stabilization is used during emergent moves.
  - Emergent moves should be made by lifting or dragging the patient on the long axis to avoid aggravating possible spinal injuries.
  - Emergent moves include blanket drags, firefighter's carry, cradle carry, and one- or two-rescuer assists.
- **Urgent moves** are performed when the scene is safe, but the patient needs to be moved to treat a life-threatening condition.
  - Urgent moves include spinal injury precautions.
    - Use a long spine board if time allows.
    - Use the rapid extraction technique if the patient needs to be moved quickly.
- **Non-urgent moves** are patient transfers in which there is no immediate threat to the life or safety of the patient or EMT.
  - Choose a method that minimizes pain and discomfort for the patient.
  - Always use spinal stabilization if a spinal injury is suspected.
  - Possible methods include extremity lift, direct carry, and direct ground lift.

HELPFUL HINT
Urgent moves are common in MVCs when patients must be rapidly removed from the vehicle to receive care.

PRACTICE QUESTION

11. A firefighter EMT finds a victim in an active house fire. What type of transfer would they use to move the patient out of the home?

AIR TRANSPORT

- **Air transport** should be used when patients require medical care that cannot be provided quickly enough by ground transport.
- Air transport may be called when:
  - a long transport would mean life-saving care is provided outside the golden hour
  - an unstable patient will require a lengthy extraction from a motor vehicle
  - the patient is in a remote location
- Local protocols will dictate when the EMT should call for a helicopter.
- Guidelines for air transports include:
  - Locate a 100 × 100 ft. flat area for the helicopter to land. The area should be free of debris and overhead obstructions.
  - Do not approach the helicopter without permission from the crew.

- ○ Approach from the front of the aircraft.
- ○ If the helicopter is on a hillside, approach from the lower side.
- ○ If the helicopter is requested at night, illuminate the landing site and any nearby hazards (e.g., power lines).

PRACTICE QUESTION

12. The EMT is caring for an MVC victim who is being extricated from the car. The patient is showing signs of shock. The time to extrication will be 20 minutes, and the distance to the hospital is 1 hour. How should the EMT plan for the patient to be transported?

ANSWER KEY

1. Possible hazards in this scenario include downed power lines, fluids leaking from the car, and traffic. Depending on the type of vehicle, the EMT may also need to check the car for hazardous cargo.

2. The EMT's priority should be to request additional resources. He should contact dispatch to request additional ambulances to the scene. He should contact police for traffic control and the fire department for extrication of victims if needed. After requesting the additional resources, the EMT should begin triaging the patients.

3. The EMT should park a safe distance away from the incident and immediately call for additional resources to handle a potential HazMat scene. The EMT should attempt to visually locate the DOT placard or other signs that may identify the truck's contents. The EMT may then begin containing the area to prevent injury to bystanders.

4. The EMT should be wearing gloves, goggles, a face shield, and a gown for this patient encounter. The spurting blood could come in contact with any uncovered clothing or skin.

5. The EMT should provide a painful stimulus, such as pinching the earlobe, to determine if the patient is responsive to pain. If he does not respond, he should be considered unresponsive, and the EMT may move on to assessing the ABCs.

6. A systolic blood pressure over 180 mm Hg is a hypertensive emergency. The patient should be transported immediately to the ED.

7. The EMT should obtain information on the history of the present illness and a SAMPLE history. The EMT should then focus the physical exam on the body system affected.

8. The patient is unstable and should receive a rapid head-to-toe assessment. The detailed assessment can be completed en route to the hospital.

9. The EMTs should acknowledge their limitations and contact dispatch to request additional EMTs to help lift the patient safely. This could also include requesting a specialized ambulance to transport the morbidly obese patient.

10. The EMT should begin transport to the hospital. If possible, they should meet the ALS intercept on the way to the hospital.

11. A house fire is an unsafe scene, so the firefighter EMT should use an emergent move to remove the patient from the hazardous environment. Depending on the scene and the patient's condition, the EMT may choose to use the blanket drag, firefighter's carry, cradle carry, or one-rescuer assist.

12. The EMT should request air transport to the hospital to ensure the patient arrives within the golden hour.

THREE: RESPIRATORY EMERGENCIES

Airway, Respiration, and Ventilation
OPENING AND SUCTIONING THE AIRWAY

- The EMT's priority task is establishing a **patent airway** (open and clear); this should always take precedence over other medical care.

- A conscious patient who is able to speak can help the EMT determine if their airway is open.

  - Conscious patients with a patent airway may remain in a comfortable position during assessment.

- Unconscious patients with a potentially compromised airway should be placed in the supine position so the EMT can assess and open their airway.

- Establishing a patent airway takes priority over the immobilization of the patient's head, neck, and spine: provide as much spinal immobilization to the trauma victim as possible without delaying assessment of the patient's airway.

- There are two common methods of manually opening the patient's airway: the head tilt–chin lift maneuver and the jaw-thrust maneuver.

- The **head tilt–chin lift maneuver** is the preferred method for opening the airway and correcting blockage.

  - Perform by placing one hand on the patient's forehead and tilting it back while simultaneously using the fingertips of the other hand to lift beneath the patient's chin.

  - This maneuver is contraindicated in patients with suspected head, neck, or spine injury.

- The **jaw-thrust maneuver** is used for suspected trauma patients to minimize movement of the cervical spine.

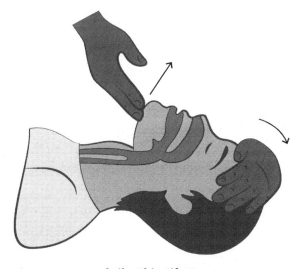

Figure 3.1. Head Tilt–Chin Lift Maneuver

○ From a kneeling position at the top of the patient's head, place fingers behind the angles of the patient's jaw and lift the jaw without moving the patient's head, neck, or spine.

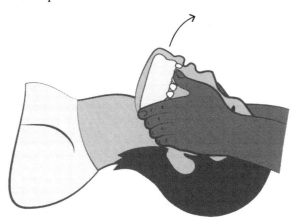

Figure 3.2. Jaw-Thrust Maneuver

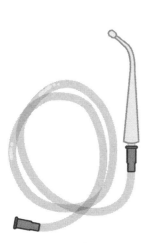

Rigid catheter

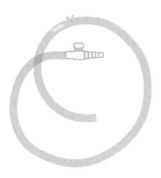

French catheter

Figure 3.3. Types of Catheters

• Excess secretions (including mucus, vomit, or blood) or foreign objects can block the patient's airway or be aspirated into the lungs.

• Secretions and foreign material should be **suctioned** after opening the airway but before inserting an airway adjunct.

• Suction devices consist of a catheter and/or tubing, a source of vacuum (such as a pump), and a collection canister.

○ Suction units can be portable or fixed (usually mounted inside the ambulance).

○ Suction devices should be able to generate at least 300 mm Hg of vacuum.

○ The disposable catheter, tubing, and collection canister are for single-patient use only.

• The two most common suction catheters are the rigid suction catheter and French tip.

○ **Rigid catheter:** Also called the Yankauer or tonsil-tip catheter, it has a large bore suitable for suctioning the oral airway.

○ **French catheter:** A flexible tip appropriate for suctioning lighter secretions such as those found in a nasal airway or stoma.

• The techniques for suctioning include:

○ Only place the tip of the catheter where it can be seen.

○ Position the tip of the catheter prior to applying suction.

○ Begin suctioning while withdrawing the catheter.

○ To reduce the risk of hypoxia, limit suction to 15 seconds for an adult, 10 seconds for a child, and 5 seconds for an infant.

1. A patient is found unresponsive at the base of a ladder with blood dripping from his mouth. How should the EMT assess and open the airway?

AIRWAY ADJUNCTS

- **Airway adjuncts** assist in maintaining the patient's airway. They are used when:
  - ○ The tongue is obstructing the airway.
  - ○ More room is needed for suctioning.
- Airway adjuncts include oropharyngeal and nasopharyngeal airways.
- The **oropharyngeal airway (OPA)** is indicated in unconscious patients with no gag reflex.
  - ○ Select the correctly sized OPA by measuring from the corner of the mouth to the earlobe.
  - ○ For adult patients, begin by inserting the OPA upside-down with the tip toward the roof of the mouth, then rotate 180 degrees.
  - ○ For pediatric patients, use a tongue depressor to move the tongue down while inserting the OPA with the tip at a 90-degree angle, and then rotate.

DID YOU KNOW?
The tongue is the most common airway obstruction, particularly in unconscious patients. When the muscles of the tongue relax, the tongue collapses and can block the airway.

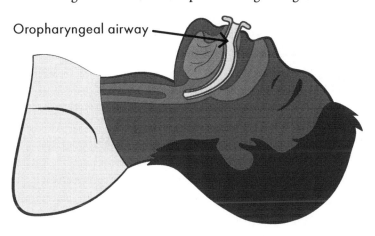
Oropharyngeal airway

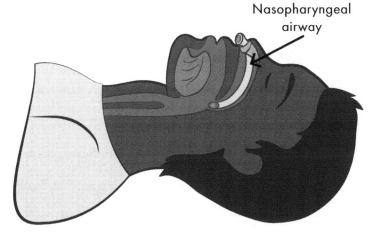
Nasopharyngeal airway

Figure 3.4. Airway Adjuncts

- If the patient gags while the OPA is being inserted, remove the OPA, log roll the patient, and suction in case of vomiting.

- The **nasopharyngeal airway (NPA)** may be used when a patient's gag reflex prevents the insertion of an OPA.

  - Contraindications include severe facial trauma and significant resistance from both nostrils during insertion.

  - Select the correctly sized NPA by measuring from the nostril opening to the earlobe.

  - Apply a water-based lubricant to the NPA before insertion (do not use petroleum jelly).

  - Place the **bevel** (angled portion) of the tip of the NPA toward the **septum** (wall separating the two nostrils).

  - If resistance is met during insertion, attempt to use the other nostril.

PRACTICE QUESTION

2. An adult patient is found with a respiratory rate of 6 breaths per minute and is only responsive to painful stimuli in the form of a trapezius pinch. How should the patient's airway be managed?

ARTIFICIAL VENTILATION

- The EMT must provide **artificial ventilation**, also referred to as assisted or positive pressure ventilation, for patients with inadequate breathing resulting from severe respiratory distress, failure, or arrest.

  - **Respiratory distress**: labored breathing or shortness of breath

  - **Respiratory failure**: breathing that does not support life due to insufficient oxygen intake

  - **Respiratory arrest** or **apnea**: complete cessation of breathing

- Deliver 10 breaths per minute for adult patients and 12 – 20 breaths per minute for children and infants, with each breath delivered over a period of 1 second.

- Artificial ventilation techniques for the EMT, in order of preference, include:

  - mouth-to-mask

  - two-person bag-valve mask (BVM)

  - flow-restricted, oxygen-powered ventilation device (FROPVD)

  - automatic transport ventilator (ATV)

  - mouth-to-mouth

- **Mouth-to-mask**, preferably with high-flow supplemental oxygen, is the NREMT-preferred method due to the ease in which a single rescuer can achieve proper face seal and tidal volume.

  - Utilizing a pocket face mask, ensure an adequate seal to the patient's face while maintaining an open airway.

  - If available, connect oxygen to the mask inlet and flow at 15 liters per minute (lpm).

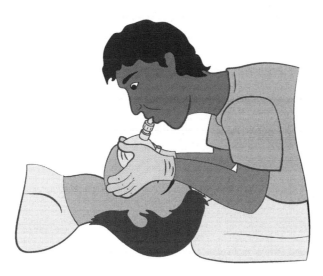

Figure 3.5. Mouth-to-Mask

- To conduct two-rescuer **bag-valve mask (BVM)** ventilation:

  ○ One rescuer at the top of the patient's head uses both hands to achieve a proper mask seal.

  ○ From either side of the patient, the second rescuer uses both hands to squeeze the bag.

  ○ Two-rescuer BVM ventilation is preferred over one-rescuer BVM.

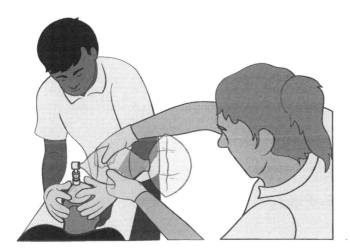

Figure 3.6. Two-Rescuer Bag-Valve Mask Ventilation

- One-rescuer BVM ventilation is problematic due to the difficulties of maintaining a patent airway and proper mask seal with one hand and achieving adequate tidal volume with the other.

  ○ The "EC" clamp technique is preferred for one-rescuer BVM ventilation: the EMT forms a "C" with the thumb and index finger surrounding the mask while the remaining three fingers form an "E" that clamps the patient's lower jaw.

- A **flow-restricted, oxygen-powered ventilation device (FROPVD)** uses pressurized oxygen to deliver ventilations when the EMT depresses a trigger attached to the face mask.
  - Using a FROPVD increases the risk of gastric distention.
  - FROPVD generally cannot be used on children.
  - The use of FROPVDs is less common, and protocols are specific to each EMS system.
- An **automatic transport ventilator (ATV)** is similar to a FROPVD, except the EMT sets the ventilation rate and tidal volume rather than triggering each breath manually.
  - Special training is required to use an ATV.
- **Mouth-to-mouth** is not recommended unless no other methods are available.
- If artificial ventilation is effective:
  - The chest will gently rise and fall.
  - Lung sounds will be heard by auscultation.
  - Pulse oximetry will trend upwards.
- EMTs in some jurisdictions may be given advanced training in the use of **continuous positive airway pressure (CPAP)**.
  - CPAP is used for patients in respiratory distress.
  - Follow local protocol.
- A **stoma** is a permanent surgical opening in the patient's neck as the result of a laryngectomy, or larynx removal.
  - Patients with a **stoma** do not breathe through their mouth or nose.
  - Provide artificial ventilation for patients with a stoma by sealing the facepiece of a BVM or pocket mask over the stoma.
  - Close the mouth and nose of a stoma patient to prevent air escape while providing artificial ventilation.
- A **tracheostomy** is similar to a stoma, but it is typically temporary and found in patients who are on a ventilator or had recent trachea trauma.
  - Patients with a **tracheostomy tube** can be ventilated by removing the facepiece of a BVM or pocket mask and attaching the one-way valve directly to the end of the universal fitting of the trach tube.

PRACTICE QUESTION

3. An 8-year-old female patient with a clear airway is responsive and breathing at a rate of 38 breaths per minute. What intervention should the EMT perform next?

OXYGEN DELIVERY

- **Supplemental oxygen** administration is intended to maintain a pulse oximetry (SpO_2) level of 94% or greater.

- In recent years there has been a fundamental shift away from routinely giving oxygen to all patients.

- Indications for prehospital supplemental oxygen administration include:
  - SpO_2 < 94%
  - cardiac arrest
  - shock
  - altered LOC
  - any patient requiring artificial ventilation

- When indicated, supplemental oxygen delivery should be **titrated** (adjusted) to maintain SpO_2 levels of 94 – 96%, guided by a pulse oximeter.

- Oxygen delivery systems consist of a cylinder with an attached valve, a removable pressure regulator with a flow meter, and a delivery device typically consisting of flexible tubing connected to a facemask.

- The amount of oxygen in a cylinder is monitored by pressure, not volume.
  - Most cylinders, regardless of size, will hold approximately 2,000 **pounds per square inch (psi)** of oxygen when full.
  - Oxygen cylinders should be removed from service to be refilled once they reach 200 psi.

- To use an oxygen delivery system:
  - Slightly open or "crack" the valve on the cylinder to purge any debris.
  - Attach the regulator to the oxygen cylinder.
  - Open the cylinder valve, verify the pressure at the gauge, and check for leaks.
  - Attach the delivery device tubing, set the flow meter to the desired lpm, and titrate based on pulse oximetry.

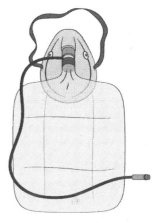

Figure 3.7. Non-rebreathing Mask

- The **non-rebreathing mask** is the preferred method of prehospital oxygen administration.
  - Flow rate is 12 – 15 lpm.
  - Pre-fill the reservoir bag by placing a finger over the connection port prior to applying the mask to the patient.
  - For pediatric patients, choose a facepiece specific to infants or children.

- The **nasal cannula** is a low-flow option that may be used for patients who do not tolerate a non-rebreathing mask.
  - flow rate: 1 – 6 lpm

- The **Venturi mask** delivers specific amounts of oxygen and is not commonly used in the prehospital setting.
  - Flow rate varies.
  - The Venturi mask is most often used on COPD patients.
  - Follow local protocol.

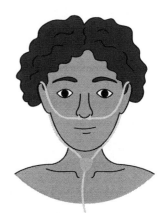

Figure 3.8. Nasal Cannula

- To provide supplemental oxygen to patients with a tracheostomy, place a non-rebreathing mask over the stoma opening.
- Oxygen administration hazards:
  - Oxygen is not a flammable gas, but it does accelerate combustion of other materials.
    - Never use or handle oxygen near ignition sources.
  - Oxygen cylinders are under significant pressure.
    - Always store oxygen cylinders on their side.

PRACTICE QUESTION

4. An awake and alert adult patient complains of nausea and a headache after accidentally leaving their car running in the garage for an extended period. The SpO_2 reading is 99% on ambient outside air, and the patient is not experiencing any difficulty breathing. Should the EMT administer supplemental oxygen? Why or why not?

Acute Pulmonary Edema

Pathophysiology

Acute pulmonary edema is the accumulation of fluid in the alveoli and lung tissue. This fluid inhibits gas exchange. Patients with pulmonary edema will struggle to breathe and will show symptoms related to hypoxia. Acute pulmonary edema is a life-threatening emergency that may lead to respiratory or cardiac arrest.

Pulmonary edema can be caused by a wide range of injuries and underlying disorders:

- Cardiogenic pulmonary edema occurs secondary to left-sided heart failure, also known as **congestive heart failure (CHF)**.
- Neurogenic pulmonary edema occurs secondary to a CNS injury.
- High-altitude pulmonary edema occurs after rapid ascent to altitudes greater than 8,200 feet.
- Inhalation of toxic gases or immersion injuries can also cause pulmonary edema.

What to Look For

KEY FINDINGS

- tachycardia
- dyspnea
- orthopnea
- crackles or wheezes
- cyanosis
- frothy pink sputum
- history of heart failure

OTHER FINDINGS

- chest pain
- pedal edema
- cough (dry or productive)
- fatigue and weakness
- dizziness

Medical Care

- Provide 100% oxygen.
- Use suction to keep airway clear.
- Keep the patient in a comfortable position.
- Use airway adjuncts as needed to maintain an airway.
- Transport the patient to the closest ED per protocols.
- Use CPAP if within local protocols.

PRACTICE QUESTION

5. Why does cardiogenic pulmonary edema cause hypoxia?

Airway Obstruction
Pathophysiology

Airway obstruction, or blockage of the upper airway, can be caused by a foreign body (e.g., teeth, food, marbles), the tongue, vomit, blood, or other secretions. Possible causes of airway obstruction include traumatic injuries to the face, edema in the airway, peritonsillar abscess, allergic reaction, and burns to the airway. Small children may also place foreign objects in their mouths. Patients or bystanders may be able to report the source of the obstruction to the EMT.

A complete airway obstruction is a life-threatening emergency that should be addressed immediately.

DID YOU KNOW?

Airway obstruction and respiratory distress account for approximately 13% of all EMS calls.

What to Look For

KEY FINDINGS

- visually observed obstruction in airway
- grasping at throat or mouth
- dyspnea
- stridor
- agitation or panic

OTHER FINDINGS

- excessive drooling in infants

- trouble swallowing

- loss of consciousness or altered LOC

- respiratory arrest

Medical Care

- If the patient can breathe and is stable:
  - ○ Provide supplemental oxygen.
  - ○ Suction as needed.
  - ○ Transport the patient to the ED per protocols.

- For complete obstruction:
  - ○ Follow BLS guidelines.
  - ○ Suction as needed.
  - ○ Use airway adjunct.
  - ○ Provide rapid transport to the ED.

- Follow allergic reaction treatment guidelines if allergic reaction is suspected.

> ### PRACTICE QUESTION
> **6.** What are some common causes of upper airway obstruction?

Asthma
Pathophysiology

Asthma, an obstructive disease of the lungs, is characterized by long-term inflammation and constriction of the bronchial airways. Patients with asthma often experience exacerbations triggered by lung irritants, exercise, stress, or allergies. Asthma cannot be cured but can be managed through pharmacological measures and lifestyle changes.

Status asthmaticus is a severe condition in which the patient experiences intractable asthma exacerbations with limited pauses or no pause between the exacerbations. The symptoms are unresponsive to initial treatment, including prescribed medications, and can ultimately lead to acute respiratory failure. Status asthmaticus can develop over hours or days.

Patients with asthma may have a **prescribed inhaler** that contains a bronchodilator (usually albuterol). The most common prescribed inhaler for asthma is the **metered-dose inhaler (MDI)**.

To administer an MDI:

- Confirm the medication is prescribed to the patient.

- Verify how many doses the patient took prior to EMS arrival.

- Follow local protocols to obtain permission from medical control.

- Prepare the inhaler by shaking it vigorously.

- Coach the patient to exhale completely and then breathe in slowly and deeply while pressing down on the medication canister.

- If there is a spacer (valved holding chamber) with the MDI, the medication is first sprayed into the chamber.

    - If available, spacers should always be used because they typically increase the amount of medication that enters the patient's respiratory system.

What to Look For

KEY FINDINGS

- wheezing, particularly during exhalation

- frequent cough

- chest tightness

- dyspnea

- history of recent exposure to asthma triggers

- difficulty speaking full sentences

OTHER FINDINGS

- tachycardia

- hypertension

- abdominal pain due to overuse of abdominal accessory muscles

Medical Care

- Provide supplemental oxygen.

- Suction mucus from airway.

    - Do not take patient off oxygen for more than 15 seconds (adult) or 10 seconds (child).

- If the patient has their own inhaler, help administer the medication.

- Patients may require airway management with BVM.

- Use CPAP if within local protocols.

- Transport the patient to the ED per protocol.

PRACTICE QUESTION

7. An EMT is assessing a 4-year-old patient complaining of difficulty breathing after playing outside. The EMT hears wheezes during lung auscultation, and the child is struggling to speak. The child's mother states that both her children have asthma, and she always has an inhaler with her. She hands the EMT the patient's brother's MDI. What should the EMT do next with the medication?

Chronic Obstructive Pulmonary Disease (COPD)

Pathophysiology

Chronic obstructive pulmonary disease (COPD) is characterized by a breakdown in alveolar tissue (emphysema) and long-term obstruction of the airways by inflammation and edema (chronic bronchitis). The most common cause of COPD is smoking, although the disease can be caused by other inhaled irritants (e.g., smoke, industrial chemicals, air pollution).

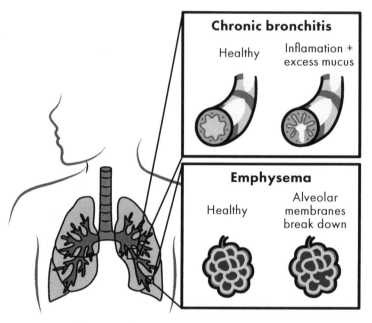

Figure 3.9. Chronic Obstructive Pulmonary Disease (COPD)

Patients with COPD may experience exacerbations characterized by increased sputum production, cough, and dyspnea. Exacerbations are most commonly caused by respiratory infections.

Many patients diagnosed with COPD will have a prescribed metered-dose inhaler. Some COPD patients will have multiple MDIs containing different medications. Follow the same protocols as outlined in the asthma section for assisting patients with MDI administration.

What to Look For

KEY FINDINGS

- chronic, productive cough
- dyspnea
- "dry" wheezing
- prolonged expiration
- history of COPD, recent respiratory infection, or smoking

OTHER FINDINGS

- crackles

- cyanosis

- altered mental status due to hypercapnia

Medical Care

- If the patient has an in-home inhaler, help administer medication.

- Provide supplemental oxygen.

  - Titrate supplemental oxygen to achieve 88 – 92% SpO_2 levels.

- Consider using CPAP if within local protocols.

- Keep the patient comfortable, and transport to the ED per protocols.

> PRACTICE QUESTION
>
> **8.** What are the common causes of COPD?

Pulmonary Aspiration
Pathophysiology

Pulmonary aspiration is the entry of foreign bodies, or material from the mouth or gastrointestinal tract, into the upper and/or lower respiratory tract. Aspiration is most common in young children and adults > 65, who have weaker muscles and less ability to expel objects from the airway. When patients report foreign body airway obstruction, EMTs should consider aspiration. Patients with an altered LOC are also at risk for aspirating fluids.

What to Look For

- dyspnea

- cough

- decreased lung sounds

- crackles if fluid was aspirated

- vomit, blood, or other fluid near the airway

- recent history of foreign body airway obstruction

Medical Care

- Suction or finger sweep the airway as appropriate.

- Provide oxygen as necessary, and keep the patient comfortable.

- Transport the patient to the ED per protocol.

Hyperventilation
Pathophysiology

Hyperventilation is an increased breathing rate (> 20 breaths per minute). During hyperventilation, more carbon dioxide (CO_2) is expelled than is produced, decreasing the amount of CO_2 found in the blood below normal (a condition known as **hypocapnia**). Hyperventilation may occur due to an underlying medical condition and functions as a way for the body to expel excess CO_2. It most commonly occurs for psychological reasons, a condition called **hyperventilation syndrome**. Patients experiencing hyperventilation syndrome typically describe the experience as a panic or anxiety attack.

Most episodes of hyperventilation syndrome resolve without injury or medical intervention. However, because the underlying cause of hyperventilation cannot be determined in the field, hyperventilation should be treated as an emergent condition.

What to Look For

- tachypnea
- dyspnea
- chest tightness
- dizziness or lightheadedness
- medical history of anxiety
- paresthesia in the hands, feet, or lips
- spasms in the hands or feet

Medical Care

- Provide reassurance to the patient.
- Evaluate the patient in a comfortable setting away from loud noise, emotional family members, and other stress-inducing elements.
- Provide verbal directions to the patient to help decrease their breathing rate.
- Provide supplemental oxygen if the breathing rate cannot be controlled.
- Transport the patient to the ED per protocols.

PRACTICE QUESTION

10. What is the most effective treatment for hyperventilation syndrome?

Pleural Effusion

Pathophysiology

A **pleural effusion** is the buildup of fluid around the lungs in the pleural space. (The pleurae are layers of tissue between the lungs and chest wall that normally have a small amount of fluid that acts as a lubricant during thoracic movement.) Excess fluid buildup can displace lung tissue and inhibit lung expansion. Pleural effusion occurs secondary to various other conditions, including heart failure, cancer, and infections.

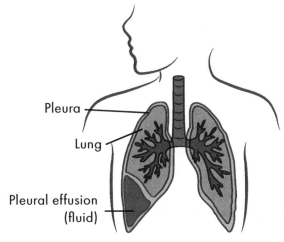

Pleura

Lung

Pleural effusion
(fluid)

Figure 3.10. Pleural Effusion

What to Look For

- dyspnea
- dullness upon percussion of the lung area
- decreased breath sounds on affected side
- asymmetrical chest expansion
- pleuritic chest pain

Medical Care

- Provide oxygen if necessary and keep the patient comfortable.
- Transport the patient to the ED per protocols.

PRACTICE QUESTION

11. How does pleural effusion prevent lung expansion?

Pneumothorax

Pathophysiology

Pneumothorax is the collection of air between the chest wall and the lung (in the pleural space). It can occur due to a blunt or penetrative chest-wall injury, medical injury, underlying lung tissue disease, or hereditary factors. Pneumothorax is classified according to its underlying cause:

- **Primary spontaneous pneumothorax (PSP)** occurs spontaneously in the absence of lung disease and often presents with only minor symptoms.

- **Secondary spontaneous pneumothorax (SSP)** occurs in patients with an underlying lung disease and presents with more severe symptoms.

- **Traumatic pneumothorax** occurs when the chest wall is penetrated or when fractured ribs puncture a lung or the pleura.

- **Tension pneumothorax** is the late progression of a pneumothorax in which the increased pressure from the air in the pleural space causes the affected lung and eventually the heart and vena cava to be compressed. It causes significant respiratory distress in the patient and requires immediate intervention.

What to Look For

KEY FINDINGS

- sudden, unilateral pleuritic chest pain

- dyspnea

- tachycardia

- unequal chest rise and fall

- thoracic trauma or recent thoracic surgery

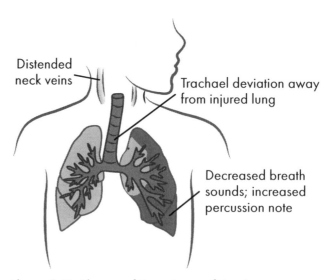

Figure 3.11. Signs and Symptoms of Tension Pneumothorax

KEY FINDINGS

- penetrating thoracic injury
- decreased breath sounds over the affected lung
- increased percussion note
- distended neck veins (late stage)
- tracheal deviation away from the side of the tension (late stage)

Medical Care

- Provide supplemental oxygen.
- Keep the patient in a comfortable position.
- Be prepared to manage the airway and provide respirations as needed.
- Apply an occlusive dressing to any open chest wounds.
- Transport the patient to the ED per protocols.

PRACTICE QUESTION

12. What is the primary difference between a simple pneumothorax and a tension pneumothorax?

Pulmonary Embolism

Pathophysiology

A **pulmonary embolism (PE)** occurs when an **embolus** (usually a blood clot or an air bubble) occludes an artery of the lungs. The occlusion prevents blood flow to affected areas of the lungs, preventing gas exchange.

The most common embolus is a blood clot caused by deep vein thrombosis (DVT). Other occlusions, such as tumor emboli, fat emboli, and amniotic fluid emboli, can also reach the lungs. People who are immobilized for long periods of time, pregnant, recently had surgery, or have a history of blood clots are at a higher risk of PE. PE is a life-threatening condition that requires immediate medical treatment. However, it can be difficult to diagnose in the field, and prehospital care is mostly supportive.

What to Look For

- pleuritic chest pain
- dyspnea
- tachypnea
- tachycardia
- hemoptysis
- hypotension

- hypoxia
- anxiety

Medical Care

- Provide supplemental oxygen.
- Place the patient in a comfortable position.
- Transport the patient promptly to the ED per protocols.

> ### PRACTICE QUESTION
> **13.** How does a DVT lead to a pulmonary embolism?

Respiratory Infections
Pathophysiology

The respiratory system is prone to **respiratory tract infections**. Upper respiratory tract infections affect air inputs in the nose and throat, and lower respiratory tract infections affect the lungs and their immediate pulmonary inputs.

- Viral infections of the respiratory system include influenza and the common cold; bacterial infections include tuberculosis and pertussis (whooping cough).
- **Pneumonia**, the inflammation of the lungs that affects alveoli, can be caused by bacteria, viruses, fungi, or parasites. It is often seen in people whose respiratory system has been weakened by other conditions.

Respiratory tract infections rarely require emergency medical care. However, they may exacerbate chronic conditions such as COPD, asthma, and heart failure. In addition, young children and older patients may require medical treatment for fever or dyspnea related to respiratory infections.

What to Look For

KEY FINDINGS

- fever
- dyspnea
- pleuritic chest pain
- difficulty swallowing
- dehydration

OTHER FINDINGS

- wheezing and crackles
- rhinorrhea

- congestion
- dry or wet cough

Medical Care

- Provide supplemental oxygen if necessary.
- Suction excess secretions if they are compromising the airway.
- Place the patient in a comfortable position.
- Transport the patient to the ED per protocols.

PRACTICE QUESTION

14. What is the difference between upper and lower respiratory tract infections?

ANSWER KEY

1. Open the airway using the jaw-thrust maneuver. The head tilt–chin lift maneuver is contraindicated due to suspected head, neck, or back injury. The blood in the patient's mouth should not be suctioned until after the airway has been opened.

2. Insert a nasopharyngeal airway. An OPA is contraindicated because the patient is responsive to painful stimuli and therefore not unconscious.

3. Although the patient is breathing, the rate is too fast and therefore inadequate. Perform assisted ventilations using the mouth-to-mask technique. (NREMT prefers mouth-to-mask over BVM, particularly when only one rescuer is present.) The insertion of an airway adjunct (OPA or NPA) is contraindicated in responsive patients. Suction is not needed because the airway is clear.

4. The EMT should administer oxygen with a non-rebreathing mask. The patient's signs and symptoms suggest the patient may have carbon monoxide poisoning. The pulse oximeter is likely mistaking carbon monoxide saturation for oxygen saturation, resulting in a false reading.

5. Cardiogenic pulmonary edema is an accumulation of fluid in the alveoli that results from congestive heart failure. The fluid interrupts gas exchange and prevents oxygen from passing into the blood, causing hypoxia.

6. Common objects that may obstruct the airway include the tongue, teeth, blood, saliva, vomit, food, and small toys. Edema can also cause airway obstruction.

7. Although the patient would likely benefit from an MDI treatment, the EMT cannot assist in the administration of medication that is not prescribed to the patient. This is true even if the patient is a child and the EMT has permission from the parents.

8. Most COPD cases are the result of long-term cigarette smoking. COPD may also be caused by lung irritants such as dust, chemicals, or smog.

9. Young children and the elderly are at higher risk for aspiration due to weaker muscles and a diminished ability to expel foreign body obstructions. Also, patients with an altered mental status are at risk for aspirating fluids such as blood or vomit.

10. Because most cases of hyperventilation syndrome involve anxiety, the preferred treatment is to reassure the patient and provide coaching to decrease the breathing rate.

11. The pleural space is made up of layers of tissue between the lungs and inner chest wall that move with the lungs as they expand and contract. During a pleural effusion, excess fluid in the pleural cavity compresses the lungs and prevents them from fully expanding.

12. The term *pneumothorax* applies to any case involving air in the pleural space. *Tension pneumothorax* is an advanced and dangerous stage in which the amount of air in the pleura causes the lung to completely collapse and the heart and vena cava to become compressed.

13. A DVT is a blood clot that forms in the deep veins, usually in the extremities. When a piece of the clot is dislodged, it travels through the veins to the heart, which then pushes it into the pulmonary arteries. As the pulmonary arteries branch and narrow, the clot will eventually stop and occlude the artery, a condition called a pulmonary embolism (PE).

14. An upper respiratory tract infection affects the structures of the nose and throat, while a lower respiratory tract infection primarily affects the lungs.

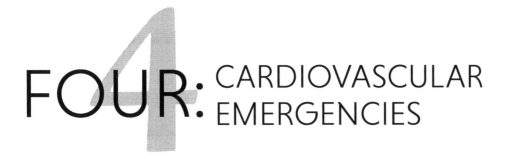

FOUR: CARDIOVASCULAR EMERGENCIES

The Role of EMTs in Cardiovascular Emergencies

- The American Heart Association (AHA) and the European Resuscitation Council have developed guidelines for two levels of care that can be provided during cardiac emergencies.

  - **Basic Life Support (BLS)** includes rescue breathing, CPR, and use of an AED. The purpose of BLS is to maintain the circulation of oxygenated blood until more advanced medical care can be provided.

  - **Advanced Cardiac Life Support (ACLS)** or **Advanced Life Support (ALS)** includes all the elements of BLS and also includes an invasive procedure such as IV administration of medications or endotracheal intubation. The purpose of ALS is to restart the heart's normal rhythm.

- EMTs are certified to provide BLS. During a cardiac emergency, the EMT may perform the following procedures:

  - rescue breathing

  - CPR

  - defibrillation with an AED

  - administration of nitroglycerin and aspirin (per local protocols)

- An **ALS intercept** is a unit staffed with ALS-certified personnel who are dispatched to meet BLS units when the patient requires advanced life support.

CARDIOPULMONARY RESUSCITATION (CPR)

- **Cardiopulmonary resuscitation (CPR)** consists of ventilations and chest compressions that keep oxygen-rich blood flowing to the brain and other vital organs during cardiac arrest.

- The process of providing CPR starts with the initial assessment.

DID YOU KNOW?
Chest pain and cardiac conditions account for approximately 13% of EMS calls.

○ Assess scene safety: Start CPR only when the scene is safe for both the EMT and the patient.

○ Wear appropriate PPE (usually gloves, but other equipment may be required depending on the scene and patient).

○ Determine the patient's responsiveness.
- For adults and children, kneel next to the patient and shake their shoulders. For infants, tap their foot.
- Simultaneously ask the patient if they are OK.
- If the patient is unresponsive, request an ALS intercept and bring the AED to the scene.

○ Check for breathing and pulse at the same time for no more than 10 seconds.
- Look, listen, and feel for breathing and pulse.
- Lean over the patient placing your ear over the patient's mouth and nose while looking down the patient's chest, watching for breathing.
- At the same time, place your fingers on the patient's carotid artery on the same side of the neck where you are kneeling.
- If the patient is not breathing and has no pulse, start CPR.

● The EMT should start **compressions** while their partner attaches the AED.

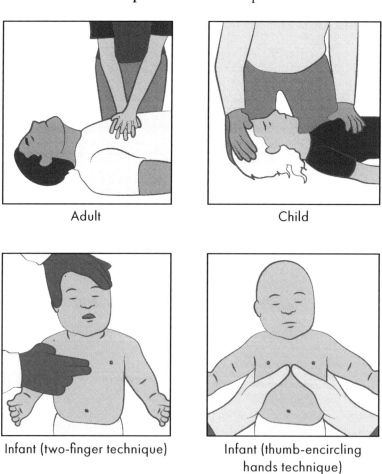

Adult

Child

Infant (two-finger technique)

Infant (thumb-encircling hands technique)

Figure 4.1. Hand Placement During CPR

- ○ Move the patient to the supine position on a hard surface.
  - • Use caution in moving a patient who may have a spinal injury.
- ○ Place hands in the center of the chest on the lower half of the sternum.
  - • Use the two-handed method for adults.
  - • Use the one-handed method for children aged 1 to 8.
  - • For infants, use the two-finger technique (for one EMT) or thumb-encircling hands technique (for two EMTs).
- ○ Allow for full chest recoil between compressions.
- ○ Interrupt compressions for no more than 10 seconds.
- **Ventilations** are given via bag-valve mask (BVM) or through a barrier device. (See chapter 3, "Respiratory Emergencies," for detailed instructions on providing artificial ventilation.)
- One cycle of CPR is five sets of 30 compressions and 2 breaths.
  - ○ When two EMTs are performing CPR, they should switch roles every five cycles (roughly 2 minutes).
  - ○ The patient's breathing and pulse should be reassessed after every five cycles of CPR.

Table 4.1. Compression and Ventilation Guidelines for CPR

	Adult	Child	Infant
Compressions per minute	100 – 120		
Depth	2 – 2.4 inches	2 inches	1.5 inches
Compression-to-ventilation ratio	30:2	1 EMT: 30:2 2 EMTs: 15:2	1 EMT: 30:2 2 EMTs: 15:2

- An oropharyngeal airway (OPA) can be inserted in between cycles of CPR.
  - ○ Do not insert an OPA if CPR compressions will be delayed.
  - ○ If there is good compliance with BVM, the airway can be delayed.
- The EMT should continue CPR until the patient has **return of spontaneous circulation (ROSC)**, the patient is delivered to the hospital emergency department, or the patient is transferred to an ALS ambulance.

PRACTICE QUESTION

1. An EMT arrives on scene to find a 3-month-old infant who is pulseless and apneic. He and his partner call for an ALS intercept and begin providing CPR. What compression-to-ventilation ratio should they use?

AUTOMATED EXTERNAL DEFIBRILLATORS (AED)

- During **defibrillation**, also known as **unsynchronized cardioversion**, electrical current is used to reset the heart to a normal sinus rhythm.

- The electrical current is supplied randomly during the cardiac cycle, disrupting the heart's electrical rhythm and allowing normal sinus rhythm to restart.

- The automated external defibrillator (AED) will defibrillate ventricular fibrillation (V-fib) and ventricular tachycardia (V-tach). The AED will not defibrillate any other heart rhythms.

- Electrical defibrillators can be **monophasic** (unidirectional current) or **biphasic** (bidirectional current).
  - Monophasic devices deliver current at a more consistent magnitude and are more effective at lower energies.

- EDs can be semi-automatic or automatic.
  - When using a **semi-automatic defibrillator**, the EMT must depress the shock button to deliver a shock.
  - **Automatic defibrillators** will deliver the shock if indicated after a countdown.
  - Both defibrillators can be shut off to disarm a shock.

- The EMT should retrieve the AED as soon as the patient is found to be unconscious.

- When using a defibrillator, consider the safety of the EMT, their crew, and the patient.
  - Do not use an AED in an explosive or flammable atmosphere.
  - Make sure no one is touching the patient when the AED defibrillates the patient.
  - Do not use an AED in water; if patient is wet, dry patient's chest before use.

- As soon as the AED is available, attach it to the patient.
  - While one EMT is providing CPR, the another can attach the AED to the patient.
    - Remove clothes and jewelry from the patient's chest.
    - Dry the chest if the patient is wet.
    - If the patient has a hairy chest, shave the AED pad locations before application.
    - Turn on the AED.
    - Peel the pads off the plastic.
    - Place one pad on the upper-right chest.
    - Place the second pad on the lower-left chest (look at the picture on the pad or packaging).
    - For infants and small children, place one pad in the center of the chest and the other in the center of the back.
    - Plug the pads into the AED if they are not already attached.
    - While the AED is analyzing, briefly discontinue CPR.
    - If no defibrillation is indicated, continue CPR.
    - If defibrillation is indicated, provide CPR while the AED is charging.

HELPFUL HINT

Do not place the defibrillator pad over an implanted pacemaker or defibrillator. Place the pad at least 1 inch below the implanted device.

- Defibrillate the patient and immediately resume CPR.
- After two minutes of CPR, check for a pulse.
- The AED will automatically re-analyze the patient.
- Defibrillate if indicated; continue to provide CPR if a shock is not indicated.
- Repeat until ALS arrives or arrival at the hospital.

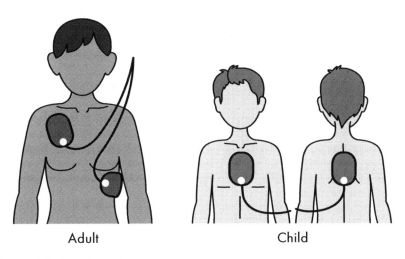

Adult   Child

Figure 4.2. AED Pad Placement

- Document the time and response of AED application and defibrillations on the patient care report.

PRACTICE QUESTION

2. The EMT arrives and finds a 92-year-old male pulseless and apneic. CPR has been started and the AED was just brought to the patient's side. While one EMT is attaching the AED, what should the other EMT be doing?

ADMINISTERING MEDICATIONS IN CARDIAC EMERGENCIES

- Most EMS systems allow EMTs to administer nitroglycerin and aspirin to patients with chest pain.
  - **Nitroglycerin** dilates blood vessels and decreases the work of the left ventricle, allowing more blood to reach the heart muscle.
  - **Aspirin** is an antiplatelet that slows blood clotting and can help prevent further damage to the heart muscle caused by occluded blood vessels.
- Patients complaining of cardiac chest pain should be given nitroglycerin.
- Nitroglycerin is available in tablets or as a spray.
- Contraindications for giving nitroglycerin include:
  - BP < 100 mm Hg
  - head injury

HELPFUL HINT

Always check the expiration date on the medication before administering it.

- infant or pediatric patient

- patient use of vasodilators within the last 24 hours, particularly those prescribed for erectile dysfunction (e.g., sildenafil [Viagra] or vardenafil [Levitra])

- Procedures for administering nitroglycerin:
  - Determine the patient's baseline pain level (usually done on a scale of 1 to 10).
  - Administer the tablet or spray under the patient's tongue.
  - One tablet or spray can be given every 5 minutes for up to three doses.
  - Check blood pressure between each dose.
  - Reassess using the pain scale after 5 minutes to determine the effectiveness of the medication administration.

- Possible side effects of nitroglycerin include:
  - severe headache
  - drop in blood pressure
  - dizziness
  - flushing
  - tachycardia

- Patients with cardiac chest pain should also be given 324 mg of aspirin.

- Contraindications for aspirin include:
  - history of asthma
  - aspirin allergy
  - internal abdominal bleeding
  - bleeding disorders
  - pregnancy
  - recent surgery
  - recent administration of medication to slow clotting (e.g., aspirin or anticoagulant)

- Give the patient the aspirin by mouth. Patient should be told to chew and swallow the tablets.

- Side effects of aspirin may include:
  - nausea
  - vomiting
  - bronchospasm
  - bleeding

PRACTICE QUESTION

3. An EMT arrives on scene to find a 76-year-old male with chest pain. The EMT determines that the patient has a history of angina and asthma. The patient also

Acute Coronary Syndrome

Pathophysiology

Acute coronary syndrome (ACS) is an umbrella term for cardiac conditions in which blood flow to the heart is impaired. ACS is usually the result of atherosclerotic plaque or clots that partially or fully occlude the coronary arteries. ACS includes unstable angina, non-ST-elevation myocardial infarction (NSTEMI), and ST-elevation myocardial infarction (STEMI).

In **angina pectoris** (commonly called angina), the coronary arteries are temporarily unable to supply an appropriate amount of oxygenated blood to meet the oxygen needs of the heart. Angina can be classified into two categories: stable angina or unstable angina.

- **Stable angina** usually resolves in about 5 minutes, is resolved with medications or with rest, and can be triggered by exertional activities, large meals, and extremely hot or cold temperatures.

- **Unstable angina** can occur at any time and typically lasts longer (> 15 or 20 minutes). The pain is usually rated as more severe than stable angina and is not easily relieved by taking nitrates.

- A **myocardial infarction (MI)** is ischemia of the heart muscle that occurs when the coronary arteries are partially or completely occluded. MI is classified by the behavior of the ST wave.

- A **non-ST-elevation myocardial infarction (NSTEMI)** includes an ST depression, which reflects ischemia resulting from a partial blockage of the coronary artery.

- An **ST-elevation myocardial infarction (STEMI)** includes an elevated ST wave, indicating a complete occlusion of a coronary artery. STEMI is a life-threatening emergency that requires immediate intervention.

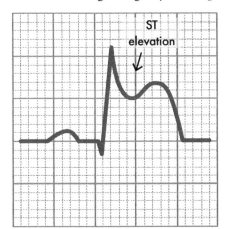
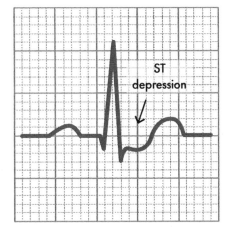

Figure 4.3. ST Depression and ST Elevation

What to Look For

KEY FINDINGS

- continuous chest discomfort or pain that may radiate to the back, arm, or jaw

- chest pressure or tightness

- syncope

- diaphoresis

- nausea or vomiting

- dyspnea

- pallor

- anxiety or feeling of impending doom

OTHER PRESENTATIONS OF MI

- Upper abdominal pain is more common in people > 65, people with diabetes, and women.

- Women are more likely to present with back pain or indigestion.

- Patients with a "silent" MI have no symptoms.

Care and Transport

- All patients who report chest pain should be thoroughly assessed for symptoms of MI.

- Provide supplemental oxygen; titrate to 95 – 99%.

- Use adjuncts as needed to manage the airway.

- Administer aspirin and nitroglycerin per local protocols (see "Administering Medications" on page 83 for details).

- Provide rapid transport to ED.

- If the patient enters cardiac arrest during transport:
  - Stop the vehicle and begin performing CPR.
  - Administer one shock via AED as soon as possible.
  - Resume CPR.
  - Follow local protocols for calling ALS support and transporting patients.

PRACTICE QUESTION

4. What symptom, identified by the patient, is the most common and consistent with an MI?

Cardiac Arrest

Pathophysiology

Cardiac arrest (also called sudden cardiac arrest) refers to the complete cessation of all cardiac activity. Most cardiac arrests are caused by sustained V-fib following an MI. Cardiac arrest can also be caused by structural abnormalities in the heart (e.g., cardiomyopathies or valve dysfunction) or abnormalities in the heart's electrical systems. Most cardiac arrests in infants and children are caused by respiratory arrest.

What to Look For

- sudden loss of consciousness
- no pulse
- respiratory arrest or apnea

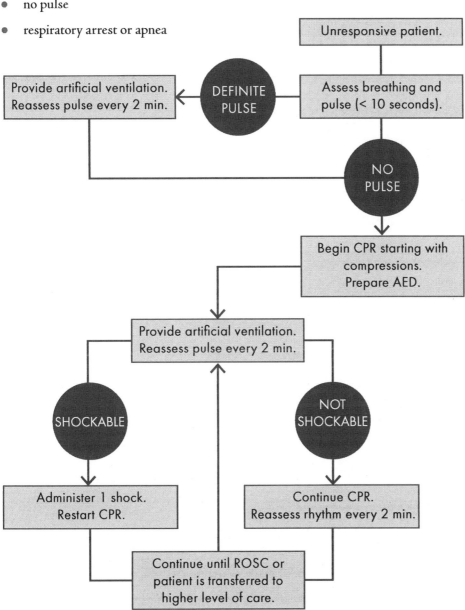

Figure 4.4. Basic Life Support (BLS) Algorithm

Care and Transport

- Follow BLS algorithm (see Figure 4.4).
- Patient will require immediate transfer to ALS care (ALS intercept or transport to hospital).

PRACTICE QUESTION

5. EMTs arrive on the scene to find a 68-year-old male who is unresponsive with agonal breathing and no pulse. The EMTs begin CPR and attach the AED to the patient. The AED indicates that no shock is needed. What should the EMTs do next?

Aortic Aneurysm
Pathophysiology

An **abdominal aortic aneurysm (AAA)**, often called a triple A, occurs when the lower aorta is enlarged. The AAA is the most common type of aneurysm. A **thoracic aneurysm** occurs when the portion of the aorta in the chest is enlarged.

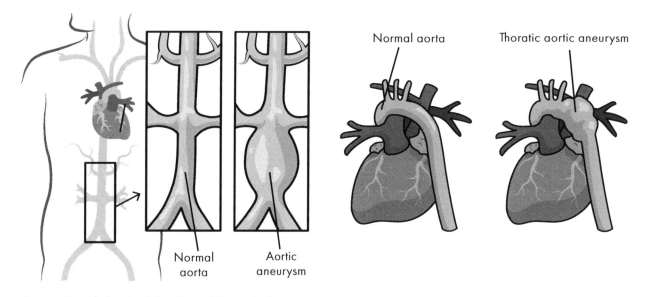

Normal aorta

Thoratic aortic aneurysm

Normal aorta

Aortic aneurysm

Figure 4.5. Abdominal Aortic and Thoracic Aneurysm

DID YOU KNOW?
Approximately 75% of aortic aneurysms occur in men.

Many patients with aortic aneurysms do not have any symptoms at all. The main concern for people with aortic aneurysms is **aortic rupture**, a complete tear in the wall of the aorta, or **dissection**, a tear in the innermost layer of the aorta that allows blood to enter the aortic media. Patients with an aortic rupture or dissection will rapidly enter hemorrhagic shock, and most will die within minutes.

Rupture or dissection in a thoracic aneurysm may present with similar symptoms to an MI and should be considered for patients with severe chest pain.

What to Look For

KEY FINDINGS

- sudden abdominal pain that radiates to the back (abdominal aneurysm)
- sudden chest pain (thoracic aneurysm)
- pain often described as "tearing"
- signs and symptoms of hemorrhagic shock

OTHER FINDINGS

- a pulsating feeling by the umbilicus (abdominal aneurysm)
- a blood pressure difference of greater than 20 mm Hg between the left and right arms
- anxiety or a feeling of impending doom

Care and Transport

- Provide oxygen.
- Gently move the patient.
- Transport the patient to the ED immediately.
- Prevent further damage to the artery.
  - Minimize patient movement.
  - If a rupture or dissected artery is suspected, do not palpate the abdomen or provide aggressive treatment.

PRACTICE QUESTION

6. EMTs respond to a call for a 77-year-old male with chest pain. They arrive to find the patient curled on the floor. He describes the pain as tearing and says it started suddenly about 15 minutes ago. He rates the pain at 10 out of 10. Assessment shows a BP of 175/112 mm Hg in the right arm and 197/125 mm Hg in the left. How should the EMTs manage this patient?

Hypertensive Crisis
Pathophysiology

Hypertensive crises include hypertensive urgency and hypertensive emergencies. **Hypertensive urgency** is a BP greater than 180/120 mm Hg without evidence of organ dysfunction. A **hypertensive emergency** is a BP greater than 180/120 mm Hg accompanied by evidence of progressive organ dysfunction.

HELPFUL HINT

Life-threatening conditions that can cause chest pain include:
- MI
- aortic dissection
- pulmonary embolism
- pneumothorax

Non-life-threatening sources of chest pain include:
- heartburn
- costochondritis
- muscle strains
- rib fractures

DID YOU KNOW?

Hypertensive crises increase the risk of stroke because of the potential damage to blood vessels in the brain.

What to Look For

KEY FINDINGS

- systolic blood pressure greater than 180 mm Hg
- diastolic blood pressure greater than 120 mm Hg

OTHER FINDINGS

- may be asymptomatic
- severe headache
- blurred vision
- bounding pulse
- ear ringing
- nausea and vomiting
- altered mental status

Care and Transport

- Continually monitor blood pressure.
- Keep patient calm and comfortable.
- Stable, asymptomatic patients may choose not to receive further care.
- Symptomatic patients require rapid transport to the ED.
- Request an ALS intercept for unstable patients who need immediate intervention to lower BP.

PRACTICE QUESTION

7. EMTs respond to a call for a 55-year-old male with a severe headache and an altered mental status. During assessment, they find the patient is dyspneic and has a BP of 202/130 mm Hg. How should the EMTs manage this patient?

Shock

Shock occurs when there is inadequate tissue perfusion. The resulting lack of oxygen circulating to major organs can lead to organ failure and death. Shock is classified by the underlying cause of the inadequate perfusion. The most common type of shock is hypovolemic.

Table 4.2. Types of Shock

Type	Description	Common Causes	Key Findings
Cardiogenic shock	occurs when the heart can no longer pump effectively, reducing blood flow and available oxygen throughout the body	• MI • dysrhythmias • inflammation or infection in the heart	• tachycardia • hypotension • cool, pale, moist skin
Hypovolemic shock (hypovolemia)	occurs when rapid fluid loss decreases circulating blood volume and cardiac output, resulting in inadequate tissue perfusion	• trauma • excessive fluid loss through vomiting, diarrhea, or urination	
Hemorrhagic shock	a type of hypovolemic shock in which blood is lost rapidly	trauma	
Septic shock	occurs when a massive infection damages blood vessels	infection, most often in the urinary tract or respiratory tract	• tachycardia • hypotension • warm, flushed skin
Neurogenic shock	caused by an injury or trauma to the spinal cord, typically above the level of T6, which disrupts the functioning of the automatic nervous system, producing massive vasodilation	trauma to neck	• bradycardia • hypotension • warm, dry skin
Anaphylactic shock	caused by a severe histamine reaction causing dilated blood vessels, flushed skin, and respiratory compromise	allergen	• tachycardia • flushed skin • hypotension • urticaria

Care and Transport

- Administer oxygen.
- Manage the airway as needed.
- Keep the patient warm.
- Transport to the ED immediately.
- Request an ALS intercept for unstable patients.

8. A 27-year-old woman was found lying on the couch complaining of the flu. The patient has had diarrhea and vomiting for the last 24 hours. During assessment, the EMTs find that she is hypotensive with cool, pale skin. What type of shock does the patient most likely have?

ANSWER KEY

1. The compression-to-ventilation ratio for 2-person infant CPR is 15 compressions to 2 ventilations.

2. While one EMT is attaching the AED, the other EMT should be continuing CPR. CPR should not be interrupted for more than 10 seconds.

3. The EMT cannot administer aspirin or nitroglycerin. The patient has a history of asthma, which prevents him from receiving aspirin. He has taken a vasodilator within the last 24 hours, which prevents him from receiving nitroglycerin.

4. An uncomfortable feeling of pressure, squeezing, fullness, or pain in the center of the chest is the predominant symptom of an MI.

5. The EMTs should continue CPR until the patient can be transferred to ALS providers. Depending on local protocols, an ALS intercept might be called to the scene or the patient may be transported to the ED.

6. The patient has signs and symptoms of an aortic aneurysm or dissection, including sudden, tearing chest pain and a blood pressure difference between the right and left arm. The patient needs oxygen and must be immediately transported to the hospital. During transport, the EMTs should be prepared for possible hemorrhagic shock and cardiac arrest in the patient.

7. The EMTs should keep the patient calm and provide oxygen if indicated. The patient is symptomatic and unstable, so he should be transported immediately to the hospital. Depending on local protocols, the EMTs may choose to request an ALS intercept.

8. The patient likely has hypovolemic shock due to fluid loss from vomiting and diarrhea.

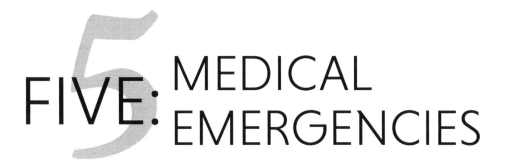

FIVE: MEDICAL EMERGENCIES

Abdominal Pain

Abdominal pain is a common reason for calls to EMS systems. Most calls will be cases of **acute abdomen,** the medical term for sudden, severe abdominal pain. Acute abdomen is frequently accompanied by nausea and vomiting. EMTs should wear the appropriate PPE when handling vomit.

Patients with acute abdomen may also have **referred pain** in other locations, such as the shoulders or hands. Referred pain is caused by the proximity of nerves carrying pain signals to and from the spinal cord.

The specific cause of abdominal pain will be almost impossible to diagnose in the field. However, the EMT should be aware of possible causes of abdominal pain, particularly those that qualify as life-threatening emergencies.

Table 5.1. Causes of Acute Abdomen

Condition	Pathophysiology	Symptoms
Abdominal aortic aneurysm (AAA)	widening of the aorta in the abdomen	See chapter 4 for more information on symptoms and care of ruptured or dissected AAA.
Appendicitis	inflammation of the appendix	right lower quadrant pain; rebound tenderness; fever
Gallstones	blockage in the duct of the gallbladder leading to inflammation (cholecystitis)	right upper quadrant pain that is exacerbated by fatty meals; fever
Kidney stones	blockage in the urethra leading to inflammation of the kidney	unilateral flank pain (can be severe); hematuria
Pancreatitis	inflammation of the pancreas	upper abdominal and back pain; distension of abdomen
Peptic ulcer	erosion of the stomach by stomach acid	upper abdomen and back pain; heartburn
Ruptured ectopic pregnancy	rupture of the fallopian tube due to ectopic pregnancy	See chapter 9 for more information on symptoms and care of ruptured ectopic pregnancy.
Ruptured ovarian cyst	rupture of cyst in the ovary	sudden, severe, unilateral pelvic pain

Care and Transport

- Manage airway.
  - Patients with vomiting may require repositioning or suctioning.
- Provide oxygen as needed.
- Transport to ED per protocols.

PRACTICE QUESTION

1. What are some conditions occurring outside the gastrointestinal system that may cause acute abdomen?

Anaphylactic Shock

Pathophysiology

Anaphylactic shock (or anaphylaxis) is a life-threatening allergic reaction that causes symptomatic vasodilation and bronchoconstriction. The most common causes of anaphylactic shock are food allergens, medications, and insect venom.

The definitive treatment for anaphylaxis is an IM injection of epinephrine. Patients with known allergies may carry an epinephrine auto-injector (EpiPen). The EMT should know how to administer an EpiPen injection.

Mild cases of anaphylaxis may present with itching and urticaria (hives) with no accompanying respiratory compromise. These patients do not usually require emergency care and transport.

What to Look For

KEY FINDINGS

- respiratory distress (can be severe)
- wheezing
- throat tightness
- edema in face, lips, or tongue
- skin pallor or flushing
- hypotension
- history of recent exposure to allergen

OTHER FINDINGS

- weak thread pulse
- syncope or presyncope
- vomiting or diarrhea
- altered mental status
- sense of doom

Care and Transport

- Anaphylaxis requires immediate transport to ED.

- Provide high-flow oxygen and manage airway as needed.

- Follow local protocols when administering patient's epinephrine (EpiPen).

- ALS intercept may be called to administer epinephrine if needed.

PRACTICE QUESTION

2. What medication is used to treat anaphylactic shock and how does it work?

Gastrointestinal Bleeding

An **upper GI bleed** is bleeding that occurs between the esophagus and duodenum. A **lower GI bleed** is any bleeding that occurs below the duodenum. Lower GI bleeds occur less frequently than upper GI bleeds.

Upper GI bleeds can lead to **hematemesis**, the vomiting of blood. The blood may be bright red or brown and clotted (commonly referred to as coffee ground emesis). Lower GI bleeds can result in **hematochezia**, bright red blood in the stool. When blood is partially digested in the lower GI tract, it produces **melena**—dark, thick stools that contain the partially digested blood.

DID YOU KNOW?
More than 70% of GI bleeds occur in the upper GI tract.

HELPFUL HINT
Pregnant people with morning sickness or hyperemesis gravidarum (severe and persistent vomiting) are at risk for Boerhaave syndrome and Mallory-Weiss tears.

Table 5.2. Causes of Gastrointestinal Bleeding

Location	Condition	Pathophysiology
Upper GI bleeding	esophageal varices	Veins in the esophagus dilate and rupture from the pressure caused by obstruction to venous flow, usually due to liver disease. Substantial bleeding can occur.
	esophagitis	Inflammation in the esophagus from infection or stomach acid that ruptures blood vessels. Often caused by **gastroesophageal reflux disease (GERD)**, a chronic condition in which stomach acid leaks into the esophagus.
	Boerhaave syndrome	Bleeding caused by rupture or perforation of the esophagus caused by forceful vomiting. Substantial bleeding can occur.
	Mallory-Weiss tear	Bleeding caused by small tears that occur at the gastroesophageal junction from forceful vomiting. The bleeding usually resolves on its own but may be substantial.
Lower GI bleeding	diverticulitis	Inflammation of the diverticula (small outpouchings in the GI tract) cause inflammation that can lead to necrosis and perforation.
	hemorrhoids	Inflammation of the blood vessels in the rectum that may present as bright red blood in stools. The bleeding is not usually substantial.

Care and Transport

- Manage airway.
    - Patients who are vomiting or have hematemesis may require repositioning or suctioning.
- Provide oxygen as needed.
- Patients with signs and symptoms of a GI bleed should be transported immediately to the ED.

> ### PRACTICE QUESTION
>
> **3.** EMTs arrive at a call to find a 54-year-old woman vomiting bright red blood. While taking her history, the EMTs learn that she has recently been diagnosed with cirrhosis secondary to a chronic hepatitis C infection. What is the most likely location of the patient's bleed?

Headache

Pathophysiology

Headaches are pain caused by pressure or inflammation in the blood vessels and muscles of the head and neck. Most headaches do not require emergency care. However, headache can be a symptom of a serious underlying medical condition, including hemorrhagic stroke and hypertensive crisis. For this reason, patients complaining of headache should be transported to the hospital for further assessment.

Patients should be considered to have a possible life-threatening condition and transported immediately to the ED when headache is:

- severe with a sudden onset
- accompanied by other symptoms such as seizure, fever, or altered mental status
- accompanied by a stiff neck (indicates possible meningitis)

Table 5.3. Types of Headaches

Pathophysiology	Presentation
A **migraine** is a neurovascular condition caused by neurological changes that result in vasoconstriction or vasodilation of the intracranial vessels.	intense or debilitating headache; **prodrome** (changes in mood or bodily sensation) or **aura** (sensory disturbance) may precede migraine; nausea and vomiting; sensitivity to light and sound; paresthesia
Tension headaches are headaches caused by muscle tightness in the head and neck.	generalized mild pain without any of the symptoms associated with migraines, such as nausea or sensitivity to light
In **temporal arteritis**, the arteries in the temporal area become inflamed or damaged.	severe, throbbing headache in the temporal or forehead region combined with scalp pain that is exacerbated with touch; visual disturbances

Pathophysiology	Presentation
Post-traumatic headaches (PTHs) are headaches that begin within 7 days of a traumatic injury or upon the patient's regaining consciousness after a traumatic injury. They typically resolve within 3 months but can become chronic headaches.	signs and symptoms of migraine with recent history of head trauma
Cluster headaches are usually episodic, lasting from 1 to 3 months, with more than 1 episode of headaches a day. They can go into remission for months to years.	intense, recurring unilateral pain that often occurs at the same time every day; agitation; nasal congestion and excessive tear production
Sinus headaches are caused by fluid that builds up in the sinus cavities during an infection.	pain (described as pressure) in areas around sinus cavities; signs and symptoms of cold or allergies

PRACTICE QUESTION

4. What signs and symptoms accompany migraines but are not found with other types of headaches?

Hyperglycemia
Pathophysiology

Hyperglycemia occurs when serum glucose concentrations are elevated in response to a decrease in available insulin or to insulin resistance. The condition is most often associated with diabetes mellitus but can also be caused by medications (such as corticosteroids and amphetamines), infection, sepsis, and endocrine disorders.

Diabetic ketoacidosis (DKA) is a hyperglycemic state characterized by an insulin deficiency that stimulates the breakdown of adipose tissues. This process results in the production of ketones and leads to metabolic acidosis. DKA develops quickly (< 24 hours) and is most common in people with type 1 diabetes.

Hyperosmolar hyperglycemic state (HHS) is a severe hyperglycemic state characterized by extreme dehydration and the absence of acidosis. HHS develops gradually over days to weeks. HHS is more common in persons with type 2 diabetes and has a much higher mortality rate than DKA.

What to Look For

KEY FINDINGS FOR HYPERGLYCEMIA

- blood glucose > 200 mg/dL
- polyphagia
- polydipsia

DID YOU KNOW?

When assessing a patient with suspected hyperglycemia, look for signs of dehydration and take a detailed history of their fluid intake and output.

- polyuria
- dehydration
- weakness and fatigue
- altered mental status

KEY FINDINGS FOR DKA

- blood glucose 350 – 800 mg/dL
- Kussmaul respirations
- fruity odor on breath
- abdominal pain
- nausea and vomiting

KEY FINDING FOR HHS

- blood glucose > 800 mg/dL
- severe dehydration
- delirium
- seizure
- coma

Care and Transport

- Patients with hyperglycemia require insulin and IV fluids and should be transported immediately to the ED.
- Severely dehydrated patients may require an ALS intercept to begin fluid replacement and to monitor for dysrhythmias caused by electrolyte imbalances.

> PRACTICE QUESTION
>
> **5.** What signs and symptoms should the EMT look for to differentiate between diabetic ketoacidosis (DKA) and hyperosmolar hyperglycemic state (HHS)?

Hypoglycemia
Pathophysiology

Hypoglycemia occurs when blood sugar (glucose) concentrations fall below normal. Patients will typically show symptoms when serum glucose is < 70 mg/dL, but the onset of symptoms will depend on the patient's tolerance.

What to Look For

KEY FINDINGS

- blood glucose < 70 mg/dL

- tachycardia
- cold, clammy skin
- altered mental status
- presyncope or dizziness

OTHER FINDINGS

- shakes/tremors
- blurred vision
- fatigue or sleepiness
- lack of coordination or impaired gait
- seizures

Care and Transport

- Administer oral glucose per protocols.
- Transport to ED.

PRACTICE QUESTION

6. An EMT receives a call for an unconscious 34-year-old female. An EMT arrives on scene to find the patient unresponsive with regular, shallow breathing. The patient has a blood sugar of 38 mg/dL. How should the EMT manage this patient?

Sudden Infant Death Syndrome (SIDS)

Sudden infant death syndrome (SIDS) refers to the death of an infant where no cause is found. These infants are usually found in the morning and may have been deceased for several hours at the time of the call. These are among the most challenging calls that an EMT will face.

What to Look For

- The infant will be blue, unresponsive, and not breathing.
- The infant may show signs of rigor mortis or dependent lividity.

Care and Transport

- Because of the sensitive nature of these types of calls, each EMS system has its own protocols that mandate varying levels of treatment.
  - The most aggressive guidelines will allow for providers to "call" a death in the field with no resuscitation efforts if there are signs that resuscitation will be futile.

- - Other guidelines are much more conservative and encourage resuscitation of all full-arrest pediatric patients with immediate transport to the ED, even if there are signs of death.

  - If there are no obvious signs of death, resuscitation efforts should be initiated.

- Attend to grieving parents.

  - Allow parents to stay with the child during resuscitation efforts.

  - If no resuscitation efforts are made, explain why.

  - Do not offer speculation as to the infant's cause of death.

  - Provide support for parents by explaining what will happen next and calling other family members.

PRACTICE QUESTION

7. EMTs have responded to a call for an unresponsive 2-month-old infant. On arrival they find that the infant is blue and not breathing with obvious rigor mortis; they decide not to provide resuscitation. The parents ask the EMTs what happened to their baby. How should the EMTs respond?

Seizure

Pathophysiology

A **seizure** is caused by abnormal electrical discharges in the cortical gray matter of the brain; the discharges interrupt normal brain function.

- **Tonic-clonic seizures** start with a tonic, or contracted, state in which the patient stiffens and loses consciousness; this phase usually lasts less than 1 minute. The tonic phase is followed by the clonic phase, in which the patient's muscles rapidly contract and relax. The clonic phase can last up to several minutes.

- **Status epilepticus** occurs when a seizure lasts longer than 5 minutes or when seizures occur repeatedly without a period of recovered consciousness between them.

- **Atonic seizures** are characterized by a sudden loss of muscle tone, which causes the patient to suddenly fall. These seizures have been called "fall attacks" as the patient has no warning prior to falling.

- An **absence seizure** is characterized by a brief lapse in attention where the patient stares off into space and has no cognitive function. The period of "absentness" is brief, and the patient usually regains cognitive awareness within a few seconds.

Seizures may be caused by **epilepsy**, a chronic condition characterized by recurrent seizures. Seizures may also be caused by trauma or other medical conditions, including:

- fever

- hyper/hypoglycemia

- dysrhythmias
- intracranial hemorrhages
- electrolyte imbalances
- poisoning

What to Look For

- loss of consciousness
- alternating muscle contraction and relaxation
- urinary and fecal incontinence
- tongue biting and frothing at the mouth

Care and Transport

- Maintain a safe environment for the patient.
    - Clear possible hazards.
    - Loosen the patient's clothing around the neck.
    - Do not place anything inside the patient's mouth.
- Prevent aspiration.
    - Roll patient on their side (if no spinal injury is suspected).
    - Suction airway as necessary.
- Provide oxygen and artificial ventilation as needed.
- Transport to ED.
- ALS intercept may be needed for status epilepticus.

> PRACTICE QUESTION
>
> **8.** An EMT is documenting a call for a 34-year-old woman who required transport to a hospital for multiple seizures. What information about the seizure should the EMT document?

Stroke

Pathophysiology

A **stroke** occurs when blood flow to the brain is interrupted.

- An **ischemic stroke** occurs when blood flow within an artery in the brain is blocked, leading to ischemia and damage to brain tissue. The lack of blood flow can be caused by a thrombosis or an embolus.
- A **transient ischemic attack (TIA)**, is a sudden, transient neurological deficit resulting from brain ischemia. It does not cause permanent damage or infarction. Symptoms will vary depending on the area of the brain affected. Most

TIAs last less than 5 minutes and are resolved within 1 hour. A majority are caused by emboli in the carotid or vertebral arteries.

- A **hemorrhagic stroke** occurs when a vessel ruptures in the brain or when an aneurysm bursts. The blood that accumulates in the brain leads to increased intracranial pressure (ICP) and edema, which damages brain tissue and causes neurological impairment. The symptoms of hemorrhagic stroke usually develop over a few minutes or hours.

What to Look For

KEY FINDING FOR ISCHEMIC STROKE

- facial drooping, usually on one side
- numbness, paralysis, or weakness on one side of the body
- slurred speech or inability to speak
- confusion

KEY FINDINGS FOR TIA

- signs or symptoms of ischemic stroke that resolve on their own

KEY FINDINGS FOR HEMORRHAGIC STROKE

- severe, sudden headache (often described by the patient as the worst pain they've ever experienced)
- decreased LOC
- nausea and vomiting
- sudden onset of weakness
- difficulty speaking or walking

DID YOU KNOW?

Bell's palsy is facial drooping caused by inflammation of the facial nerve (cranial nerve VII). It is not life threatening and usually resolves without medical treatment. Bell's palsy is similar to the facial droop seen in stroke patients. However, patients with Bell's palsy will not show any other signs of stroke (e.g., weakness or altered LOC).

Care and Transport

- Manage patient's airway.
- Provide oxygen as needed.
- Transport immediately to a hospital with a stroke center.
  - Ischemic strokes may be treated with thrombolytic drugs that must be administered within 4.5 hours.
  - "Time is brain": the sooner the patient receives hospital treatment, the more likely they are to retain brain function.

PRACTICE QUESTION

9. An EMT receives a call for a 68-year-old man complaining of headache, dizziness, and left arm weakness. When the EMT arrives on scene, the patient reports that the symptoms started about 20 minutes ago and are gone now. The patient has clear speech and answers questions appropriately. He states that he feels fine and does not need to go to the hospital. How should the EMT respond?

1. Acute abdomen—sudden, severe abdominal pain—may be caused by cardiovascular conditions, including a ruptured or dissected aortic aneurysm or an MI (particularly in women). It can also be caused by obstetrical or gynecological conditions, including a ruptured ectopic pregnancy or ruptured ovarian cyst.

2. Epinephrine at 0.3 mg IM (adults) is used to treat anaphylactic shock. Epinephrine is a sympathomimetic and works by dilating the airway, constricting peripheral blood vessels, and reducing swelling in the upper airways.

3. The patient most likely has esophageal varices—bleeding in the lower esophagus that is most often caused by liver cirrhosis.

4. Migraines are usually accompanied by extreme sensitivity to light and sound. They are usually preceded by a prodrome characterized by irritation or euphoria. They may also be preceded by an aura, which includes the sensation of strange lights, smells, or sounds or other sensory disturbances.

5. DKA develops rapidly and presents with hyperglycemia, Kussmaul respirations, abdominal pain, and vomiting. HHS presents with hyperglycemia and neurological changes, including delirium or coma. It may develop over many days or weeks.

6. The patient is hypoglycemic. Because she is unconscious, she cannot be administered oral glucose. She should be transported immediately to the ED where she can be given IV glucose.

7. The EMTs should explain that the infant has died, but the cause of death is still unknown. They should express sympathy and offer the parents the chance to hold the infant.

8. The EMT should include the length of the seizure, the activity witnessed during the seizure, the number of seizures, and the length of time between seizures. This information will be crucial for the physicians who will be following up with the patient.

9. The EMT should explain that the patient is showing symptoms of a transient ischemic attack (TIA), meaning he suffered a small stroke. He may have an underlying condition that is placing him at high risk for further strokes, so he should go to the hospital for further assessment.

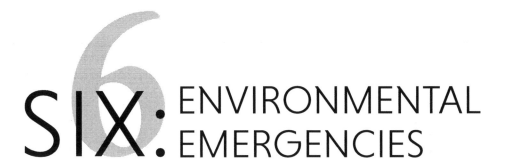

SIX: ENVIRONMENTAL EMERGENCIES

Bites

Pathophysiology

Bites and stings can come from many different sources, including domestic animals, snakes, spiders, scorpions, ants, and marine animals.

- Wild or domestic animal bites can cause punctures, lacerations, and fractured bones. Wounds caused by animal bites are also at high risk for infection.

- While some snakes are venomous, most snakes are not; most bites should be treated like other animal bites.

- Insect bites and stings (e.g., bees, wasps, fire ants) do not typically require emergency care but may cause anaphylaxis.

- Jellyfish are venomous marine animals whose stings can cause intense pain, burning, and rashes.

Care and Transport

- Assess scene safety.
    - Move patient away from source of the bite (e.g., wasp nest).
    - Have animal control remove animals that pose a risk to the patient or EMS crew.
- Uncover and clean injured area.
- Treat soft tissue injuries and fractures as needed.
- Treat allergic reactions and anaphylactic shock as needed.
- Specific interventions may be required for some bites.
    - Request shot records for domestic animals that cause injury.
    - Contact medical control to advise hospital of necessary antivenom if a poisonous snakebite is suspected.

DID YOU KNOW?

There are four common poisonous snakes in the United States: the rattlesnake, water moccasin, copperhead, and coral snake. The saying "Red on yellow kills a fellow, red on black the venom it lacks" can be used to identify coral snakes.

- If a poisonous bite is suspected, splint the extremity to slow the toxin from being absorbed into the body.

- Rinse jellyfish stings with saltwater (not fresh water).

- Patients with fractures, bleeding, anaphylaxis, or bites with high risk of infection should be transported to the appropriate level of care.

PRACTICE QUESTION

1. An EMT is assessing a 24-year-old female who was bitten by a stray dog that ran away when EMS arrived. She has minor puncture wounds with controllable bleeding and little pain. The patient says that she does not need medical care or transport. How should the EMT respond?

Cold Exposure
FROSTBITE AND IMMERSION FOOT
Pathophysiology

Frostbite is injury to the dermis and underlying tissue caused by freezing temperatures. Frostbite most commonly affects fingers and toes. **Immersion foot** is the result of prolonged exposure to cold (but not freezing) temperatures, often in wet conditions. It typically affects the feet but can affect the hands as well.

Both frostbite and immersion foot are characterized by vascular system impairment that leads to cellular damage and inflammation. While frostbite is more likely to cause permanent damage to tissue, both injuries may cause ischemia in the affected extremity.

What to Look For

- Signs and symptoms will be localized in extremities.
- early-stage frostbite:
    - cold and white waxy skin
    - numbness, tingling, or throbbing sensation
- mild-stage frostbite:
    - skin hard or frozen to the touch
    - skin red and blistered when warmed and thawed
- severe-stage frostbite:
    - damage to underlying muscle, tendons, and bone
    - blue, blotchy, or white skin
    - blood-filled blisters as skin warms
    - necrotic areas that are black in appearance
- immersion foot:
    - numbness
    - cold and clammy skin

- ○ pallor
- ○ edema

Care and Transport

- Move patient to warm area.

- Remove any wet clothing.

- Handle affected areas carefully to avoid further damaging tissue.

- Splint and cover if the frozen body part is an extremity.

- Gently warm affected area using warm passive heating or warm water.

  - ○ Do not use intense heat—the extremity will be numb, so the patient will not be able to sense burns or other injuries.

  - ○ Do not rub the affected area.

- Administer oxygen via a non-rebreathing mask.

- Transport to ED.

PRACTICE QUESTION

2. An EMT finds a 23-year-old male lying in the snow near his snowmobile. After walking for help and stepping in a creek, the man returned to his snowmobile to wait for help to arrive. On examination, the EMT finds his right foot to be pale, swollen, and clammy. How should the EMT care for this patient?

HYPOTHERMIA

Pathophysiology

Hypothermia occurs when core body temperature drops below 95°F (35°C), causing a reduction in metabolic rate and in respiratory, cardiac, and neurological functions. When body temperature drops below 86°F (30°C), thermoregulation ceases. If hypothermia persists, coma and respiratory arrest will result.

Fluid shifts during hypothermia can lead to hypovolemia, which is masked by vasoconstriction. When the patient is rewarmed and the blood vessels dilate, the patient will go into shock or cardiac arrest if the fluid volume is not replaced.

What to Look For

- intense shivering that lasts until core body temperature drops below 87.8°F (31°C)

- CNS symptoms:

  - ○ lethargy

  - ○ clumsiness

  - ○ confusion and agitation

  - ○ possible hallucinations

  - ○ unconscious in late stage

- abdomen cool to the touch
- unreactive pupils
- rapid breathing and pulse in early stages
- decreased cardiac and respiratory function in late stages

Care and Transport

- If patient is alert and oriented, the priority intervention is to slowly warm the patient.
    - ○ Remove the patient from the cold environment, and remove wet clothing.
    - ○ **Passive rewarming** is moving the patient to a warmer environment and allowing the patient to warm themselves. This is achieved by removing wet clothing and applying blankets.
    - ○ **Active rewarming** is applying heat packs to the neck, armpits, and groin. Check local protocols to determine if the EMT can utilize active rewarming.
    - ○ Administer warmed, humidified oxygen.
- If patient has an altered LOC or is unconscious, the priority intervention is to manage the airway and breathing.
    - ○ Open the airway if necessary.
    - ○ Access pulse for 30 – 45 seconds. (The pulse can slow drastically for extremely hypothermic patients.)
    - ○ If no pulse, follow BLS protocols.
    - ○ If there is a pulse, provide high-flow oxygen via bag-valve mask or a non-rebreathing mask.
    - ○ Passively rewarm the patient.
- Transport the patient to the hospital.

> PRACTICE QUESTION
>
> **3.** A 68-year-old female was shoveling the snow in her driveway and sat down to take a break. Her neighbor found her sitting in the chair outside shivering and lethargic. He took her into the house and called 911. When the EMT arrives, the woman is alert and oriented but still shivering. How should the EMT care for this patient?

Heat Exposure
Pathophysiology

Heat cramps occur when exercise or physical exertion leads to a profuse loss of fluids and sodium through sweating. When fluids are replaced but sodium is not, the resulting hyponatremia causes muscle cramps.

Heat exhaustion occurs when the body is exposed to high temperatures, leading to dehydration. It is not a result of deficits in thermoregulation or the central nervous system.

Heat stroke results when the compensatory measures for ridding the body of excess heat fail, leading to an increased core temperature. The resulting inflammatory process can cause multiple organ failure that, if not treated, leads to death.

There are two forms of heat stroke: classic and exertional. **Classic heat stroke** occurs as the result of prolonged exposure to high temperatures with no air conditioning or access to fluids. **Exertional heat stroke** occurs when exercising in extreme heat.

What to Look For

- Heat cramps cause a sudden onset of severe spasmodic muscle cramps:
  - seen in the extremity muscles
  - can last from a few minutes to hours
- heat exhaustion
  - temperature elevated but < 104°F (40°C)
  - sweating
  - dizziness or weakness
  - rapid shallow breathing
  - weak pulse
  - cold, clammy skin
- heat stroke
  - temperature > 104°F (40°C)
  - no longer sweating
  - hot, dry skin
  - confusion, delirium, or seizures

Care and Transport

- The priority intervention for heat exposure is to cool the patient.
  - Evaluate body temperature.
  - Remove the patient from the hot environment.
  - Cool the patient with cold packs in the neck, armpits, and groin; misting or fanning the skin; or cool-water immersion.
  - Cool as much of the body as possible.
  - Cool the patient first, and then transport the patient.
- Provide oral fluids if they can be tolerated.
- Provide oxygen via a non-rebreathing mask.
- Transport the patient to the hospital.
  - Patients with heat cramps that subside with cooling may not require transport.

HELPFUL HINT

Never give dehydrated or overheated patients fluids with carbonation, alcohol, or caffeine.

PRACTICE QUESTION

4. An EMT arrives at an outdoor construction site to find a 38-year-old male with hot, dry skin; rapid pulse; and a body temperature of 105°F (40.6°C). The patient is conscious and complaining of weakness. What should the EMT do first for this patient?

High-Altitude Emergencies
Pathophysiology

High-altitude illnesses are caused by rapid ascent to high altitudes. At higher altitudes, atmospheric pressure is lower, and less oxygen is available in the air. If the body is not able to compensate, less oxygen will reach tissues, resulting in hypoxia. EMTs working at high altitudes may see several types of high-altitude illnesses.

- **Acute mountain sickness** occurs 6 to 24 hours after patients quickly ascend to high altitudes (> 6,600 feet).

- **High-altitude cerebral edema (HACE)** is a rise in intercranial pressure due to increased fluid in the brain; it is often considered a progression from acute mountain sickness. HACE may be fatal if not treated promptly.

- **High-altitude pulmonary edema (HAPE)** is fluid in the lungs that occurs 2 to 4 days after ascent (> 8,000 feet).

DID YOU KNOW?

Descent is the definitive treatment for most high-altitude illnesses; symptoms will usually resolve 1 to 2 days after altitude is decreased.

What to Look For

- acute mountain sickness:
  - headache
  - dizziness
  - dyspnea
  - nausea or vomiting
- HACE:
  - often follows signs and symptoms of acute mountain sickness
  - altered mental status
  - uncoordinated motor function
  - coma
- HAPE presents with similar signs and symptoms as other types of pulmonary edema:
  - dry cough
  - dyspnea
  - crackles in lungs
  - cyanosis
  - production of frothy sputum

Care and Treatment

- Patients with signs and symptoms of high-altitude illnesses should immediately stop ascent.

  - Patients with signs and symptoms of mild acute mountain sickness may be able to stay at current altitude with support treatment.

  - Immediate descent is indicated for patients with signs and symptoms of HACE or HAPE.

- Administer oxygen via a non-rebreathing mask.

  - Be prepared to aggressively manage the airway of patients with signs and symptoms of HAPE.

PRACTICE QUESTION

5. An EMT is dispatched to a high-altitude hiking trail for a dyspneic and disoriented 25-year-old male. The patient's friend tells the EMT that the patient arrived in the area two days ago and has been complaining of severe headaches. What should the EMT expect to do for this patient?

Electrical Injuries

Pathophysiology

Generated electrical energy causes external and internal injury from the electrical current running through the body. Injuries will vary depending on the intensity of the current, voltage, resistance, the length of time exposed, entry and exit locations, and the tissue and organs affected by the electrical current.

Generated electrical injury can result in skin burns, damage to internal organs or tissue, respiratory arrest, or cardiac arrhythmias/arrest. Generated current will often cause subcutaneous or deeper tissue injury much greater than the areas indicated by the line of demarcation.

When a person is struck by **lightning**, the electrical energy can result in cardiac arrest, neurological deficits (both acute and long term), and changes in the level of consciousness. It differs from generated electrical energy in that it does not usually cause burns, rhabdomyolysis, or internal organ or tissue damage.

What to Look For

- electrical injury
  - burns with a clean line of demarcation at entry and exit points
  - involuntary muscle contractions
  - difficulty breathing or respiratory arrest
  - seizure or loss of consciousness
  - paralysis
- lightning injury

- confusion, amnesia, or loss of consciousness
- keraunoparalysis (weakness in limbs following a lightning strike)
- hearing loss due to tympanic membrane perforation
- cardiac or respiratory arrest

Care and Transport

- Ensure the safety of the crew and bystanders before caring for the patient.
  - Shut off power or remove the patient from the power source if it is safe to do so.
  - If there are downed power lines, be aware of objects in the environment that may conduct electricity (e.g., aluminum siding).
- Remove any burning or smoldering clothes.
- Check ABCs and follow BLS protocols.
- Treat burns and secondary wounds as needed.
- Transport immediately.

PRACTICE QUESTION

6. An EMT arrives at a scene to find an electrician who has been electrocuted by wires in a circuit breaker box. The patient is still in contact with the wires. What should the EMT do first?

Submersion Injuries
Pathophysiology

A **submersion injury** (drowning) is a respiratory injury or impairment that occurs as a result of being submerged in liquid. These injuries were previously known as "wet drowning" when water was aspirated or "dry drowning" when the patient had a laryngospasm but did not ingest or aspirate water. The term "near drowning" is another term that is no longer commonly used.

Diving into shallow water can cause spinal injuries. If the patient strikes their head on the bottom, the spinal injury may cause paralysis, which makes the patient unable to save themselves in the water.

DID YOU KNOW?
Only a small amount of fluid is required to cause a submersion injury. Young children, the elderly, and intoxicated persons have the highest risk of drowning and may drown in only a few inches of water.

Care and Transport

- The priority care for submersion injuries is to open the airway and follow BLS protocols.
- Assume a possible spinal injury if the patient is unconscious with no witnesses or if there is an obvious mechanism of injury (e.g., diving accident).
  - Move the patient's arms above their head and grasp their biceps to stabilize the neck while rotating them face up.

○ Open the airway and provide rescue breaths while the patient is further stabilized and removed from the water.

○ Once the patient has been immobilized and removed from the water, follow BLS protocols for CPR and AED use.

- If there is no reason to suspect a spinal injury, do not delay rescue breaths or CPR to immobilize the patient.

- Transport the patient to the hospital.

PRACTICE QUESTION

7. An EMT crew arrives at an apartment to find a pulseless, apneic 2-year-old. His parents tell the crew that they found their son with his face submerged in a bucket of mop water. What should the EMT do first for this patient?

1. The EMT should tell the patient that he will not treat her without her consent. However, he should discuss with the patient the risk of infection from dog bites, including rabies. Since the dog has not been found, the patient will likely need prophylactic care for rabies and other possible infections.

2. The EMT should move the patient to a warm area as soon as possible. The EMT should then remove the patient's wet clothing and gently warm the foot using passive warming or warm water. The foot should be splinted if the patient is transported to the hospital.

3. The neighbor has already moved the patient to a warm environment. The EMT should continue passive warming by removing any wet clothing from the patient and wrapping her in blankets. The patient should then be gently moved to the ambulance and transported to the hospital.

4. The EMT's first action should be to cool the patient. He should be moved to a cool area, and the EMT may use ice packs, fans, and/or cool water to cool the patient. Once cooling measures have been taken, the EMT can give oxygen and fluids to the patient and prepare for transport.

5. The patient is showing early signs of high-altitude cerebral edema and will need to descend to a lower altitude immediately to prevent further injury.

6. The EMT should shut off power to the wires or have someone shut off power before administering patient care.

7. The EMTs should follow BLS protocols and begin CPR.

SEVEN: PSYCHIATRIC EMERGENCIES

Pathophysiology

- A **behavioral crisis** is a change in behavior during which the patient does not act in an acceptable or normal manner (as defined by family, friends, and/or cultural norms).
  - The EMS is usually contacted when a person with a behavioral crisis becomes a threat to themselves or others.
  - Examples of a behavioral crisis include a patient sitting at a bus stop eating raw chicken while talking to themselves, or a patient yelling at a tree.

- A **psychiatric emergency** is an acute incident in which the patient is in psychological distress.
  - The patient may be a danger to themselves or others.
  - An example would be a patient that has suffered a recent loss and is having suicidal ideations.

- Behavioral crises or psychiatric emergencies can be the result of:
  - psychiatric conditions (e.g., bipolar disorder)
  - underlying medical conditions (e.g., stroke)
  - psychosocial issues (e.g., depression after divorce)

- **Organic brain syndrome** refers to behavioral or psychological issues caused by an identifiable injury or disease process (e.g., Alzheimer's disease, TBI, drug exposure).

- **Functional disorders** are psychological or behavioral issues without an obvious physiological abnormality (e.g., depression).

HELPFUL HINT

Common medical conditions that cause altered behavior may include: hypo- or hyperglycemia, hypo- or hyperthermia, hypoxia, stroke, head injury, and exposure to toxins.

PRACTICE QUESTION

1. An EMS unit is flagged by a truck driver who says that the woman in the car behind him has been following him for several hours. He confronted her, and the woman stated she is supposed to follow him home. The EMT does a primary assessment and finds a 75-year-old woman who is unable to answer alertness orientation questions. What conditions should the EMT consider during further assessments?

Psychiatric Conditions

- **Anxiety** refers to feelings of fear, apprehension, and worry. Anxiety can be characterized as mild, moderate, or severe (**panic**).
  - Anxiety will impact other functions such as the respiratory, cardiac, and gastrointestinal systems. Patients may experience palpitations, chest pain, dizziness, or shortness of breath.
  - When a patient presents with anxiety, the EMT should always look for organic causes, as other life-threatening illnesses may present with similar symptoms.

- **Bipolar disorder** (formerly known as manic-depressive illness) is characterized by extreme shifts between mania and depression.
  - **Mania** is a state of high energy, increased activity, and feelings of elation and immortality. Mania is often a manifestation of bipolar disorder but can also result from an underlying medical condition (e.g., tumor, hyperthyroidism) or drugs/medications (e.g., cocaine, corticosteroids).
  - **Depression** is a mood disorder characterized by feelings of sadness and hopelessness.

- **Delirium** is a temporary cognitive change from baseline.
  - The patient exhibits confusion and disorientation with a decreased ability to focus or hold attention.
  - Common causes of delirium include medications, hypoxia, stroke, and metabolic disorders (e.g., hypoglycemia, hyponatremia).

- **Dementia** is a broad term for progressive, cognitively debilitating symptoms that interfere with independent functioning.
  - Patients may show decline in one or more cognitive domains, including language, memory, executive function, motor skills, or social cognition.
  - The most common causes of dementia are Alzheimer's disease (most common form of dementia in geriatrics) and vascular dementia (from stroke).

- **Post-traumatic stress disorder (PTSD)** occurs as a result of exposure to traumatic events. Patients with PTSD will have heightened anxiety, anger, and fear, particularly when exposed to triggers associated with the traumatic event. They may experience nightmares or flashbacks related to the event and show heightened sympathetic nervous system activity (e.g., tachycardia, hypertension).

- **Psychosis** is a mental state characterized by delusions, hallucinations, paranoia, suicidal or homicidal ideation, and disturbances in thinking and perceptions. Schizophrenia and severe episodes of either mania or depression can also result in psychosis.

- **Schizophrenia** is a chronic psychotic condition that is characterized by bouts of psychosis, hallucinations, and disorganized speech.
  - Positive symptoms of schizophrenia are those not normally seen in healthy persons. These include delusions, hallucinations, and disorganized speech.

- Negative symptoms are disruptions of normal behaviors. These include social withdrawal, paranoia, and flattened affect.

- A **situational crisis** is an acute change or event in a patient's life that may lead to feelings of anxiety, fear, depression, or other mental or emotional illness concerns.

  - Examples of a situational crisis include divorce, sexual assault, and loss of a family member.

  - The EMT should understand that the crisis is as problematic as the patient perceives it to be: assessment should focus on the patient's response to the event, not the event itself.

- **Suicidal ideation** is characterized by feelings or thoughts of attempting or considering suicide.

  - Patients exhibiting suicidal ideation may have vague thoughts without a distinct plan, or they may have a specific plan and the means to carry it out.

  - When assessing patients having a behavioral or psychiatric emergency, the EMT should always screen for suicidal ideation.

PRACTICE QUESTION

2. What behaviors should an EMT expect to see in a patient with bipolar disorder who is having a manic episode?

Approaching a Behavioral Crisis

- When approaching a patient with altered behavior, the EMT should always be aware of scene safety.

  - Do not enter violent scenes without law enforcement.

  - Maintain situational awareness: look for patients, bystanders, exits, weapons, and other elements of the scene that may affect EMT safety.

  - EMTs should identify themselves and avoid sudden movement that may alarm the patient.

  - Watch for patient movements and never place the patient between the EMT and the exit.

  - Do not leave the patient unattended.

- When assessing patients with altered behavior, the EMT should follow these steps.

  - Complete an initial assessment (ABCs) to check for life-threatening issues.

  - Complete a full set of vital signs and look for medical issues that may have caused the emergency (e.g., low blood glucose, low blood oxygen).

  - Evaluate the patient's psychological state by asking the patient if they have:
    - tried to hurt themselves
    - a plan to commit suicide or attempted suicide
    - a history of psychiatric disorders

- recent increased stress levels or emotional trauma
- used or abused alcohol or drugs

- When communicating with patients with altered behavior, the EMT should take control of the scene and attempt to keep the patient calm.

  ○ Speak in a slow, clear voice.

  ○ Be compassionate and do not judge the patient.

  ○ Stay out of the patient's personal space except for necessary medical assessments.

  ○ Use active listening skills.

  ○ Be aware of the patient's response to bystanders (e.g., if the patient is agitated by family members, have them leave the scene).

  ○ Do not challenge or affirm patients with delusions or hallucinations. Instead, redirect the conversation toward what is real.

- Patients with psychiatric emergencies should be transported to the appropriate facility.

  ○ Cooperative patients may be transported using standard protocols.

  ○ Uncooperative patients may require restraints for transportation. (See "Using Restraints" below.)

  ○ Law enforcement or an ALS unit may be needed to restrain violent patients. Law enforcement officers may also ride in the back of the ambulance.

  ○ Document any statements the patient made about harming themselves or others and report these statements to the receiving facility.

PRACTICE QUESTION

3. EMTs respond to a call about a man shouting and behaving erratically in a park. When the EMTs arrive, they find the man lying still on a bench. Law enforcement is on the scene and tells the EMTs that the man appears to be in a stupor and won't answer questions. What should the EMTs do first?

Using Restraints

- Patient **restraints** may be used when patients are a threat to EMS personnel or to themselves.

- Restraints should only be used when other de-escalation techniques have failed (i.e., as a last resort).

- Restraints may be physical (e.g., wristlets, chest harness) or chemical (i.e., sedation, usually benzodiazepines).

  ○ EMTs may apply physical restraints when necessary (usually with approval from medical control).

  ○ **Chemical restraints** must be administered by an ALS unit.

- Law enforcement should always be requested when a violent patient needs to be restrained.
- The safety of the patient should always be the primary concern when applying restraints.
  - To prevent **positional asphyxiation**, never restrain a patient in a position that may compromise their breathing (e.g., face-down).
  - Use reasonable force (only the force necessary) to apply restraints.
  - Use soft restraints.
  - Never sit on the patient to apply the restraints.
  - Never leave a restrained patient unattended.
- Steps to restrain a violent patient:
  - Communicate and plan with other crew members before attempting to restrain the patient.
  - The patient should be restrained supine with one arm restrained above their head and one at their side. Both legs should also be secured.
  - Attach restraints to non-moving parts of the stretcher.
  - If the patient is spitting, a surgical mask may be used (ensure the patient's airway can still be monitored).
  - A cervical collar can be used when patients attempt to bite EMS personnel.
  - Check distal pulses after application of the restraints; repeat pulse checks every 10 minutes.
  - If the restraints have a lock, keep a key with the EMT in the back of the ambulance.
- Once restraints have been applied, do not remove them unless required for medical care.
- Notify the receiving facility that restraints are being used and why.
- Request additional help at the hospital to transfer the patient to the hospital stretcher.

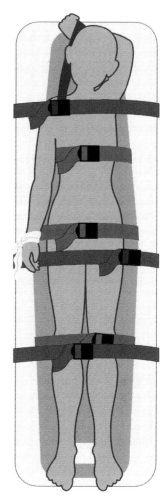

Figure 7.1. Restraint Positioning

PRACTICE QUESTION

4. EMTs respond to a call to find a patient yelling at and punching a tree. He repeatedly states he is going to hang himself from this tree. He is uncooperative and ignores all questions and direction from the EMT. What options does the EMT have to restrain and transport this patient?

1. The patient's age and altered mental status suggest dementia (e.g., Alzheimer's disease). The EMT should also assess for an underlying medical condition, such as stroke or hypoxia, that would cause altered behavior. Finally, the EMT should also consider that the woman may be having an acute exacerbation of an underlying psychological issue (e.g., bipolar disorder).

2. People with bipolar disorder who are experiencing a manic episode will be highly energetic, often accompanied by euphoria or extreme irritability. They may be loud or aggressive and will likely have trouble focusing their attention.

3. The EMTs' priority should be to cautiously approach the patient and perform an initial assessment to look for life-threatening issues with the patient's airway, breathing, or circulation. If no life-threatening issues are found, the EMTs can proceed to assess for medical or psychiatric explanations for the patient's behavior.

4. If the man continues to refuse transport, the EMT should follow local protocols for restraint use. This may include physically restraining the patient with the help of law enforcement and transporting him in an ambulance or a police vehicle. Alternatively, the EMT may contact an ALS unit for chemical restraint.

EIGHT: TRAUMA

Amputation

Pathophysiology

An **amputation** occurs when a body part is separated from the body by surgical or traumatic means. Traumatic amputations typically occur in the extremities and may include fingers, toes, hands, feet, arms, or legs. Amputations are categorized as complete or incomplete (partial).

- **Complete amputations** occur when the body part is entirely separated from the body.

- **Incomplete** or **partial amputations** occur when the body part is non-functional but still technically connected by a tendon, ligament, or other tissue.

Severe hemorrhaging may be absent in some amputations due to the tendency for severed blood vessels to spasm and retract. Partial amputations or those with significant tissue damage (such as crush injuries) will likely result in more blood loss than cleanly severed body parts.

Care and Transport

- The primary concern during a traumatic amputation is bleeding control.
  - Apply direct pressure with a sterile dressing.
  - If bleeding continues, apply a tourniquet proximal to the amputation site.

- If the completely amputated body part is located, wrap it in sterile gauze moistened with saline and put it in a clean, sealed plastic bag. Then place the bag on ice (but do not freeze it).

- If amputation sites are contaminated with dirt or debris, irrigate with saline.

- Do not place ice directly against amputation injuries as this may cause tissue damage.

- Transport patient and amputated body part immediately.

HELPFUL HINT

Trauma is often the result of situations that may be dangerous to the EMT, including violence, motor vehicle crashes (MVCs), or industrial accidents. Assess the scene both for safety and for information that may help treat the patient.

PRACTICE QUESTION

1.   What is the priority care for a patient with an amputation?

Blast Injuries

Pathophysiology

Blast injuries, or trauma caused by explosions, are grouped into four categories.

1. **Primary blast injuries** are caused by the over-pressurization shock wave that results from a high-explosive detonation (e.g., dynamite). Primary blast injuries result in **barotrauma** (injuries caused by increased air pressure) to hollow gas-filled structures such as the lungs, GI tract, and ear drums.

2. **Secondary blast injuries** occur from flying debris impacting the body and causing blunt or penetrative trauma.

3. **Tertiary blast injuries** result from the human body being thrown against a hard surface by the blast of an explosion.

4. **Quaternary blast injuries** are any symptoms not categorized as primary, secondary, or tertiary. Often, quaternary blast injuries are existing conditions (e.g., heart disease) that are exacerbated by the explosion. Quaternary blast injuries may also include burns or crush trauma.

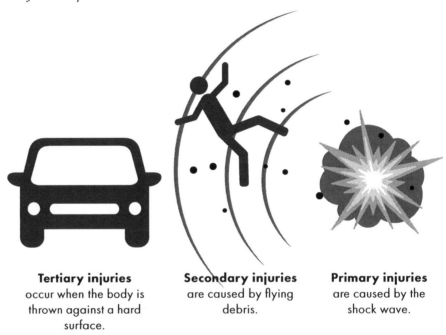

Tertiary injuries occur when the body is thrown against a hard surface.

Secondary injuries are caused by flying debris.

Primary injuries are caused by the shock wave.

Figure 8.1. Classification of Blast Injuries

Care and Transport

- Scene safety is paramount due to the risk of additional explosions.
  - Coordinate with fire, hazardous materials, and law enforcement for safety.

- If possible, move patients to a treatment area that has already been cleared by law enforcement.
- Patient care is symptomatic and often involves controlling bleeding from secondary blast injuries.
- Palpate and auscultate when primary blast injuries are suspected, as internal organs can be ruptured with no exterior signs.
  - Patients with suspected internal injury should be a priority transport to the ED.

PRACTICE QUESTION

2. What are the four types of blast injuries?

Bleeding

EXTERNAL BLEEDING

Pathophysiology

External bleeding, often caused by trauma such as lacerating or penetrating wounds, is categorized into three groups based on the source of the bleeding.

- **Arterial bleeding** is bright red blood that forcibly spurts each time the heart beats.
  - Arterial bleeding is difficult to control due to the pressure it is under.
  - As blood pressure drops, so will the force of the blood spurts.
- **Venous bleeding** is a steady flow of dark red blood.
  - The deoxygenated blood is darker in color than arterial blood.
  - The size of the vein and the wound will dictate how profuse the bleeding is.
- **Capillary bleeding** is slow and "oozing."
  - Capillary bleeding is usually from minor abrasions.
  - Capillary bleeding is easy to control, and the blood may clot on its own without intervention.

Care and Transport

- To reduce the likelihood of exposure, wear a mask, eye protection, a gown, and sleeves in addition to gloves.
- Determine severity by estimating the volume and rate of blood loss compared to the size, age, and medical history of the patient.
- The first and most effective step in controlling external bleeding is to apply direct pressure.
  - Apply temporary pressure with a gloved hand.
  - To create a pressure dressing, place sterile gauze pads over the wound and wrap tightly with a bandage.

○ Check for a distal pulse before and after applying the pressure dressing to ensure circulation has not stopped.

○ Do not remove dressing once applied. If bleeding continues, apply additional dressing.

HELPFUL HINT

Estimated blood loss for a patient with an open fracture to the femur or pelvis is 1500 to 2000 mL. These patients are at high risk for hemorrhagic shock.

• If pressure dressings do not effectively control bleeding, apply a tourniquet proximal to the wound.

• Other interventions may be used to prevent bleeding per local protocols.

○ **Hemostatic agents** are chemicals that promote coagulation. They can be applied as granules or dressings and are helpful in cases where a pressure dressing or tourniquet cannot be applied due to the location of the injury.

○ A **pelvic binder** can be used to decrease bleeding in patients with pelvic fractures.

○ **Air splints** can be used to immobilize fractures in the extremities and to slow bleeding.

○ **Traction splints** can reduce bleeding from femur fractures.

○ The effectiveness of **pneumatic anti-shock garments (PASG)**, also known as **medical/military anti-shock trousers (MAST)**, has been criticized in recent years, and their use has become increasingly less common.

• Administer high-flow oxygen to all patients with severe bleeding.

• Transport patients with arterial or uncontrolled bleeding to the ED immediately.

PRACTICE QUESTION

3. An EMT is dispatched to an MVC involving one car with a single occupant. On arrival, the EMT finds the patient in the driver's seat. He is agitated and repeatedly tells the EMT that his leg is broken and he needs to get out of the car. The EMT does a rapid head-to-toe assessment and finds an open femur fracture with significant blood loss. What is the priority EMT action for this patient?

INTERNAL BLEEDING

Pathophysiology

HELPFUL HINT

The risk of internal bleeding is elevated with some medications, particularly anticoagulants (blood thinners).

Internal bleeding describes any bleeding inside of the body. Most internal bleeding is caused by blunt trauma such as falls or MVCs; broken bones may also cause internal bleeding. There may not be any obvious external signs of internal bleeding, and the severity of internal bleeding is difficult to determine since large amounts of blood may be pooling inside internal cavities.

What to Look For

• contusions

• edema

• pain associated with internal organs

- rigid or tender abdomen
- blood in the vomit or stool
- signs of shock

Care and Transport

- Obtain an accurate history of possible traumatic mechanisms of injury in the days leading up to the symptoms.
- Treatment for internal bleeding is mostly supportive.
- Treat for shock.
- Splint and stabilize broken bones.
- Transport rapidly to an appropriate emergency center.

PRACTICE QUESTION

4. Why is internal bleeding difficult to assess?

Burns
Pathophysiology

Burns are tissue injuries caused by heat, chemicals, electricity, or radiation. In addition to the primary tissue damage, severe burns can lead to life-threatening secondary complications such as hypothermia and infection. Significant **circumferential burns,** which wrap entirely around a body part, can cause constriction of blood vessels and nerves due to edema.

External burn injuries are classified by depth.

- **Superficial** (first degree): Damage is limited to the epidermis and does not result in blisters (e.g., sunburn).
- **Partial-Thickness** (second degree): Damage includes the dermis and epidermis accompanied by severe pain.
- **Full-Thickness** (third degree): All layers of the skin are damaged and there is likely underlying tissue damage. The patient may not feel pain in areas of significant nerve damage.

The severity of external burns is also dependent on the amount of damage, known as **body surface area (BSA).** The **rule of nines** (Figure 8.2) is used to estimate BSA and is different for pediatrics than adults. The **rule of palm** (also known as the **rule of one**) may also be used to estimate BSA, particularly with smaller burns. The size of the *patient's* palm (not the EMT's) is approximately 1 percent of their body surface area.

The overall severity of burn injuries is classified based on depth and BSA plus any complicating factors.

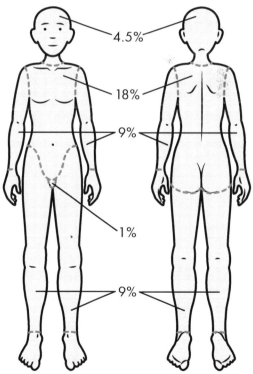

Figure 8.2. Rule of Nines for Calculating Total Body Surface Area (TBSA) of Burns

- **Minor**
  - full-thickness burns less than 2 percent
  - partial-thickness burns less than 15 percent
  - superficial burns 50 percent or less
- **Moderate**
  - full-thickness burns 2 to 10 percent
  - partial-thickness burns 15 to 30 percent
  - superficial burns greater than 50 percent
- **Severe/Critical**
  - full-thickness burns more than 10 percent
  - partial-thickness burns more than 30 percent
  - any burns to the respiratory tract
  - any full-thickness burns to the face, hands, feet, or genitals
  - any burns associated with traumatic or musculoskeletal injury
  - any circumferential burns
  - for patients under age 5 or over age 55, any burn that would otherwise be considered moderate

Care and Transport

- Look for signs of airway compromise such as burns to the face, soot in the nose or mouth, singed nasal hair, or coughing due to smoke inhalation.
- Aggressively manage the airway of any patient with possible airway burns.
- Priority care for burn injuries is to stop the burning.
  - Thermal: Remove the patient from the heat source.
  - Chemical: Brush off any dry powders or flush any liquids with water (irrigate for at least 20 minutes).
  - Electrical: Turn off electrical appliance if safe to do so or have electrical utility company isolate power.
- Dressings may be applied based on type and severity of burn.
  - Superficial and minor partial-thickness thermal burns may be treated initially with moist dressings, but apply dry sterile dressings once the skin has cooled.
  - Due to the risk of hypothermia, use only dry dressings for any burns more severe than minor partial-thickness.
  - Use sterile dressings whenever possible to lessen the risk of infection.
- Certain interventions should be avoided.
  - Do not apply ice or ointments to burn injuries.
  - For chemical burns, do not attempt to apply a "neutralizing" material.

HELPFUL HINT

For chemical burns, check the product label or safety data sheet (SDS) to ensure the chemical is not water-reactive before irrigating (if this can be done without significant delay).

○ Never attempt to remove anything that has melted to a patient's skin.

- Treat patients with high body surface area burns for shock and keep them warm.

- Transport the patient to the appropriate burn care center.

- With chemical burns, document the chemical name and its properties. Do not bring dangerous chemicals or their containers into the ambulance or hospital.

PRACTICE QUESTION

5. An EMT arrives on a scene to find a 5-year-old patient with partial-thickness thermal burns on 2 percent of his body caused by placing his hands in boiling water. The patient has an elevated heart and respiratory rate and is in obvious pain. What is the priority EMT action for this patient?

Crush Injuries
Pathophysiology

Crush injuries occur when sufficient force is applied to the exterior of the body to compress and rupture internal organs, tissues, and bones. The major risk with crush injuries is internal bleeding and associated shock.

Crushing pressure that is sustained for a long period of time (> 60 minutes) can lead to **rhabdomyolysis**, the rapid breakdown of muscle tissue that releases large amounts of waste products into the circulatory system. When reperfusion occurs, these waste products flood the rest of the body, causing kidney failure (a condition sometimes called **crush syndrome**).

HELPFUL HINT

Rhabdomyolysis caused by crush injuries is the second most common cause of death following an earthquake (second only to direct trauma).

Care and Transport

- Extract patient as soon as it can be done safely.

- Manage fractures and bleeding as needed.

- Patients at risk for crush syndrome require paramedic-level care and transport.

PRACTICE QUESTION

6. An EMT arrives on the scene of an MVC. The driver's right leg is trapped under the vehicle, but he is alert and has no complaints other than pain. The fire department will not be able to extract him until specialized equipment arrives. Why should the EMT request higher-level care for this patient?

Facial Injuries
Pathophysiology

Facial injuries are typically caused by traumatic impact with another object secondary to motor vehicle crashes, recreational or sports activity, violent incidents, or falls. Facial injuries may include penetrating trauma (e.g., stab wounds), soft tissue injuries (e.g., lacerations), broken or avulsed teeth, or fractures. Facial bones subject to fracture from blunt force trauma include:

- zygomatic bones (cheeks)
- nasal bones
- maxilla (upper jaw)
- mandible (lower jaw)
- frontal bone (forehead)

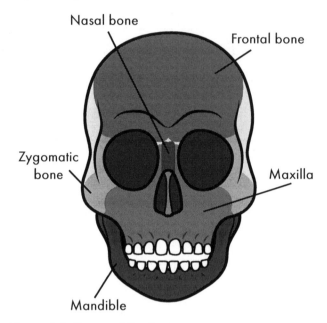

Figure 8.3. Bones of the Face

What to Look For

- The primary concern with facial injuries is airway compromise from fluid, broken bones, teeth, or swelling.
- Observe for signs of traumatic brain injury or associated head, neck, or back injury.
- Document any obvious deformities or asymmetries in the patient's facial structures.
- For dental injuries, observe the scene for any avulsed teeth.

Care and Transport

HELPFUL HINT

For **epistaxis** (nosebleeds), instruct the patient to lean forward and pinch nostrils. Do not let the patient lean back or tilt their head back as this may cause the blood to flow into the stomach.

- Follow appropriate protocol for suspected head, neck, or back injury.
- Be prepared to continuously suction the airway.
- Control any bleeding.
- Impaled objects not obstructing the airway should be secured in place.

- Avulsed teeth should be gently handled by the crown (not the root), rinsed (but not scrubbed) with sterile saline, and transported in sterile saline or in sterile gauze moistened with sterile saline.

PRACTICE QUESTION

7. Describe the process of assessing and caring for a nosebleed.

Eye Injuries

Pathophysiology

Eye injuries occur when there is direct contact with the eye and can be caused by trauma or chemical exposure. Very small foreign objects can easily disturb the **sclera** (outer surface of the eyeball), and foreign objects can cause abrasions to the **cornea** (transparent covering of the pupil and iris). The eyes are also subject to penetrative trauma.

What to Look For

- Assess eye movement by having the patient keep their head still while following the tip of a finger or pen with only their eyes.

- Ask the patient to read print of a size they can normally read without difficulty.

- Have the patient perform the eye movement and reading tasks with both eyes open, then repeat for each individual eye while keeping the other one closed.

- Check for blood or foreign objects in the eyes.

- Ask if the patient normally wears eyeglasses or contacts and if they were on at the time of injury.

Care and Transport

- For chemical exposure, irrigate the eyes immediately and continuously with copious amounts of water.

- Small amounts of debris in the eye, such as dust, can typically be removed by irrigation.

- Cover eyes injured by blunt trauma with a gauze bandage using minimal pressure.

- Do not remove objects impaled in the eye in the prehospital setting.
  - Stabilize impaled objects in place using rolled or folded gauze pads.
  - Add rigid stabilization, such as a paper cup, over the object and gauze.

- Patients with significant eye injury, such as impaled objects, may benefit from having both eyes covered in order to reduce the natural tendency for both eyes to move together.

- Transport patients with significant eye injuries to the ED.

Falls
Pathophysiology

Fall injuries vary considerably, from an elderly patient rolling out of bed to a construction worker falling 20 feet off a roof. Fall injuries may be secondary to medical conditions such as sudden cardiac arrest, syncope, or seizures. Falls greater than 15 feet or three times the patient's height are considered severe. Geriatric patients are at much higher risk for significant injury from falls of any height.

What to Look For

- Attempt to determine the scope of injury by looking for:
  - the height of the fall
  - what type of surface the patient fell on
  - if the patient braced for the fall
  - if an object interrupted the fall
  - what part(s) of the body took direct impact
- Assess for signs and symptoms of common fall injuries including:
  - loss of consciousness
  - TBI
  - internal or external bleeding
  - broken bones

Care and Transport

HELPFUL HINT
Remove jewelry or other constrictive items when swelling is likely to occur (e.g., fractures, burns, soft tissue injuries).

- Follow appropriate protocol for suspected head, neck, or back injury.
- Splint any broken bones and treat any soft tissue injuries.
- Treat for shock as needed, particularly when internal bleeding is suspected.
- Transport to an appropriate emergency facility.

PRACTICE QUESTION

9. What are the indications of a severe fall injury?

Motor Vehicle Crash
Pathophysiology

All **motor vehicle collision** incidents involve three distinct impacts: 1) the vehicle initially impacting an object, 2) the occupant(s) impacting the vehicle, and 3) the organs of the occupant(s) impacting the inner surfaces of the human body. Depending on the speed involved, patients may have multi-system trauma, brain injury, broken bones, internal bleeding, amputations, burns, or abrasions ("road rash").

Motor vehicle crashes (MVCs) are classified by the motion of the vehicle. EMTs should be familiar with the types of crashes and the most common injuries caused by each.

- **Head-On (frontal):** A vehicle in forward motion strikes a stationary object or another vehicle traveling in the opposite direction.
  - ○ Unrestrained drivers may travel up-and-over or under the steering wheel, striking either the windshield or the underside of the dashboard.
  - ○ The driver may also strike the steering wheel with their head, chest, or abdomen.
  - ○ Occupants in other seating positions may strike the dashboard or the back of the seat in front of them.
  - ○ Common injuries include trauma to the head, neck, chest, and abdomen, and fractures in the knees, femur, and pelvis.
- **Rear-End:** A vehicle at rest (or nearly at rest) is struck from behind by another vehicle.
  - ○ Occupants of the rear-ended vehicle often experience head or neck injuries (e.g., hyperextension), particularly when the headrests are not properly positioned.

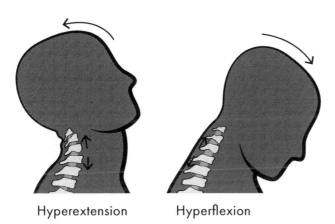

Hyperextension   Hyperflexion

Figure 8.4. Hyperextension and Hyperflexion in the Neck

- **Lateral, T-Bone, Side-Impact,** or **Broadside:** A vehicle is struck by another traveling in a perpendicular direction.
  - ○ Neck injuries are common as the head tends to remain still while the body is forced laterally.
  - ○ Direct traumatic injury due to intrusion is more likely for the occupants on the side of the vehicle where the impact occurred.
- **Rollover:** A vehicle may roll onto its side or roof, or it may roll multiple times.
  - ○ Injuries in rollover accidents are unpredictable.
  - ○ Unrestrained occupants in rollover crashes have a high potential of ejection.

HELPFUL HINT

Seatbelts protect occupants from injuries caused by impact with the vehicle. However, they may cause other injuries, including hip dislocations, lumbar fractures, and damage to abdominal organs.

- **Rotational**: A vehicle spins, while remaining upright, after striking an object or being struck.
  - ○ Rotational injuries are similar to those found in side-impact crashes.

What to Look For

- Observe the crash scene and attempt to determine the mechanism of collision and number of patients.
  - ○ In significant MVCs, unrestrained occupants who are ejected may be some distance from the impact site.
  - ○ Pedestrians, bicycle riders, and motorcyclists may become trapped underneath vehicles.
  - ○ Look for clues such as blood on a broken windshield, a bent steering wheel, or impact depressions on the dashboard.
- Attempt to determine where each occupant was sitting and whether they were properly restrained.
- Ask witnesses and occupants to estimate vehicle speed.
- Conduct a rapid trauma assessment as motor vehicle collisions often involve injury to multiple parts of the body.
- Look for signs and symptoms of underlying medical conditions exacerbated by trauma.

Care and Transport

- Follow appropriate steps for suspected spinal injury.
  - ○ Maintain manual in-line stabilization for trapped occupants requiring advanced extrication.
  - ○ The rescuer maintaining in-line stabilization during mechanical extrication should have appropriate personal protective equipment such as long sleeves and pants, eye protection, gloves, and a helmet.
  - ○ Protect the patient against sparks, broken glass, and other debris present during mechanical extrication.
- Treat patients based on signs and symptoms.
- Transport patients to an appropriate hospital based on severity and extent of injuries.

PRACTICE QUESTION
10. What are the common mechanisms of injury in a head-on motor vehicle collision?

Neck Injuries

Pathophysiology

With the exception of spinal injuries, which are discussed separately, the main source of injury to the neck is an open wound due to trauma (e.g., cutting, gunshot wound). Neck injuries may be self-inflicted or caused by an outside force; they typically include lacerations or penetrations. Neck injuries may involve the jugular veins, carotid arteries, esophagus, larynx, or trachea.

Care and Transport

- The main priorities for neck injuries are to:
  - maintain the airway
  - control significant bleeding
  - prevent air embolism
- Apply pressure to the wound to control bleeding.
  - Take care not to apply so much pressure that all veins/arteries or the airway are obstructed.
- Place an occlusive dressing over any open neck wounds to prevent an air embolus from entering the blood vessels.
- Use bandages to secure any impaled objects in place, and do not attempt to remove the objects.
- Be prepared to suction excess secretions for patients with esophageal injury who may experience difficulty swallowing.
- Transport immediately to an appropriate medical facility.

> ### PRACTICE QUESTION
>
> **11.** What is the EMT's priority when managing a patient with a penetrating neck wound?

Orthopedic Injuries

DISLOCATIONS

Pathophysiology

Dislocations involve bones being separated or "disrupted" from the joint they are a part of. Most dislocations are caused by sudden, abnormal force placed on the joint. Common causes of dislocations include falls, motor vehicle collisions, and athletics; common sites include shoulders, fingers, hips, and knees.

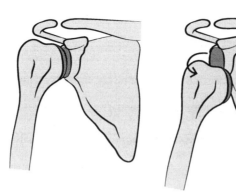 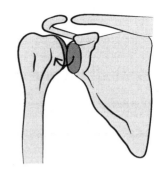

Normal anatomy   Anterior dislocation   Posterior dislocation

Figure 8.5. Shoulder Dislocation

Dislocations usually result in damage to ligaments and tendons and may damage muscles and blood vessels. Significant damage may still have occurred even if the joint was restored (sometimes done by the patient or bystanders before EMS arrival).

What to Look For

- intense, localized pain at the joint
- deformity of joint
- loss of function or range of motion
- absent pulses distal to injury (with blood vessel damage or constriction)

Care and Transport

- The primary objective for dislocations is stabilization.
- Take spinal immobilization measures if indicated.
- Assess distal pulses, motor function, and sensation.
- If distal pulses are absent, manually realign the joint and reassess for circulation.
  - Realign by applying **manual traction** (gently pulling the limb away from the body).
  - Do not attempt to correct the dislocation by putting the bones back in place.
  - If distal pulses cannot be restored by realignment, patient transport should be a high priority.
- Select an appropriate size and type of splint to immobilize above and below the joint.
  - Reassess pulses, motor function, and sensation after the splint is in place.
- Transport to an appropriate medical facility.

PRACTICE QUESTION

12. What is the goal of realigning a dislocated shoulder joint?

Pathophysiology

A **fracture** is a break in any bone. They are most commonly caused by trauma. Broken bones can cause serious internal damage, including significant blood loss and damage to nerves, tendons, or ligaments. Fractures are categorized as open or closed.

- **Open** (also known as compound): The broken bone has punctured the skin and is protruding outside of the body.

- **Closed**: The skin surrounding the break remains intact.

Compartment syndrome occurs when the pressure within a compartment (areas within the body separated by fascia tissue) becomes high enough to prevent perfusion. Most cases of compartment syndrome are caused by fractures that lead to blood collecting within the compartment. However, compartment syndrome can also be caused by hematomas, infections, or crush injuries. If left untreated, compartment syndrome can cause tissue necrosis.

HELPFUL HINT

Commonly fractured bones include the clavicle, radius/ulna, femur, and tibia/fibula. The most common area affected by compartment syndrome is the calf.

Assessment

- localized pain

- swelling

- deformation

- crepitus (grating of broken bones)

- The cardinal symptom of compartment syndrome is pain at the site that is disproportionate with the injury.

Care and Transport

- Take spinal immobilization measures if indicated.

- Control any external bleeding from open fractures.

- The care for fractures is stabilization, primarily achieved by splinting.
  - Stabilize broken bones at the joints above and below the injury.
  - Position the splinted limb as close to anatomically normal as possible.
  - Do not reposition the limb if there is resistance or evidence of further injury.
  - Reassess pulses, motor function, and sensation after the splint is in place.

- **Femur fractures** have the potential for large blood loss and are also very painful for the patient.
  - Use traction splints to stabilize femur fractures.
  - Continually reassess distal pulse, motor function, and sensation before and after splinting.
  - Transport immediately to an appropriate medical facility.
  - Contraindications for traction splints include open fracture, pelvic fracture, or any significant injury to distal bones or joints.

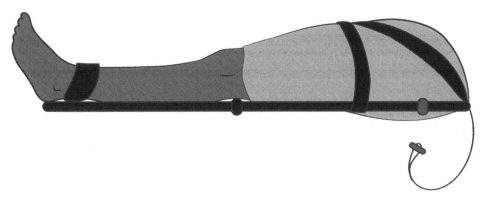

Figure 8.6. Traction Splint for Femur Fracture

PRACTICE QUESTION

13. A 6-year-old boy fell while running and caught himself with outstretched hands. He is now complaining of intense pain in his shoulder and is holding his arm across his chest. What possible injuries should the EMT suspect?

SKULL FRACTURES

Pathophysiology

Skull fractures are caused by trauma such as falls, violent incidents, motor vehicle collisions, and recreational activity. Skull fractures are subdivided into several categories:

- **Linear:** A single fracture line with no accompanying depression or movement of cranial bones.

- **Depressed:** The skull is indented, and the patient is at high risk for brain damage.

- **Basilar:** A fracture located at the base of the skull.

- **Compound:** A skull fracture that breaks the skin.

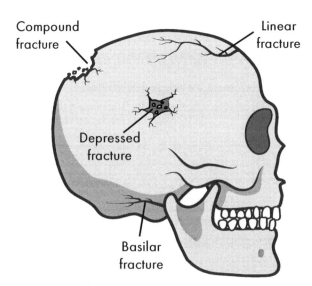

Figure 8.7. Types of Skull Fractures

- **Diastatic:** Limited to infants, the fracture widens the suture lines of the cranial bones before they fuse together.

What to Look For

- Skull fractures and brain injuries are assessed similarly since the two often accompany each other.
- The most obvious sign of skull fracture is deformity.
- It may be difficult or impossible to assess the difference between a skull fracture and a head laceration without fracture.

Care and Transport

- Initiate spinal immobilization measures.
- Control bleeding.
    - Do not apply pressure to depressed skull fractures.
- Keep the patient calm and treat for shock.
- Transport patients with known or suspected skull fracture to the ED immediately.

> PRACTICE QUESTION
>
> **14.** What is a diastatic skull fracture?

STRAINS AND SPRAINS

Pathophysiology

A **strain** is the overstretching or tearing of muscles and/or tendons. The most common strains are the hamstring and lower back, with the latter often resulting from improper lifting technique. A **sprain** is the overstretching or tearing of ligaments. The most common sprains are the ankle, wrist, and knee.

Both injuries are usually caused by general overuse, a sudden force, or manual stretching. While strains and sprains are not life-threatening, improper care can lead to long-term joint or muscle complications and loss of quality of life.

What to Look For

- localized pain
- delayed swelling
- loss of range of motion
- Patients can usually attribute their injury to a specific activity.
- Strains may result in muscle twitching or spasm.
- Sprains are more likely to include discoloration or bruising.

- Complete tears may result in the patient feeling a "pop" at the time of injury and a deformity due to the tissues contracting or "rolling up."

Care and Transport

- Priority care for strains and sprains is splinting and immobilization.

- If the patient requests transport to a medical facility, provide supportive care and place in a position of comfort.

PRACTICE QUESTION

15. What is the difference between a sprain and a strain?

Penetration Injuries and Impaled Objects
Pathophysiology

Penetration injuries and impaled objects involve any foreign object completely puncturing the skin of the body. **Penetrating injuries** may be objects that have entered and remain in the body, leaving only an entrance wound. The object may also enter and pass through the body, leaving both entrance and exit wounds (**perforating wound** or **perforation**). **Impaled objects** are a subset of penetration injuries and describe objects that have punctured the skin and remain protruding from the body.

Penetration injuries are classified by velocity:

- **Low-Velocity:** Typically limited to objects propelled by hand or a bodyweight fall onto an object.

- **Medium-Velocity:** Handguns, shotguns, some rifles (including air rifles), and bows and arrows will produce medium-velocity wounds.

- **High-Velocity:** Limited to high-powered rifles, high-velocity projectiles will likely produce secondary internal damage known as **cavitation** or pressure-related damage resulting from the pressure wave that accompanies very fast-moving projectiles.

Regardless of velocity or location on the body, penetration injuries may be difficult to locate and are not always accompanied by pain or profuse external bleeding.

Care and Transport

HELPFUL HINT

The rapid trauma assessment should always include anterior and posterior portions of the body to verify the total number of entrance and exit wounds.

- Attempt to determine the size and characteristics of penetrating objects no longer in the body (e.g., caliber of firearm, length of knife).

- Expose the patient (remove clothing and equipment), taking care not to cut or tear through holes in clothing created by the penetrating object.

  - For violent incidents, the victim's clothing is considered evidence and should be left in the custody of law enforcement after being removed from the patient.

- Secure in place foreign objects that have impaled or otherwise penetrated the body, with the following exceptions:
  - objects that are obstructing the patient's airway
  - objects that are preventing the EMT from performing CPR when CPR is necessary
- Control bleeding with direct pressure and sterile dressings.
- Impaled objects that are too large or stationary to allow the patient to be moved will require specialized personnel and tools to cut the object. Follow medical direction and local protocol.
- Treat for shock as needed and transport to an appropriate facility as soon as possible.

PRACTICE QUESTION

16. What is the difference between perforating and non-perforating puncture wounds?

Sexual Assault

Pathophysiology

Sexual assault includes any sexual contact to which an individual does not explicitly consent. It can happen to people of any age, race, sex, gender identity, sexual orientation, marital status, or mental status. Sexual assault may result in injuries to the anus or genital regions and may be accompanied by trauma to other areas of the body (e.g., damage to airway caused by strangulation).

Care and Transport

- Notify the appropriate law enforcement agency in every case of known or suspected sexual assault.
- Most sexual assault survivors know their attackers. Ensure law enforcement has declared the scene safe for first responders if there is a risk the attacker may return.
- Provide a safe and private environment for the patient.
  - Remove any bystanders or non-essential persons from the area where the sexual assault patient is to be assessed.
  - Do not separate pediatric sexual assault patients from parents or guardians. If the pediatric patient accuses a parent of sexual assault, follow the direction of law enforcement and do not leave the child alone with the parent.
  - Sexual assault patients may be uncomfortable discussing what happened or allowing the EMT to examine them.
  - The EMT and the sexual assault patient should never be left alone together.

○ If possible, the EMT and the sexual assault patient should be the same gender unless the patient specifically requests otherwise.

- Encourage victims of sexual assault to refrain from showering/bathing or discarding clothing, which should be treated as evidence.

- Control any external bleeding.

  ○ Sexual assault patients who are conscious and alert may wish to apply their own dressings, particularly to trauma of the genitalia.

  ○ Do not dispose of dressings or similar medical equipment used on sexual assault patients as it may be considered evidence.

- Provide supportive care.

- If possible, transport the patient to a medical facility with an on-duty **sexual assault nurse examiner (SANE)**, a registered nurse (or advanced practitioner) certified to treat victims of sexual assault.

PRACTICE QUESTION

17. A male EMT is the first responder on scene and approaches a woman who has been sexually assaulted. The woman refuses care and states that she just wants to take a shower and go to sleep. How should the EMT respond?

Soft Tissue Injuries
Pathophysiology

Closed soft tissue injuries are mainly caused by blunt force trauma that does not result in broken skin. A **contusion**, also referred to as a bruise, is temporary and indicates minor damage to the blood vessels in the dermis that will heal on its own. **Hematomas** are similar to contusions: they involve the collection of blood underneath the unbroken skin. However, hematomas involve larger amounts of blood and often need surgical intervention to heal. If left untreated, the internal pressure created from hematomas can be life threatening.

Open soft-tissue injuries are those in which the skin has been broken.

- An **abrasion**, often called a "scrape" or "scratch" by the layperson, involves only the outer layer of skin being damaged by friction. Bleeding may be minimal, but pain can be significant.

- A **laceration** is a tearing of the skin. They are commonly referred to as a "cut" but may also result from blunt trauma.

- **Avulsions** are flaps of skin that have been partially or completely severed.

  ○ **Degloving** describes an avulsion where the skin surrounding an appendage has been peeled or rolled back onto itself.

  ○ Degloving is often the result of constrictive jewelry being forcefully removed, such as after getting caught on an external object.

Assessment

- discoloration
- swelling
- pain at site
- Deep hematomas might not have visible discoloration.

Care and Transport

- Care for soft tissue injuries is supportive.
  - Splint the injury site, checking for distal pulses, motor function, and sensation before and after.
  - Treat for shock and transport to an appropriate medical facility.
- The priority care for open soft-tissue injuries is to control bleeding and help prevent infection.
  - Expose the open soft-tissue injury.
  - Control any major bleeding with direct pressure and sterile dressing.
  - Quickly yet gently clean minor bleeds by using sterile gauze to wipe away debris that could lead to infection.
  - Minimize movement or completely stabilize the injury site to reduce bleeding and further injury.
  - Gently put back in place partial avulsions after cleaning the wound site.
  - Total avulsions should be packaged separately in the same manner as a total amputation.

> PRACTICE QUESTION
>
> **18.** An EMT arrives on the scene of an industrial accident in which the skin on the patient's left finger was totally avulsed after his wedding ring became caught in equipment. What interventions should the EMT plan to provide?

Spine Injuries
Pathophysiology

Spinal injuries may occur by different means, such as MVCs, falls, sports or recreational activities, and blunt or penetrative trauma. Spinal injury can result in the fracture, dislocation, compression, bruising, or severing of the spinal anatomy. Spine injuries are classified by mechanism.

- **Compression** occurs when the head is pressed down onto the spine (e.g., diving injury, unrestrained occupants in MVCs).
- **Extension** occurs when the head is forced backward (e.g., rear-end MVC with an improperly set headrest).

- **Flexion** occurs when the head is forced forward (e.g., frontal collision when the torso is secured but the head is not).

- **Rotation** occurs when the head is moved in a sideways motion (e.g., hard collisions in contact sports).

- **Distraction** is the elongation or stretching of the spine; it typically only occurs in hangings.

What to Look For

- loss or reduction of motor or sensory function in the extremities

- paralysis

- pain, tenderness, or deformities along the spine

- signs and symptoms of complications caused by damage to spinal nerves
  - impaired breathing
  - priapism
  - loss of bowel or bladder control
  - neurogenic shock (hypotension with a normal or slightly low heart rate)

HELPFUL HINT
The treatment of life-threatening conditions, including the removal of the patient from an imminently dangerous scene, takes priority over spinal stabilization.

Care and Transport

- Follow protocols for spinal immobilization. (See chapter 12, "The Psychomotor Exam," for detailed instruction on spinal immobilization.)

- Patients with suspected spinal injury should be transported to an appropriate receiving facility, such as a trauma hospital.

PRACTICE QUESTION

19. What are the most reliable indications of spinal cord injury?

Traumatic Brain Injuries
Pathophysiology

Traumatic brain injury (TBI) is caused by direct or indirect contact with the brain. Direct contact with the brain typically happens as the result of a penetrating head wound or blunt force head trauma resulting in cranial fracture. Indirect brain contact involves an impact to the head wherein the force is transferred to the brain.

TBI may result in **intracranial hemorrhage** (bleeding within the skull). This bleeding is named for its location:

- **Epidural hematoma**: blood between the skull and the dura mater (usually associated with skull fracture)

- **Subdural hematoma**: blood between the brain and the dura mater

- **Subarachnoid hematoma**: bleeding within the subarachnoid space

- **Intracerebral hemorrhage**: blood pooling within the brain tissue

The brain is tightly encased within the skull, and there is minimal room for swelling or blood. Significant brain injury will cause increased **intercranial pressure (ICP)**, the pressure within the skull. In severe cases of increased ICP, the brain may shift into the **foramen magnum** (the opening in the base of the skull where the spinal cord enters) in a process known as **cerebral herniation syndrome**.

A **concussion** is a mild brain function disruption in which the acute symptoms have a rapid onset but gradually improve.

What to Look For

- signs and symptoms of TBI:
  - altered LOC or mental status
  - headache
  - trismus (clenched teeth/jaw)
  - cerebrospinal fluid (CSF) leaking from the ears or nose
  - Battle's sign (bruising behind the ears) (associated with skull fracture)
  - discoloration under the eyes ("raccoon eyes")
- signs and symptoms of intercranial hematoma:
  - posturing (stiff legs, arms stiff or drawn up toward the chest, fists or fingers clenched)
  - unequal or unreactive pupils
  - seizure
  - hypertension
  - decreased respiratory effort
- **Cushing's triad** is a sign of increased ICP and/or herniation syndrome:
  - hypertension
  - bradycardia
  - altered respiratory pattern
- signs and symptoms of concussion:
  - briefly altered LOC
  - headache
  - nausea or vomiting
  - amnesia
  - general disorientation

Care and Transport

- Patients with suspected head injury are unreliable witnesses, so look for bystanders or rely on context clues.

- Provide manual stabilization of the head and neck.

- Reverse Trendelenburg position (head elevated) may be indicated by local protocol or medical direction.

- Aggressively manage airway and oxygen saturation.
  - ○ Have suction ready in case patient vomits.

- Do not apply pressure to the skull if fracture is suspected.

- Do not apply pressure to areas with CSF leakage.

- Transport immediately to the ED.

PRACTICE QUESTION

20. What is Cushing's triad, and what interventions should the EMT expect to provide for patients with the symptoms associated with it?

ANSWER KEY

1. The EMT's primary concern with an amputation is controlling bleeding. While cleanly severed amputations may bleed less due to the blood vessels contracting, incomplete amputation or amputations involving arteries can lead to hemorrhage and shock.

2. Primary blast injuries are caused by the shock wave from a high-explosive detonation. Secondary blast injuries are from explosion fragments impacting the body. Tertiary blast injuries are from the body being thrown by the blast, and quaternary blast injuries are all of those not otherwise categorized.

3. Significant bleeding from an open femur fracture is a life-threatening injury that must be addressed before the patient can be moved or further assessed. If possible, the EMT should apply a pressure dressing to the patient before he is removed from the car. A tourniquet or hemostatic agent may also be used depending on the position of the patient and local protocols. The patient should then be removed from the car using a rapid extraction technique and immediately loaded for transport.

4. Assessing internal bleeding is challenging because the cause and the source of the bleed cannot be seen and may be unknown. The amount of blood hemorrhaging into internal cavities cannot be determined in a prehospital setting. Signs and symptoms may be minimal and are consistent with other conditions, such as shock or simple blunt force trauma.

5. The priority action for the EMT is to stop the burning process by cooling the area with a cool, wet dressing. Once the area is cool, the burn should be covered with a dry, sterile dressing, and the patient should be transported to the ED.

6. Because the driver's leg will be trapped under the car for an extended period of time, he is at high risk for crush syndrome. He will require fluids and analgesics while he remains trapped, and paramedics will need to monitor for and treat damage to the kidneys once he has been extracted.

7. For patients with epistaxis (nosebleed), have the patient lean forward and pinch the nostrils if this can be done without further pain or injury. The patient should never be instructed to lean back or tilt their head back as this could cause blood to drain into the stomach, leading to vomiting.

8. Eye movement is assessed by having the patient keep their head still while following an object, such as the tip of the EMT's finger, side-to-side as well as up and down using only their eyes. This assessment should be performed using both eyes followed by each eye individually while the other is covered.

9. Falls from greater than 15 feet or more than three times the patient's height are automatically considered severe. However, elderly patients may experience a severe fall from much lower height. Any fall resulting in spinal injury, loss of consciousness, significant internal or external bleeding, or brain injury should also be considered severe.

10. The driver of a vehicle in a head-on collision may travel up-and-over the steering wheel, striking the windshield and causing injury to the head or neck. The driver may also travel under the steering wheel, striking the underside of the dashboard and causing fractures of the knee, femur, or pelvis. The chest or abdomen may strike the steering wheel, causing rib fractures or trauma to the lungs or heart.

11. The EMT's priority should be maintaining the airway. The EMT will also need to control bleeding and prevent air emboli from entering the venous system.

12. The EMT should attempt to realign a dislocated shoulder if the pulse distal to the injury is absent. The goal of realigning the joint is to return circulation to the affected extremity. Realignment may also help alleviate pain.

13. The mechanism of injury and the patient's complaint could be consistent with either a fracture or a dislocation. The EMT should suspect either a shoulder dislocation or a fracture to the clavicle, humerus, or scapula.

14. A diastatic skull fracture is the widening or enlargement of the cranial sutures present in newborns and infants. Since the cranial bones fuse together in early childhood, diastatic skull fractures are only found in infants.

15. Sprains and strains are differentiated by the part of the anatomy they affect. Sprains are injuries to the ligaments, which connect bone to bone. Strains are injuries to either the muscles or tendons, the latter of which connect bone to muscle.

16. A perforating puncture injury is the result of an object that has left an entrance wound and an exit wound. A perforating wound may be caused by an object that entered and exited the body completely, such as a "through-and-through" gunshot wound. Impaled objects can also be perforating. A non-perforating puncture injury only has an entrance wound.

17. The EMT should assure the woman that he will not assess or treat her without her consent. He or his partner should then call for a female EMT to examine the woman and should ensure that the appropriate law enforcement personnel are en route. While he waits for further resources, he should suggest to the woman that she refrain from removing her clothes or showering, but he should not attempt to restrain her if she wants to leave.

18. The EMT should gently remove debris from the wound and control bleeding with direct pressure and a sterile dressing. The avulsed skin should be packaged in sterile moist dressing and transported with the patient.

19. In conscious patients, the most reliable signs of spinal cord injury are paralysis, loss or reduction in motor function, and/or loss or reduction in sensory function in the extremities.

20. Cushing's triad consists of hypotension, bradycardia, and irregular change in breathing. Cushing's triad is a sign of increased ICP and impending or actual cerebral herniation. Treatment may include positioning the patient in reverse Trendelenburg and hyperventilation with supplemental oxygen.

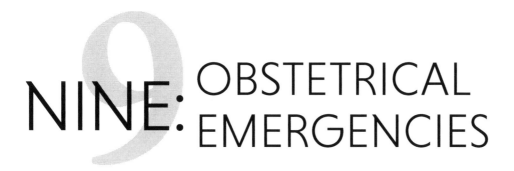

NINE: OBSTETRICAL EMERGENCIES

Anatomy and Physiology of Pregnancy

- After an egg is fertilized with sperm, it develops into an embryo, which implants itself on the wall of the uterus.

- After approximately eight weeks, the embryo is described as a **fetus**.

- The fetus is surrounded by a fluid-filled membrane called the **amniotic sac**.

- The **placenta** is a blood-rich temporary organ attached to the wall of the uterus that provides nutrients and gas exchange for the fetus and eliminates waste.

- The placenta is attached to the fetus by the **umbilical cord**.

- During **labor**, the cervix dilates and thins to allow the fetus to pass. Then, **contractions** of the muscular walls of the uterus push the fetus through the cervix and out the birth canal (**delivery**).

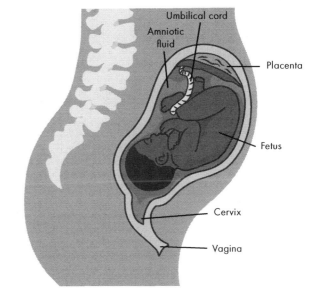

Figure 9.1. Fetus in Third Trimester

- Labor and delivery occurs in 3 stages.

  - Stage 1: cervix dilates and contractions begin (12 – 16 hours).

  - Stage 2: cervical dilation is complete, pushing begins, and the fetus is delivered (2 – 3 hours).

  - Stage 3: the placenta is delivered (10 – 12 minutes).

- **Full-term pregnancy** is 40 weeks and is divided into the first trimester (1 – 12 weeks), second trimester (13 – 26 weeks), and third trimester (27 – 40 weeks).

  - **Preterm labor** occurs between 20 and 37 weeks.

  - Post-term pregnancy occurs when the fetus has not been delivered by 42 weeks.

- The likelihood of survival is very low for fetuses delivered before 24 weeks but increases with gestational age.
- With access to appropriate neonatal care, around 90 percent of fetuses delivered at 27 weeks survive.

- Normal position for the fetus during delivery is head down. **Breech** position is when the fetus has its feet or buttocks downward.
- During pregnancy, the woman will experience physiological changes that may affect the delivery of medical care. These changes include:
  - increased blood volume (as much as 50 percent by the end of pregnancy)
  - increased heart rate (normal increase is around 15 beats per minute)
  - increased respiratory rate
  - increased oxygen demand and decreased lung capacity
  - increased clotting speed
  - displaced GI and respiratory organs

PRACTICE QUESTION

1. What changes from normal should the EMT expect to see when taking vital signs for a patient who is 38 weeks pregnant?

Labor and Delivery

- Start assessment of a pregnant patient by assessing ABCs. Conditions that threaten the life of the mother should be addressed before any further assessment is done.
- If the patient has no life-threatening conditions, take vital signs and assess the status of the pregnancy by asking the patient:
  - the due date
  - how many pregnancies the patient has had
  - if the patient has received prenatal care
  - how far apart the contractions are (time the contractions as well)
  - if their "water broke" (did the amniotic sac rupture)
  - if they feel the need to push or move their bowels
- Physically examine the vaginal opening for **crowning** (the emergence of any part of the baby from the vaginal opening).
- EMTs must assess pregnant patients to decide whether to load and go or stay to deliver the baby.
- Load and go if birth is not imminent.
- The EMT should stay and deliver the baby if birth is imminent. Signs that birth is imminent include:
  - crowning

- contractions 2 minutes apart or less
- feeling the urge to push or having a bowel movement
- if the mother has had multiple births and expresses that the baby is coming

- Load and go and call for an ALS intercept for complicated deliveries, which include:
  - crowning that reveals a body part other than the head (including the umbilical cord)
  - unstable patient vital signs
  - the birth is not progressing
  - preterm labor
  - no prenatal care
  - labor induced by trauma or drugs
  - multiple births (twins or triplets)
  - meconium staining

- Follow these steps to prepare the patient for birth.
  - Move the patient to a private area.
  - Use PPE (face masks, gloves, gown, face shield, and eye protection).
  - Remove patient's clothes and undergarments that obstruct the view of the vaginal opening.
  - Use sterile sheets when available to drape the patient.
  - Elevate the mother's buttocks with the knees drawn up.

- During delivery:
  - The EMT should allow the patient to push out the child while the EMT gently guides the head and shoulders out.
  - Place the newborn on the patient to warm the baby before the cord is cut.
  - When the cord is no longer pulsing, clamp 10 inches and 7 inches from the baby, and cut between the clamps.
  - Deliver the placenta; do not pull on the cord.

- After delivery, assess the mother and address any bleeding or tearing.
  - If the placenta delivers, massage the mother's abdomen to help contract the uterus (this will slow vaginal bleeding).
  - Control bleeding by placing a 5 × 9 gauze on the vaginal opening, and instruct the mother to lower and put her legs together.
  - There may be torn tissue on the perineum: advise the mother that this is normal and dress the wound with a sanitary pad.

HELPFUL HINT
ALS should always be called for a birth in the field.

DID YOU KNOW?
Meconium is the fetus's feces. If meconium is released into the amniotic fluid, the fetus may inhale it, causing asphyxiation.

PRACTICE QUESTION

2. An EMT arrives at a scene to find a 27-year-old woman having contractions. She has had four previous live births and states that she thinks the baby is about to come out. What should the EMT do?

Pregnancy and Delivery Complications

- **Umbilical cord prolapse** occurs when the cord presents alongside (occult) or ahead of (overt) the presenting fetus during delivery. Exposure of the cord makes it vulnerable to compression or rupture, which disrupts blood flow to the fetus.

- **Preeclampsia** is a syndrome caused by abnormalities in the placental vasculature that cause hypertension and proteinuria (protein in urine).
  - Signs and symptoms of preeclampsia include hypertension, edema, severe headache, and rapid weight gain.
  - Preeclampsia can lead to life-threatening complications, including eclampsia, pulmonary edema, and abruptio placentae (placental abruption).
  - In most cases, preeclampsia will resolve after delivery, but symptoms can develop up to 4 weeks postpartum.

- **Eclampsia** is the onset of tonic-clonic seizures in women with preeclampsia.

- In an **ectopic pregnancy**, the fertilized egg implants in a location other than the uterus.
  - In > 95% of cases, implantation occurs in the fallopian tubes (tubal pregnancy), but implantation can also occur in the ovaries, cervix, or abdominal cavity.
  - A tubal pregnancy may rupture the fallopian tube, causing a life-threatening hemorrhage.
  - Ectopic pregnancy should be considered for female patients with abdominal pain.

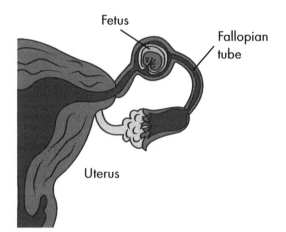

Figure 9.2. Ectopic Pregnancy (Tubal Pregnancy)

- **Hyperemesis gravidarum** is severe nausea and vomiting that occurs during pregnancy and leads to dehydration, hypovolemia, and electrolyte imbalances.

- **Abruptio placentae** (placental abruption) occurs when the placenta separates from the uterus before delivery.

- ○ Abruption can lead to life-threatening hemorrhage.
- ○ Blood loss due to abruption can be difficult to quantify as blood may accumulate behind the placenta (concealed abruption) rather than exiting through the vagina.

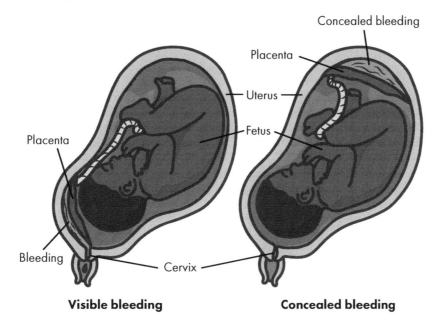

Visible bleeding   **Concealed bleeding**

Figure 9.3. Abruptio Placentae

- **Placenta previa** occurs when the placenta partially or completely covers the cervix.
  - ○ Placenta previa is usually asymptomatic and is found on routine prenatal ultrasounds.
  - ○ The presence of previa makes the placenta susceptible to rupture or hemorrhage and necessitates a cesarean delivery.
- In **placenta accreta**, the placenta attaches abnormally deeply in the uterine lining and cannot detach following delivery. Placenta accreta can lead to hemorrhage and requires a hysterectomy.
- **Postpartum hemorrhage** is bleeding that occurs any time after delivery up to 12 weeks postpartum and exceeds 1000 ml or that causes symptoms of hypovolemia.
  - ○ Primary hemorrhage occurs during the first 24 hours after delivery, usually as the result of trauma, retained tissue in the uterus, or failure of the uterus to contract.
  - ○ Secondary hemorrhage occurs between 24 hours and 12 weeks postpartum, usually as the result of dilated arteries in the uterus, retained tissue, or infection.
- Postpartum patients are frequently discharged soon after delivery and may develop **postpartum infections** at home that require further treatment. Possible

sites of infection include the endometrium (endometritis), surgical incisions, breasts (mastitis), and urinary tract.

- **Spontaneous abortion** (miscarriage) is the loss of a pregnancy before the twentieth week of gestation. (Death of the fetus after the twentieth week is commonly referred to as a stillbirth.)

  o Spontaneous abortions are a common complication of early pregnancy. They can occur because of chromosomal or congenital abnormalities, material infection or disorders, or trauma.

  o **Septic abortion** occurs when the abortion is accompanied by uterine infection; it is a life-threatening condition that requires immediate medical intervention.

- Patients with pregnancy complications should always be transported to the appropriate facility and may require an ALS intercept.

  o Manage bleeding and hypovolemic shock as needed.

  o Provide oxygenation and airway management as needed.

PRACTICE QUESTION

3. A 24-year-old patient is 28 weeks pregnant and is complaining of severe headache. During assessment, the EMT finds that her blood pressure is 170/95 mm Hg, and she has pitting edema on her ankles. What condition should the EMT suspect?

Care of the Neonate

- Dry and stimulate the infant, and then wrap them in a blanket to keep them warm.

- Assess the neonate.

  o Evaluate the airway, and suction mouth and then nose as needed.

  o If the neonate's HR is less than 100 bpm, provide assisted ventilation via BVM with room air.

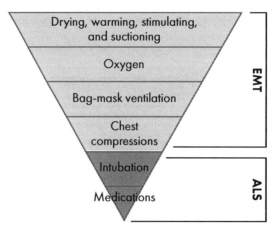

Figure 9.4. Inverted Pyramid of Neonatal Care

○ Use BVM with 100% oxygen if HR and respirations do not respond.

○ Start CPR if the neonate is not breathing or has an HR less than 60 bpm.

● Evaluate the neonate's **Apgar score** at 1 minute and 5 minutes; neonates should score between 8 and 10 by the 5-minute evaluation.

Table 9.1. Apgar Scores

Criteria	Score
Appearance	0: blue 1: extremities blue, trunk pink 2: pink all over
Pulse	0: 0 1: < 100 bmp 2: > 100 bmp
Grimace	0: no reaction 1: facial grimace 2: sneeze, cough, or cry
Activity	0: no movement 1: slight activity 2: moving around
Respirations	0: none, slow 1: irregular, weak cry 2: good breathing, strong cry

PRACTICE QUESTION

4. The EMT is evaluating a neonate at 1 minute after birth. The neonate is crying loudly, with a pulse of 160, and he is moving around well. His trunk is pink, but his extremities are blue. What is the Apgar score for this neonate?

ANSWER KEY

1. The EMT should expect the patient's heart rate and respiratory rate to be increased. Some patients may also show a slight increase in BP resulting from increased cardiac output.

2. If the patient states that she believes the baby's birth is imminent, the EMT should call ALS, stay on the scene, and prepare for delivery.

3. The patient has symptoms of preeclampsia.

4. The Apgar score is 9: 1 for the appearance, 2 for the pulse, 2 for the grimace, 2 for the activity, and 2 for the respiratory effort.

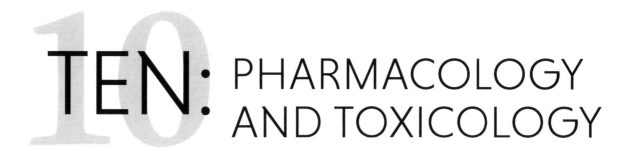

TEN: PHARMACOLOGY AND TOXICOLOGY

Pharmacology
MECHANISM OF ACTION

- **Pharmacology** is the science of drugs and their effects on the human body. **Pharmacodynamics** is the branch of pharmacology that involves how a drug affects the body.

- A drug's **mechanism of action** describes the biochemical pathways affected by the drug. The majority of drugs act on the system in two ways:
  - mimicking or suppressing normal physiological processes in the body
  - inhibiting the growth of certain microbial or parasitic organisms

- Drugs cannot change the fundamental physiological processes that occur in the body—they can only change the rate at which they occur. Drug action occurs when the drug binds to receptors on a protein molecule in the body to activate or block a physiological process.
  - An **agonist** binds to receptors and stimulates activity. For example, nitroglycerin is an agonist that results in the activation of enzymes that dilate blood vessels. Endogenous agonists (e.g., serotonin, epinephrine) are the molecules produced by the body that naturally bind to receptor sites.
  - An **antagonist** binds to a receptor to block activity. For example, ACE inhibitors block the angiotensin-converting enzyme (ACE), which normally causes blood vessels to constrict. The result is dilation in the blood vessels.
  - Some drugs are **partial agonists**, meaning they only partially activate receptors.

- The **brand name** of a drug is the name it is given by the pharmaceutical company that funded its research and development. This company holds the drug's patent for up to twenty years after its initial development, but when the patent expires, other pharmaceutical companies can produce the drug.

HELPFUL HINT
Anticholinergic drugs block activity at acetylcholine receptors in the parasympathetic nervous system. They relax smooth muscles and are used to treat conditions like asthma, overactive bladder, and tremors. Some antipsychotics and SSRIs are also anticholinergic drugs.

- A **generic drug** is the therapeutic equivalent of the brand-name drug.
  - It must have the same active ingredient, strength, and dosage form as the brand-name drug, but the inactive ingredients do not need to be the same.
  - The names of generic drugs are often shortened versions of a drug's **chemical name**, which describes its molecular structure.

QUICK REVIEW QUESTION

1. Naloxone is an opioid antagonist. How does it reverse the effects of opioid overdose?

Common Medications

Drugs are grouped into **classes** based on their chemical structures and the conditions they treat. The major drug classes, their general purpose, and examples of each are given in the table below.

Table 10.1. The Fifty Most Commonly Prescribed Medications in the United States

Generic Name (Brand Name)	Drug Class (Indication)	Adverse Effects and Contraindications
atorvastatin (Lipitor) simvastatin (FloLipid, Zocor) rosuvastatin (Crestor) pravastatin (Pravachol)	HMG-CoA reductase inhibitors (high cholesterol)	**ADR**: muscle/joint pain **Pregnancy**: Category X
levothyroxine (Synthroid)	synthetic hormone (hypothyroidism)	**BBW**: weight reduction **ADR**: dysrhythmias, dyspnea, headache, nervousness, irritability, weight loss
lisinopril (Prinivil, Zestril)	ACE inhibitor (hypertension)	**BBW**: fetal toxicity **ADR**: cough, hypotension, dizziness **Interactions**: other drugs that lower BP
metformin (Fortamet, Glucophage) glipizide (Glucotrol)	antidiabetic (type 2 diabetes)	**ADR**: hypoglycemia, diarrhea, nausea, headache
amlodipine (Amvaz, Norvasc)	calcium channel blocker (hypertension, dysrhythmias)	**ADR**: headache, edema, tiredness, dizziness **Interactions**: other drugs that lower BP

Generic Name (Brand Name)	Drug Class (Indication)	Adverse Effects and Contraindications
metoprolol (Toprol XL, Lopressor) carvedilol (Coreg) atenolol (Tenormin)	beta blocker (hypertension)	**ADR**: dizziness, fatigue, weight gain **Interactions**: other drugs that lower BP
albuterol (Ventolin HFA, Proventil HFA, Combivent Respimat, DuoNeb, ProAir HFA)	bronchodilator (asthma, COPD)	**ADR**: headache, tachycardia, dizziness, sore throat, nasal congestion **Interactions**: beta blockers, digoxin, MAOI, tricyclic antidepressants
omeprazole (Prilosec) pantoprazole (Protonix)	proton pump inhibitor (acid reflux)	**ADR**: headache, abdominal pain, nausea, diarrhea, vomiting **Interactions**: digoxin, clopidogrel, benzodiazepines, warfarin
losartan (Cozaar)	angiotensin II receptor blocker (hypertension)	**BBW**: fetal toxicity **ADR**: dizziness, headache, fatigue **Interactions**: potassium supplements, other drugs that lower BP
gabapentin (Gralise, Neurontin)	anticonvulsant (seizures, neuropathy)	**ADR**: drowsiness, dizziness, edema, angioedema (pregabalin), suicidal thoughts, emotional changes **Interactions**: alcohol, other CNS depressants
acetaminophen and hydrocodone (Norco, Vicodin, Lortab) tramadol (Ultram) oxycodone (OxyContin)	opioid (pain)	**ADR**: constipation, light-headedness, dizziness, nausea and vomiting **Interactions**: other CNS depressants
hydrochlorothiazide (Microzide) furosemide (Lasix)	diuretic (hypertension, edema)	**ADR**: hypotension, weakness, dizziness, blurred vision **Interactions**: alcohol, other antihypertensive drugs, NSAIDs

continued

Generic Name (Brand Name)	Drug Class (Indication)	Adverse Effects and Contraindications
sertraline (Zoloft) escitalopram (Lexapro) fluoxetine (Prozac) trazodone (Desyrel) citalopram (Celexa)	selective serotonin reuptake inhibitor [SSRI] (mood disorders)	**BBW**: increased risk of suicidal thoughts/behaviors **ADR**: insomnia, headache, agitation, dizziness, drowsiness, dry mouth, nausea, vomiting
bupropion (Wellbutrin, Zyban)	dopamine/norepinephrine-reuptake inhibitor (mood disorders, smoking cessation)	
duloxetine (Cymbalta) venlafaxine (Effexor)	serotonin-norepinephrine reuptake inhibitor (mood disorders)	
montelukast (Singulair)	bronchodilator (asthma)	**BBW**: neuropsychiatric symptoms **ADR**: respiratory infection, fever, headache, sore throat, cough
fluticasone (Flonase, Flovent)	nasal/oral corticosteroid (asthma, allergies)	**ADR**: headache, nasal/throat irritation, nosebleed, cough, worsening of infections
amoxicillin (Augmentin)	antibiotic [penicillin]	**ADR**: diarrhea, nausea
acetaminophen (Tylenol)	analgesic, antipyretic (pain, fever)	**BBW**: hepatotoxicity **ADR**: nausea and vomiting
prednisone (Sterapred)	oral corticosteroid (inflammatory or auto-immune conditions)	**ADR**: fluid retention, hyper/hypoglycemia, hypertension, changes in behavior/mood, weight gain, worsening of infections
amphetamine and dextroamphetamine (Adderall) methylphenidate (Ritalin)	ADHD treatment	**ADR**: insomnia, headache, tachycardia, mood changes, decreased appetite, vomiting, dry mouth

Generic Name (Brand Name)	Drug Class (Indication)	Adverse Effects and Contraindications
insulin glargine (Lantus)	insulin (diabetes)	**ADR**: hypoglycemia, injection site reactions
ibuprofen (Advil, Motrin) meloxicam (Mobic)	NSAID (pain, fever)	**BBW**: cardiovascular thrombotic events, GI bleeding **ADR**: abdominal pain, diarrhea, upset stomach **Pregnancy**: Category D (> 30 weeks)
tamsulosin (Flomax)	alpha-1 blocker (BPH)	**ADR**: orthostatic hypotension, sexual disorder, dizziness, headache
alprazolam (Xanax) clonazepam (Klonopin)	benzodiazepine (anxiety)	**ADR**: drowsiness, sedation, fatigue, memory impairment **Interactions**: other CNS depressants
potassium	supplement	**ADR**: nausea, vomiting, flatulence, abdominal pain/discomfort, diarrhea
clopidogrel (Plavix) aspirin	anticoagulant	**ADR**: bleeding **Interactions**: omeprazole/esomeprazole (clopidogrel), NSAIDs
ranitidine (Zantac)	histamine H2 antagonist (acid reflux)	**ADR**: headache, constipation, diarrhea, nausea, vomiting **Interactions**: warfarin
cyclobenzaprine (Flexeril)	muscle relaxant	**ADR**: drowsiness, dizziness, dry mouth, nausea and vomiting **Interactions**: other CNS depressants
azithromycin (Zithromax)	antibiotic [macrolide]	**ADR**: diarrhea, nausea
allopurinol (Lopurin, Zyloprim, Aloprim)	antigout	**ADR**: rash, nausea, vomiting, drowsiness

BBW: black box warning

ADR: adverse drug reactions

HELPFUL HINT

Aspirin is an NSAID that also slows platelet aggregation, which prevents clotting. It is often prescribed to prevent thrombus formation (e.g., MI, stroke), but it can also be taken for pain, fever, or inflammation.

QUICK REVIEW QUESTION

2. What adverse drug reaction should EMTs be aware of when caring for a patient taking clopidogrel (Plavix)?

Adverse Drug Reactions

- **Intended effects** are the desired or expected responses to a drug.

- **Adverse drug reactions** are unwanted responses to a drug. Adverse drug reactions can range from mild (e.g., drowsiness) to lethal (e.g., liver failure).

- Adverse drug reactions are classified into six types, which are described in the table below.

HELPFUL HINT

The term side effects is sometimes used to refer to mild adverse drug reactions, like fatigue or weight gain.

Table 10.2. Adverse Drug Reactions

Type	Description	Example
A augmented	predictable reactions arising from the pharmacological effects of the drug; dependent on dose	diarrhea due to antibiotics; hypoglycemia due to insulin
B bizarre	unpredictable reactions; independent of dose	hypersensitivity (anaphylaxis) due to penicillin
C chronic	reactions caused by the cumulative dose (the dose taken over a long period of time)	osteoporosis with oral steroids
D delayed	reactions that occur after the drug is no longer being taken	teratogenic effects with anticonvulsants
E end of use	reactions caused by withdrawal from a drug	withdrawal syndrome with benzodiazepines
F failure	unexpected failure of the drug to work; often caused by dose or drug interactions	resistance to antimicrobials

QUICK REVIEW QUESTION

3. A patient who has recently started taking lisinopril to treat hypertension is reporting dizziness and weakness. How would this adverse drug reaction be categorized?

Drug Interactions

- Medications may interact with other medications or health conditions. These **drug interactions** can increase or decrease the action of the drug, which changes the therapeutic effects of the medication.

- There are three main types of drug interactions: drug-drug, drug-disease, and drug-nutrient.

- In a **drug-drug interaction**, a person takes multiple medications.
  - The drugs may be duplicates, resulting in toxicity or increased effect.
  - Combining drugs with opposite effects may reduce the effectiveness of one or both medications.

- **Drug-disease interaction** occurs when a medication taken for one disease causes or exacerbates a different disease. For example, calcium channel blockers (to treat hypertension) must be used cautiously in patients with chronic kidney disease because they can impair kidney function.

- **Drug-nutrient interactions** occur when drugs interact with other consumable substances, including foods, alcohol, and nutritional supplements. For example, alcohol and grapefruit juice both change the absorption and effectiveness of antibiotics.

QUICK REVIEW QUESTION

4. What concern should an EMT have when a patient reports taking monoamine oxidase inhibitors (MAOIs) for depression?

Drug Administration

- **Indications** are the signs and symptoms that make it appropriate for a patient to receive a medication. For example, nitroglycerin is indicated for patients with chest pain or suspected MI.

- **Contraindications** are specific signs, symptoms, or situations that make it unsafe to administer a medication. Contraindications for nitroglycerin administration include hypotension and recent use of erectile dysfunction medications.

- **Dose** is the amount of medication given in a single administration. Manufacturers carefully gauge medication dosages to balance the desired therapeutic effect against possible adverse reactions.

- Drugs are available in many different forms.
  - **Pill** is a general term for a solid medication that is ingested.
  - Specific types of pills include **tablets** (compressed powders) and **capsules** (medication enclosed in a dissolvable container).
  - Liquid medications may be ingested (**enteral**) or injected (**parenteral**).
  - Drugs may also be given as a gas or solid powder to be inhaled.

- **Route** is how the medication enters the body. The following routes are used to administer medications:
  - **buccal** (BUC): in the cheek
  - **inhalational** (INH): through the mouth

HELPFUL HINT

Drug-drug interactions are common when patients take medications that contain multiple drugs. For example, a patient taking Norco and OTC Nyquil might not realize that both medications contain acetaminophen.

HELPFUL HINT

Monoamine oxidase inhibitors (MAOIs) are a class of antidepressants that are effective in treating mood disorders, but they are rarely used due to their potential for drug-drug interactions. Most drugs that affect serotonin, norepinephrine, or dopamine levels are contraindicated for patients taking MAOIs.

- o **intramuscular** (IM): into the muscle
- o **intranasal** (NAS): through the nose
- o **intravenous** (IV): into the vein
- o **oral** (PO): by mouth
- o **rectal** (PR): into the rectum
- o **subcutaneous** (subcut): under the skin
- o **sublingual** (SL): under the tongue
- o **transdermal** (TOP): through the skin
- o **vaginal** (PV): into the vagina

HELPFUL HINT

EMTs are only able to administer a limited list of specific drugs (per local protocols). Usually these include:

- nitroglycerin and aspirin for cardiac chest pain
- prescribed inhaled bronchodilators (e.g., albuterol) for asthma
- epinephrine (EpiPen) for anaphylaxis
- oral glucose for hypoglycemia

- EMTs should follow the six rights of medication administration to prevent medication errors.

  - o Right Patient—Is this the appropriate patient for the medication? Is this the appropriate situation to use the medication?

  - o Right Medication—Is this physically the correct medication?

  - o Right Dose—Is the amount of medication appropriate for this patient?

  - o Right Route—Is the way the medication is entering the body correct and appropriate?

  - o Right Time—Is this the right time in the sequence of the care of this patient to give the medication?

  - o Right Documentation—Have the indications for giving the medication been documented? Have the vital signs before and after administration been documented? Has the response to the medication been documented?

QUICK REVIEW QUESTION

5. A patient has a prescription for nitroglycerin 0.4 mg SL. How should the patient take this medication?

Drug Overdose

Assessment and Care for Patients with Suspected Poisoning

- During scene size-up, determine scene safety and look for clues that suggest what substance may have led to the emergency.

  - o The patient may have left drugs, medication bottles, or drug paraphernalia (e.g., syringes) nearby.

  - o Look for sources of inhaled pollutants, and unusual odors, such as those indoor fires, natural gas valves, or open chemical containers (e.g., chlorine).

  - o Industrial settings should have material safety data sheets for on-site chemicals and may also have specific emergency care equipment (e.g., eye wash station, antidotes).

- For suspected hazardous substances, request a HazMat team.
  - Do not treat the patient until they have been decontaminated. The HazMat team will move and decontaminate the patient.
  - A HazMat team should always enter the scene first when toxic gas (e.g., carbon monoxide) is suspected.
- For ingested poisons or medications, contact medical control and poison control (if permitted by local protocol). They can be contacted enroute to expedite care at the scene.
- Perform a primary assessment and manage ABCs. Provide immediate transport to patients with life-threatening issues.
- Take a history focusing on the suspected poison.
  - What poison or drug was involved?
  - When did the exposure occur?
  - How much of the poison or drug was the patient exposed to?
  - What route did the poison take to enter the body (ingestion, inhalation, absorption, or injection)?
  - How long was the patient exposed to the poison or drug?
  - What treatments has the patient or family attempted?
  - What are the patients' signs and symptoms?
- Get a complete set of vitals, including a glucose reading.
- Transport the patient to the hospital.

QUICK REVIEW QUESTION

6. The EMT sees three patients lying outside of a industrial facility with a green mist coming from a tank close to the patients. The patients have green residue covering their clothes and skin. What should the EMT do first?

Toxidromes

- **Drug overdose** occurs when a patient has taken a toxic amount of a drug.
- The most common drugs involved in overdoses requiring medical care are opioids (both legal and illegal), psychostimulants (e.g., cocaine, methamphetamine), and benzodiazepines.
- **Toxidromes** are groups of signs and symptoms present in patients who have large amounts of toxins or poisons in the body. General signs and symptoms are given below, but these may vary based on the specific drug (or combination of drugs) ingested.

Table 10.3. Signs and Symptoms of Toxidromes

Toxidrome	HR	BP	RR	Temp	Bowel Sounds	Pupils	Skin	Mental Status
Anticholinergic antihistamines, antipsychotics, tricyclic antidepressants (TCA), scopolamine, atropine, some medications used for COPD and asthma	↑	↑	—	↑	↓	↑	dry	agitated and delirious
Cholinergic anticholinesterase, insecticides and pesticides, nerve agents (e.g., sarin)	—	—	—	—	↑	↓	moist	—
Hallucinogenic LSD, psilocybin ("magic mushrooms"), mescaline, DMT, *salvia divinorum*, dextromethorphan (DXM), PCP	↑	↑	↑	—	↑	↑	—	disoriented
Sympathomimetic cocaine, amphetamines, methamphetamines, hallucinogenic amphetamines (MDMA, MDA), khat and related substances (methcathinone, "bath salts"), cold medications, diet supplements containing ephedrine	↑	↑	↑	↑	↑	↑	moist	agitated and delirious
Sedative-hypnotic benzodiazepines, barbiturates, antipsychotics, zolpidem (Ambien), clonidine, GHB	↓	↓	↓	↓	↓	—	dry	lethargic and confused

HELPFUL HINT

Presentation of anticholinergic overdose:

hot as a hare: hyperthermia

red as a beet: flushing

blind as a bat: blurred vision

dry as a bone: dry skin

mad as a hatter: agitation or delirium

full as a flask: urinary retention

HELPFUL HINT

Presentation of cholinergic overdose:

DUMBELS

Diarrhea

Urination

Miosis

Bronchorrhea, Bradycardia, Bronchoconstriction

Emesis

Lacrimation

Salivation

QUICK REVIEW QUESTION

7. What symptoms should the EMT expect to see in a patient who has overdosed on amphetamines?

OPIOID OVERDOSE

Pathophysiology

Opioids depress the CNS and lower the perception of pain by stimulating dopamine release. Opioid overdose depresses respiration and can be fatal.

What to Look For

- opioid overdose triad: pinpoint pupils, respiratory depression, decreased LOC
- hypotension
- wheezing or dyspnea
- nausea or vomiting
- seizure

HELPFUL HINT

Common opioids include codeine, fentanyl, heroin, hydrocodone, morphine, and oxycodone.

Care and Transport

- Priority is airway management and supplemental oxygen.
- Narcan (**naloxone**) is an opioid antagonist administered via IV, IM, or intranasally.
  - Naloxone is indicated for patients with agonal breathing or apnea to restore respiratory status.
  - Naloxone is <u>not intended</u> to restore consciousness or cardiac activity, although patients may regain consciousness after administration.
  - Place a nasopharyngeal airway and adequately ventilate patient with BVM before and after administration.
  - Initial IM dose is 0.4 mg; initial intranasal dose is 2 mg.
  - Closely monitor patients who respond to naloxone. The effects of naloxone may wear off while opioids remain in the patient's system, resulting in the reappearance of overdose symptoms.
  - A side effect of Narcan is vomiting. An oropharyngeal airway may also induce vomiting when the patient's gag reflex returns.
- If the patient is pulseless, follow BLS protocols for patients in cardiac arrest.

HELPFUL HINT

Do not delay BLS measures to administer naloxone.

QUICK REVIEW QUESTION

8. A patient has overdosed on fentanyl. He has pinpoint pupils, has a respiratory rate of 20, and is alert to painful stimuli. What should the EMT do?

Other Drug Overdoses

- **Alcohol** is a central nervous system (CNS) depressant.

  - Overconsumption of alcohol can lead to respiratory depression and excessive vomiting.

  - Alcohol interacts with many prescription and OTC medications, particularly other drugs that also suppress the CNS (e.g., benzodiazepines, antihistamines).

  - Alcohol use can mask other health conditions, such as TBI and hypoglycemia. Patients who appear intoxicated should be thoroughly evaluated for other conditions.

  - Patients who are intoxicated by alcohol are not considered competent and cannot refuse care.

- **Benzodiazepines** are CNS depressants. Overdose depresses respiratory and cardiac activity. The care priority is to provide oxygen and ventilations as needed and transport promptly.

- During **acetaminophen (Tylenol)** overdose, toxic metabolites accumulate in the liver causing hepatotoxicity.

  - Acetaminophen toxicity occurs at single doses higher than 250 mg/kg. (A single OTC Tylenol tablet is 500 mg).

  - Gastritis symptoms usually appear within hours; symptoms of hepatotoxicity do not appear until 24 – 72 hours after ingestion.

  - The antidote for acetaminophen overdose (N-acetylcysteine [Mucomyst]) is most effective when delivered within 8 hours, so patients with suspected acetaminophen overdose should always be transported promptly.

- **Inhalant abuse** (huffing) is the process of inhaling substances to experience a short high.

  - Many common household products release gases that can be inhaled, including freon, gasoline, paint, glue, and cleaning products.

  - Propellants in aerosols, such as **nitrous oxide**, can also be inhaled.

  - Inhalant abuse is most common in children and young adults because inhalants are cheap and easily accessible.

  - Overuse of inhalants can lead to respiratory distress, altered LOC, and cardiac dysrhythmias. Inhaled aerosols can also cause burns in or around the mouth.

- An overdose of cardiac medications, including beta blockers, calcium channel blockers, and digitalis, can cause hemodynamic instability and cardiac dysrhythmias.

  - These overdoses are most common with elderly patients who have mistakenly taken too much of a prescribed medication. Cardiac medications are also taken during suicide attempts by young people with access to these drugs in their households.

○ Care includes management of ABCs and prompt transport. ALS intercept may be required for patients with severe symptoms.

Substance Withdrawal

- Chronic **alcohol abuse** alters the sensitivity of CNS receptors, and cessation of drinking causes hyperactivity in the CNS.

  ○ Alcohol withdrawal can be fatal and requires hospitalization for treatment.

  ○ Symptoms develop 6 to 24 hours after last consuming alcohol.

  ○ Symptoms of alcohol withdrawal: tachycardia, hypertension, agitation and restlessness, nausea and vomiting, sweating, seizures

  ○ **Delirium tremens (DTs)** is a type of severe alcohol withdrawal characterized by hallucinations and hyperthermia. Symptoms occur 2 to 4 days after stopping alcohol intake.

- Chronic use of **opioids** increases excitability of CNS neurons, and withdrawal leads to hypersensitivity of the CNS.

  ○ Symptoms of opioid withdrawal: drug craving, tachycardia, tachypnea, hypertension, GI upset, anxiety, yawning, rhinorrhea and lacrimation, pupil dilation, piloerection, sweating, muscle pain and twitching

  ○ The onset, length, and severity of symptoms will depend on the type of drug used. Withdrawal symptoms make take several weeks to completely resolve.

  ○ Opioid withdrawal is rarely fatal, but death can occur, usually as a result of hemodynamic instability or electrolyte imbalances.

- Care and transport for patients in alcohol and opioid withdrawal:

  ○ Manage patient ABCs.

  ○ Patients with dyspnea may require oxygen.

  ○ Be prepared to suction the airway if vomiting occurs.

  ○ Manage related medical conditions, including seizures, hallucinations, and hypovolemic shock (secondary to vomiting).

Carbon Monoxide and Cyanide Poisoning

Pathophysiology

Carbon monoxide (CO) displaces oxygen from hemoglobin, which prevents the transport and utilization of oxygen throughout the body. Mild CO poisoning can be resolved with oxygen; severe CO poisoning can lead to myocardial ischemia, dysrhythmias, pulmonary edema, and coma. Sources of CO include smoke from fires, malfunctioning heaters and generators, and motor vehicle exhaust.

<Helpful Hint: CO poisoning and cyanide poisoning often occur together.>

Cyanide interferes with the production of ATP in mitochondria. Cyanide poisoning is rare, but it is usually fatal without medical intervention. Sources of cyanide include smoke from fires, medications (e.g., sodium nitroprusside), and pits/seeds from the family *Rosaceae* (which includes bitter almonds, apricots, peaches, and apples).

HELPFUL HINT

Pulse oximeters should be used cautiously on patients with suspected carbon monoxide poisoning. They cannot differentiate between oxygen and carbon monoxide on hemoglobin, so they will show a high SpO_2 even if the patient's oxygen levels are actually low.

What to Look For

Table 10.4. Signs and Symptoms of CO and Cyanide Poisoning

Carbon Monoxide Poisoning	Cyanide Poisoning
headache	bitter almond smell on breath
altered LOC or confusion	anxiety, agitation, or confusion
dizziness	headache
visual disturbances	hematemesis
dyspnea on exertion	diarrhea
vomiting	flushed, red skin
muscle weakness and cramps	tachycardia and tachypnea
syncope	hypertension
	seizure

Care and Treatment

- Ensure scene safety before entering.

- Remove patient from the source of poisoning.

- For mild symptoms, provide high-flow oxygen through a non-rebreathing mask.

- For unconscious patients, insert airway adjunct and provide ventilations.

- Transport promptly.

QUICK REVIEW QUESTION

11. A patient's carbon monoxide detector went off, and the fire department was called to the scene. EMTs arrive to find the patient alert and sitting outside the home. They report a headache earlier in the day that has resolved. How should the EMTs treat the patient?

ANSWER KEY

1. Naloxone binds to opioid receptors and prevents opioid agonists (such as morphine and oxycodone) from binding to those sites.

2. Excessive bleeding may occur.

3. Augmented (A): Dizziness and weakness are predictable reactions arising from the pharmacological effects of the lisinopril, which lowers blood pressure.

4. MAOIs have a high risk for potential drug-drug interactions.

5. SL is the abbreviation for sublingual, meaning "under the tongue."

6. The EMT should request a HazMat team and move to a safe area.

7. Symptoms of amphetamine overdose include increased blood pressure and respiratory rate; hypertension; dilated pupils; moist, hot skin; agitation; and delirium.

8. The EMT should monitor the patient. (Naloxone should not be used unless there is respiratory depression.)

9. Acetaminophen is hepatotoxic, but symptoms of liver failure will not appear for 24 to 72 hours; the patient should be transported promptly so she can receive an antidote.

10. The patient is showing signs of delirium tremens (DTs). The patient should be transported immediately to the hospital because DTs can be life-threatening.

11. The CO poisoning is not severe: the EMTs should provide oxygen to the patient and encourage the patient to go to the hospital for further evaluation.

ELEVEN: SPECIAL POPULATIONS

Geriatric Patients

- **Geriatric** patients are those 65 years of age or older.

- Currently more than 40 million Americans are 65 or older, and 5.5 million people are 85 or older.

- The geriatric population is more than twice as likely to use EMS than other age groups and make up a significant percentage of call volume.

  - Geriatric patients are more likely to have chronic diseases that require complex care.

  - They may require emergency care due to poor management of chronic conditions or acute exacerbations of chronic conditions.

  - Due to underlying physiology, geriatric patients may experience more severe symptoms of common acute illnesses.

- Every physical system is affected by the aging process, though the degree of diminishment depends on the individual.

Table 11.1. Physiological Effects of Aging

System	Physiological Changes	Outcome of Physiological Changes
Cardiovascular	degeneration of valves, muscle, and conduction system systemic thickening and narrowing of arteries decreased cardiac output and stroke volume	high risk for MI, CVA, aneurysm, PAD, and DVT cardiac dysrhythmias orthostatic hypotension decreased cerebral perfusion lowered tolerance for physical activity
Respiratory	diminished lung volume, elasticity, and cilia activity decreased cough and gag reflex	increased risk of pneumonia lowered ability to increase oxygen intake as needed increased choking and aspiration risk

Table 11.1. Physiological Effects of Aging (continued)

System	Physiological Changes	Outcome of Physiological Changes
Gastrointestinal	decreased GI motility decreased production of stomach acid decreased sense of taste decreased ability to chew and swallow degrading of GI lining and sphincters	constipation bowel obstruction malnutrition dehydration incontinence high risk of GI bleeding, GERD, and GI cancers
Liver and kidneys	decreased ability to process and clear medications decrease in clotting factor production	significantly higher risk of medication toxicity and negative interactions higher risk of edema and bleeding disorders
Endocrine	gradual loss of thyroid and pancreatic function	lowered energy and metabolism poor body temperature regulation higher risk for type 2 diabetes
Musculoskeletal	decreases in mass and strength	general weakness decreased mobility and ability to care for self more prone to falling, often unable to pick themselves up higher probability of fractures, even from minimal impact development of arthritis and spinal curvatures
Nervous	decrease in number of neurons	decreased pain sensation increased reaction time decreased visual acuity and hearing dementia and depression sleep disorders
Integumentary	loss of subcutaneous fat	thin and frail skin susceptible to burns, bruising, and skin tears chilled very easily

- Treat geriatric patients with respect and dignity.
  - Do not assume that the patient cannot hear or understand you.
  - Speak slowly, clearly, and with adequate volume for the patient to understand.

- ○ Give patients enough time to respond to questions.
- ○ Begin by speaking directly to the patient, not to caretakers or bystanders.
- ● Take care when determining LOC and alertness.
  - ○ Geriatric patients are more likely to have dementia or delirium.
  - ○ If the patient seems to have altered mental status, attempt to determine the baseline from a caretaker or family member. (Confusion may be normal for a dementia patient.)
  - ○ Geriatric patients often have less need to track the days of the week as closely as other demographics. A broader question such as, "What year is it?" or "What season is it?" may be more appropriate.
- ● Considerations for taking a SAMPLE history from geriatric patients:
  - ○ Geriatric patients often have their medical history and medication lists in writing. Confirm whether the information is up to date or has been adjusted.
  - ○ Determining degree of compliance with dosing schedule is critical: symptoms may be related to missing or extra doses of medications.
  - ○ Dehydration is a very common cause of illness in geriatrics, so get an estimated amount of daily water consumption.
  - ○ Gather and examine legal documents such as a DNR or living will during the SAMPLE history.
- ● Considerations during the physical examination of geriatric patients:
  - ○ Keep the patient as warm as possible during the examination, both for patient comfort and to get the most accurate readings from your instruments.
  - ○ Handle the patient carefully to avoid injuring the patient and minimize the pain of existing injuries, such as arthritic joints or bruised extremities.
  - ○ Inform the patient of what you are doing as you are doing it to minimize fear or panic.
  - ○ Maintain a high level of suspicion of any injury, even if the mechanism of injury would be less concerning for a younger patient.
- ● Considerations for the transport of geriatric patients:
  - ○ Pressure ulcers and other injuries can develop quickly in geriatric patients, so take care when positioning the patient.
  - ○ When a geriatric patient is immobilized, pad the void spaces and provide cushioning.
  - ○ Drive as gently as possible to avoid further injury to the patient and to reduce panic.
- ● Use the acronym GEMS to remember special considerations for geriatric patients.
  - ○ **G**eriatric patients present atypically.
  - ○ Assess the **E**nvironment to look for signs of neglect or inadequate medical care.

HELPFUL HINT

UTIs are a common cause of delirium in geriatrics.

DID YOU KNOW?

Geriatric patients tend to have higher blood pressure and are more prone to postural blood pressure changes.

○ Perform a thorough **Medical** assessment regardless of the chief complaint.

○ Perform a **Social** assessment to determine if the patient's needs related to activities of daily living (ADLs) are being met.

- Be aware of the signs of **elder abuse**. These should be documented and handled per local protocols.

  ○ frequent visits to ED or urgent care

  ○ apathy or aggression from the caregiver

  ○ vague or inconsistent explanations for injuries or poor medical management

  ○ psychosocial issues such as depression, sleep disorders, or eating disorders

PRACTICE QUESTION

1. An EMT is dispatched to an assisted living facility for a 74-year-old female who had a ground-level fall (GLF) after standing up to walk to the restroom. She was assisted back into her bed by the staff members and is now complaining of left hip pain. Why is a full medical and trauma assessment necessary for this patient?

Pediatric Patients

- **Pediatrics** refers to the care of young children and adolescents.

- The parent must provide consent for any interventions performed on pediatric patients, with very few exceptions.

  ○ Necessary emergency care can be given if the legally responsible parent cannot be reached.

  ○ **Emancipated minors**, who are not legally bound to a caregiver, may make their own medical decisions.

  ○ Teachers or other professional caregivers may act *in loco parentis* when parents are not available.

- Significant variation can be seen in the growth and development of children, but they can be put into six general age groups.

  ○ **Newborns** (neonates) are in their first month of life. They may sleep up to 18 hours a day and must eat every 2 to 3 hours. They communicate through crying; a newborn that cries inconsolably should be transported immediately for further assessment.

  ○ **Infants** are between 1 month and 1 year old. During this stage, children grow rapidly. They develop social skills, including smiling, laughing, and making eye contact. Physically, they will learn to lift their heads, use their hands, sit up, and crawl. Infants older than 6 months may show anxiety when separated from their caregivers.

  ○ **Toddlers** are between 1 and 3 years old. Most children will learn to walk around the age of 1 and will begin exploring their environment. Common calls for toddlers include environmental injuries such as falls, poisonings, and airway obstruction. Children will begin to talk around age 2 and may be able to communicate basic ideas to their caregiver or the EMT. However, they will not have developed the language to communicate precisely.

- ○ **Preschool** children are between 3 and 5 years old. They will be able to perform complex physical tasks such as running, jumping, and kicking. Preschool children will also have a large vocabulary and can communicate effectively. However, they will not understand medical terms and have vivid imaginations, so information should still be gathered from caregivers or bystanders when possible.

- ○ **School-aged** children are between 6 and 12 years old. They will be able to communicate effectively with the EMT and will have an understanding of basic medical terms and procedures. Children in this age group will have a basic understanding of concepts such as privacy, pain, and death. Explain procedures to them in plain language and respect their autonomy.

- ○ **Adolescents** are between 13 and 18 years old. They will be able to think abstractly and understand complex concepts. Adolescents should be actively involved in their care. Puberty begins in adolescence, and many adolescents will be involved in behaviors that put them at risk of injury.

- The younger the patient, the more dissimilar the normal vital signs will be compared to the average adult vital signs.

  - ○ For patients younger than 3 years old, **NIBP** (non-invasive blood pressure) is rarely taken. **Capillary refill time (CRT)** is the primary method of determining adequate perfusion.

  - ○ The following chart demonstrates the range of normal vital signs for pediatrics based on age grouping.

Table 11.2. Normal Pediatric Vital Signs (Ranges)				
Age Range	**Pulse Range**	**Respiratory Range**	**Systolic BP Range**	**Diastolic BP Average**
Newborn	120 – 160	30 – 50	N/A	N/A
0 – 5 months	90 – 140	25 – 40	N/A	N/A
6 – 12 months	80 – 140	20 – 30	N/A	N/A
1 – 3 years	80 – 130	20 – 30	N/A	N/A
3 – 5 years	80 – 120	20 – 30	78 – 104	65
6 – 12 years	70 – 110	15 – 30	80 – 122	69
13 – 18 years	60 – 105	12 – 20	88 – 140	76

DID YOU KNOW?

Capillary refill time (CRT) is determined by pressing the nail bed, or the top of the hand or foot, until it turns white and then releasing. If circulation is adequate, normal color should return in less than 2 seconds.

- The anatomical differences between pediatrics and adults are naturally most profound in the earliest years of life. The EMT should be aware of how these differences may impact care, expressed in Table 11.3.

- How a pediatric patient is assessed will depend on the age of the child.

  - ○ For very young patients, the EMT will need to get a history and MOI/NOI from the caregivers or bystanders.

  - ○ School-aged children may be able to provide critical information to the EMT.

- Adolescents may be assessed much like adult patients. However, the EMT should be aware that adolescents may be less likely to share some information in the presence of caregivers or peers.

- Use visual cues, such as pointing or the Wong-Baker faces pain scale, for patients too young to effectively communicate verbally.

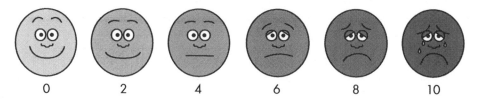

Figure 11.1. Wong-Baker Faces Pain Scale

Table 11.3. Important Anatomical Features of Pediatrics	
Region	**Description**
Head	The head is disproportionally larger and heavier than the rest of their body until roughly age 4, causing children to often fall headfirst.
	Fontanelles, or soft spots, occur in infants due to the incomplete fusing of the skull plates until after birth. A bulging fontanelle may indicate increased intracranial pressure, and a sunken fontanelle may indicate dehydration.
Airway and upper body	The mouth and nose are smaller and the tongue is proportionally larger, causing a higher risk of airway obstruction.
	The trachea is narrower, softer, and more flexible, increasing the risk of obstruction due to inflammation or foreign bodies.
	Hyperextending the neck or allowing the head to fall forward can obstruct the airway in small children. Padding the shoulders of a pediatric patient helps maintain an inline neutral position.
	The thorax and chest wall are shorter and softer, forcing the patient to rely on the diaphragm for deeper breathing. This makes the use of accessory muscles very apparent.
Body surface area (BSA)	BSA is disproportionally larger than the body mass, making temperature regulation more difficult.
Blood	Children have a lower blood volume than adults. They will show signs of dehydration and hypovolemic shock after losing a smaller proportion of blood or fluids than adults.

- Use the **Pediatric Assessment Triangle (PAT)** to rapidly assess pediatric patients. The PAT can be done within the first 30 seconds of meeting the patient.

  - appearance: tone, interactiveness, consolability, look/gaze, speech/cry (**TICLS**)

  - work of breathing: airway noises, accessory muscle use, head bobbing, nasal flares

- circulation to skin: pallor, mottling, cyanosis
- Show care and consideration when interacting with pediatric patients and their families.
  - Children will be less likely to become anxious or scared if their caregivers are allowed to remain present and involved in their care.
  - Allow parents to hold young children until it is time for transport.
  - Unless it is going to interfere with patient care or the caregiver is a safety risk, have the caregiver ride in the back with the patient.
  - Always explain to the child and the parent what you are doing and why.
  - Use a calm, gentle voice, and attempt to communicate on their visual level.
  - Adolescents often wish to be treated as an adult and respond poorly to being patronized. However, they may revert to more child-like behaviors when injured or ill.

DID YOU KNOW?
Cardiac arrest in pediatrics is almost always due to respiratory arrest and hypoxia. Aggressive respiratory intervention is the key to a positive outcome.

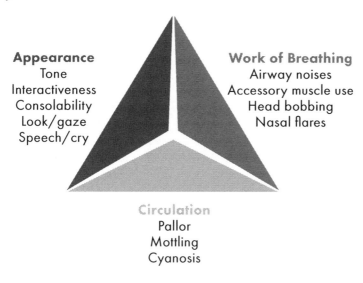

Appearance
Tone
Interactiveness
Consolability
Look/gaze
Speech/cry

Work of Breathing
Airway noises
Accessory muscle use
Head bobbing
Nasal flares

Circulation
Pallor
Mottling
Cyanosis

Figure 11.2. Pediatric Assessment Triangle (PAT)

- Below is a list of the most common injuries and medical conditions seen on pediatric calls.
  - trauma (MVC is most common)
  - foreign body airway obstruction
  - poisonings (usually from medications or household chemicals)
  - infections (e.g., pneumonia, croup)
  - anaphylaxis
  - dehydration

PRACTICE QUESTION

2. An EMT is dispatched to a single-family dwelling for a 6-month-old infant male who has been ill for two days. The patient is in his mother's arms in the living room, and the EMT can see and hear obvious signs of respiratory distress as she approaches them. What should be the EMT's priority?

ANSWER KEY

1. A full head-to-toe examination is imperative in geriatric patients, even on a simple GLF. The patient may have injured her upper extremities attempting to catch herself, hit her head, or injured her neck. The EMT should also perform a full medical assessment to look for underlying medical conditions that may have caused the fall.

2. The EMT's priority should be a rapid assessment and a decision to transport or upgrade to ALS. If an ALS intercept is called, the EMT may administer oxygen or ventilation while waiting and take a history. If the decision is made to transport, oxygen delivery and history should be done en route.

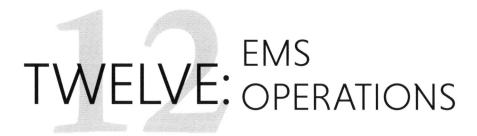

TWELVE: EMS OPERATIONS

EMT Scope of Practice

- EMTs are governed by protocols and legal guidelines created by the state, county, city, and local medical director.

- The National Highway Traffic Safety Administration (NHTSA) Office of EMS developed a **scope of practice** for EMTs that is followed nationwide.

  - The EMT provides basic acute care and transportation for critical and emergent patients.

  - The EMT provides only non-invasive care.

  - The EMT may assist patients with taking prescribed medications or provide patients with oral glucose, aspirin, or nitroglycerin (per local protocols). They do not provide any other pharmacological interventions.

  - The EMT must consult medical control when making decisions about patient disposition.

- The **standard of care** describes the type of care that a trained EMT should be expected to provide.

- EMTs can lose their certification/licensure or face legal consequences for working outside their scope of practice or not meeting the standard of care.

- The care provided by EMTs is guided by **medical control**, which is run by a **medical director**.

  - **Online medical control** (or direct medical control) is the direct communication between on-site EMTs and physicians via phone or radio. These physicians are usually on duty in emergency departments, but they may also be specialized personnel within larger EMS systems.

  - **Offline medical control** (or indirect medical control) includes guidelines and protocols written by the medical director who oversees EMS operations.

- **Protocols** are parameters written by medical control to guide EMTs. In some cases, the department that oversees EMS operations within a state writes the protocols.

HELPFUL HINT

Scope of practice describes what the EMT is allowed to do. Standard of care describes what the EMT should do.

HELPFUL HINT

State laws regulate what specific procedures EMTs can perform. The medical director can limit that scope, but they cannot expand it.

- Protocols provide detailed guidance for EMTs on the duties they perform and describe permissions given to them by medical control.
- Violation of standard protocols can lead to termination and possible legal liability.

PRACTICE QUESTION

1. EMTs are caring for a 37-year-old patient with a closed humerus fracture. The patient is agitated and asks the EMTs for something to help with the pain. What medications can the EMT administer?

Patient Communication

- Communication with the patient is a critical component of effective medical care and allows the EMT to identify the patient's complaint.
- Communication should be direct, non-threatening, and calm.
- EMTs should be aware of their tone and address patients properly. There are situations that require an EMT to be forceful or direct, while other situations may require the EMT to be supportive and nurturing.
- The EMT should be aware of their body language; negative body language can lead to patient mistrust and can affect care.
  - Work on the same level as the patient (e.g., crouch to speak to a seated patient).
  - Do not make facial expressions that suggest frustration, anger, confusion, or fear.
  - Face the patient when communicating with them.

Table 12.1. Dos and Don'ts of Patient Communication	
Do	**Don't**
<ul><li>Make eye contact with the patient</li><li>Introduce yourself and use the patient's name</li><li>Speak directly to the patient when possible</li><li>Ask open-ended questions</li><li>Speak slowly and clearly</li><li>Show empathy for the patient</li><li>Be silent when appropriate to allow patients time to think and process emotions</li></ul>	<ul><li>Use medical jargon</li><li>Threaten or intimidate the patient</li><li>Lie or provide false hope</li><li>Interrupt the patient</li><li>Show frustration or anger</li><li>Make judgmental statements</li></ul>

- When treating a young patient:
  - Crouch or lie down at the patient's level.
  - Be honest and direct when speaking with them.
  - Ask parents for permission to communicate directly with the patient.

- When treating patients who are blind or have low vision, describe what actions are being taken throughout assessment, treatment, and transport so that the client understands what is occurring.

- EMTs should be prepared to communicate with patients who do not speak English or who have language impairments.

  ○ Address patients using short, simple sentences to gauge their level of English.

  ○ Learn basic medical terms in languages commonly used in the service area.

  ○ Carry tools such as communication boards and translation apps on phones or tablets.

  ○ Use family members as translators when necessary.

PRACTICE QUESTION

2. An EMT is caring for a 6-year-old patient with acute abdomen and vomiting. The patient's mother is aggressively questioning the child about what he recently ate and when he started feeling sick. The patient is withdrawn and is not speaking to his parents or the EMT. What techniques can the EMT use to communicate with this patient?

Professional Communication and Documentation

- EMS systems use a combination of radios and cell phones for communication.

  ○ EMTs usually communicate with dispatch using **mobile radios** located in the ambulance or **hand-held radios** that can be carried to the site of care.

  ○ EMTs usually communicate with receiving facilities via cell phone.

- An EMS call starts with a call to an **EMS dispatcher**. These calls usually come through 911 but may also come from automated systems (e.g., OnStar).

  ○ The 911 operator questions the caller to collect as much information as possible and may give directions of care including bystander CPR.

  ○ The EMS dispatcher dispatches the appropriate personnel and help (e.g., fire apparatus, rescue teams).

- The EMS dispatcher communicates with the EMS unit assigned to the call.

  ○ The EMS unit should report to dispatch when they arrive at the scene, leave the scene, and arrive at the point of transfer.

  ○ The dispatcher must give the crew the address of the call and the complaint of the patient.

  ○ The dispatcher may also give directions or follow-up information to the crew as the call continues.

  ○ The crew should always repeat information back to the dispatcher for confirmation and should ask for clarification if they are unsure.

DID YOU KNOW?

Cell phones and tablets are used to communicate with medical control and to pass images for notification. EMS-issued phones or tablets may have apps or programs that allow the EMT to communicate directly with the emergency department.

- The EMS unit should communicate with the receiving facility before their arrival to provide a **prehospital radio report**. The report should include:
  - unit ID and level of service
  - estimated time of arrival (ETA)
  - patient's age and gender
  - chief complaint and relevant history
  - mechanism of injury
  - patient's mental status
  - relevant physical findings and vital signs
  - treatment and patient response to treatment
- All aspects of patient care—from dispatch to transfer of care—should be documented in the **patient care report (PCR)**.
  - The PCR may be used in legal proceedings, billing, research, or as a reference for further medical care.
  - Errors committed by the EMT should be carefully documented in the PCR.
  - Mistakes in the PCR should be crossed out and amended; content should never be erased from a PCR.

PRACTICE QUESTION

3. An EMT calls in the following report to the receiving hospital.

Ambulance 714-BLS to the hospital: we are inbound with a 76-year-old male with chest pain radiating to jaw beginning at approximately 1:30 a.m. He has a history of stable angina. Patient is alert and oriented. Treatment was 325 mg aspirin and one sublingual nitroglycerin. ETA 6 minutes.

What information is missing from the report?

Maintaining the Truck

- EMS crews use vehicles to get to the scene and transport the crew and their patient to their destination.
- It is vital that all parts of the vehicle are in good working order.
  - At the beginning of each shift, check and top off fluids to the level set by the vehicle manufacturer. Fluids include motor oil, steering fluid, transmission fluid, and radiator fluid.
  - Check vehicle tires to ensure they have proper tread, there is no unusual wear or damage, and they are at the proper pressure.
  - Ensure that the vehicle has a full tank of fuel at the beginning of the shift so that the crew can make calls without running out of fuel.
  - Check that all lights are properly working.
  - Check that windows are clear and clean to ensure that the crew has an unobstructed view.

- If there are any issues that may affect safety, the vehicle should be placed out of service.

- Maintenance also includes ensuring that the EMS crew has the proper equipment to do their job.
  - Before each shift, check the truck to ensure it is stocked with the proper type and amount of supplies and equipment.
  - Check equipment to make sure it has not expired, is operational, and is fully charged.
  - Replace all equipment and supplies as used or at the end of the shift to ensure the next crew is ready for their shift.

- Every EMT truck should include in stock:
  - oxygen masks and airway adjuncts
  - bandaging materials
  - blood pressure cuffs
  - AED
  - thermal blankets
  - thermometers
  - personal protective and safety equipment (e.g., gloves, sharps container)
  - pharmaceuticals as allowed by protocols
  - stabilization devices (e.g., C-collars)
  - other supplies specified by local requirements

- Maintenance of the vehicle and the requirements for supplies and their amounts may be set by the governing body within the jurisdiction or state where the vehicle is operated.

PRACTICE QUESTION

4.   Why is it important to ensure all vehicle fluids are topped off at the start of every shift?

Driving to the Scene and Receiving Facility

- Driving the emergency vehicle in a safe manner ensures the safety of the crew, the passengers, and the public.

- When transporting a patient, one member of the unit is the driver and the other will attend to the patient.

- Protect crew and passengers by correctly using seat belts and restraints.
  - EMT personnel should wear seat belts at all times unless providing emergency care.
  - Patients should be appropriately restrained.
  - Equipment should be stowed properly.

- The operation of emergency vehicles, such as ambulances and fire apparatus, differs greatly from driving a personal vehicle.
  - EMS vehicles are usually much larger and heavier than personal vehicles. Their size means they require greater stopping distances and more space to turn corners.
  - EMS vehicles usually have larger blind spots that can make some driving maneuvers, such as backing up, more difficult.
- When operating the EMS vehicle in a **nonemergency**, the driver must adhere to all applicable motor vehicle laws where the vehicle is driven. This includes speed limits, direction of travel, and passing rules.
- During **emergency operation**, the driver uses the lights and siren and may be exempt from some traffic laws (per local regulations).
  - During emergency operation, turn on all lights and use the siren. (In some states, the law requires the use of the siren while the emergency lights are on.)
  - Use of the lights and siren give the vehicle right of way over other drivers on the road.
  - During emergency operation, the driver may proceed through red lights or stop signs, exceed the posted speed limits, drive against traffic, or drive against posted travel directions.
  - Some areas use traffic preemption devices to change traffic signals and give clear passage to emergency vehicles.
- Research has consistently shown that driving with lights and sirens is more dangerous than normal driving. Thus, driving during emergency operations should always be **defensive**.
  - Some drivers may panic or not know what to do when an emergency vehicle with lights and siren approaches. Be prepared for other drivers to behave in unexpected ways, such as stopping quickly, changing lanes, or speeding up.
  - Other drivers may not notice the approaching emergency vehicle, even if the lights and siren are on, and thus may not clear intersections or move to the side of the road.
- When arriving at a scene, the driver should park the vehicle such that it can exit the scene quickly and is not a threat to patients, bystanders, or emergency personnel.

PRACTICE QUESTION

5. The driver of an EMS vehicle is driving with lights and siren on. She approaches a red light at an intersection and cannot see cross-traffic. What should the driver do?

Postrun

- After the call is over, the crew should plan to clean up, restock, and report.

- When the call is done, clean and disinfect the stretcher and any equipment that was used.

- Restock as necessary any supplies that were used.

- Verbally give a report to the receiving facility and then follow up with a paper or electronic report as required by the jurisdiction in which the call was done.

- After the run is complete, the crew should discuss what happened and address any issues that occurred during the operation.
  - If a member of the crew is having trouble physically or mentally due to the call, contact a supervisor or chief officer to ensure the member gets the proper treatment and care for their issue.

- If necessary and appropriate, the crew should obtain insurance information from the patient, their family, or the facility to assist in the billing process.

> ### PRACTICE QUESTION
>
> **6.** Cleaning the ambulance attendant area and equipment after a call is routine. Why must this area and the equipment be cleaned after a call?

Legal and Ethical Considerations

LEGAL LIABILITY

- **Legal liability** means that a person has a legal obligation and is subject to criminal and civil penalties if they do not meet those obligations.

- EMTs have varying levels of legal liability during a run.
  - When an EMS crew has been dispatched, the driver is legally liable for their actions and must follow all federal, state, and local driving laws. However, the crew has no legal liability for the patient.
  - Liability to the patient starts when the crew makes contact with the patient.
  - Failure to use the proper equipment and follow protocols while rendering care may lead to legal action against the EMT.
  - If a dispatcher has sent out a crew and then cancels the call, the EMS crew has no liability to the patient.
  - For a canceled call, the EMT may be legally liable if the EMT should have been able to assess that the patient did not have the capacity to refuse treatment (e.g., unconscious, altered mental state). For this reason, EMS protocols often do not allow a call to be canceled unless the patient has been seen by the EMT.
  - The EMS crew is also liable for the maintenance and safety of their equipment. If it is determined that an injury was the result of faulty equipment, the EMS crew and their company may be held liable.

- **Negligence** is a type of tort (a wrongful civil act) defined as failure to offer an acceptable standard of care. There are four types of negligence:
  - Nonfeasance is a willful failure to act when required.

- Misfeasance is the incorrect or improper performance of a lawful action.
- Malfeasance is a willful and intentional action that causes harm.
- Malpractice occurs when a professional fails to properly execute their duties.

- **Malpractice** is the most common type of legal claim against EMTs. For malpractice to occur, four things must happen:
  - The patient-EMT relationship was established (duty).
  - The EMT neglected to act or acted improperly (dereliction).
  - A negative outcome occurred from an action or lack of an action (direct cause).
  - The patient sustained harm (damages).

- **Gross negligence** describes an especially reckless action that the provider should have known would result in injury.

- **Abandonment** occurs when an EMT terminates care without the patient's consent or without transferring the patient to an equal or higher level of care.

- When EMTs are legally liable and the patient sustains injury, the EMT and their employer may be sued in civil court.
  - Successful malpractice suits against EMS personnel are relatively rare.
  - The most common sources of legal liability for EMTs are vehicle accidents, patient consent or refusal of care, and poorly restrained patients.

PRACTICE QUESTION

7. An EMS crew is dispatched to a patient who has been found lying on a sidewalk in an altered mental state. On arrival, the crew determines that the patient is under the influence of alcohol. His vital signs are within normal range, and he demands to be left alone because he has a terrible headache. The EMT believes the patient is drunk and does not require treatment or transport. Later that night, the patient is admitted to the ED with a subdural hematoma and dies shortly thereafter. Is the EMT legally liable for damages to the patient?

DUTY TO ACT AND GOOD SAMARITAN LAWS

- A **duty to act** is a legal term that describes the actions a person or an organization must take, by law, to respond to and prevent harm to a person or a community as a whole.
  - An on-duty EMT has a duty to act in their jurisdiction: they are legally required to respond to dispatcher calls, assess patients, and provide treatment within their scope of practice.
  - EMTs may have a duty to act when not on a call or not on duty depending on local regulations.

DID YOU KNOW?

States with duty-to-act laws for off-duty EMS include Ohio, Massachusetts, Vermont, Hawaii, California, Florida, Rhode Island, Minnesota, Wisconsin, and Washington.

- A **Good Samaritan law** provides legal protection for people who give reasonable care to those who need assistance.

- All states and the District of Columbia have some version of a Good Samaritan law. These laws vary, but most protect people who act rationally to provide aid but do not protect people from gross negligence.

- The laws in some states cover EMS personnel who render care while off duty. The EMT must do their best to help the injured individual and must not do anything outside their scope of practice.

- Good Samaritans may be on the scene when an EMT arrives.

  - Accept any information the Good Samaritan provides, and ask the Good Samaritan to step back so you can render care.

  - In some cases, a doctor or fellow rescuer may be on the scene and try to take over care. Thank them for their service, and ask them to step back so you can continue your care. Contact medical control if they request to continue their involvement in care.

  - If a Good Samaritan refuses to back away, ask the police to remove the person from the scene.

PRACTICE QUESTION

8. An off-duty EMT is eating dinner in a restaurant when a man at a nearby table collapses. The EMT assesses the man and finds he has no pulse and is not breathing. The EMT begins compressions and rescue breathing. The man survives but is left incapacitated due to anoxic brain injury. The family sues the EMT, claiming he did not do enough to provide treatment for the man. Will the EMT be protected under Good Samaritan laws?

PATIENT CONSENT

- Patient **consent** is required before any care is rendered.

  - Permission is obtained by asking if the patient would like help and if it is okay to touch the person.

  - **Expressed consent** is an affirmative verbal or nonverbal agreement to care.

  - **Implied consent** allows the EMT to provide care to unconscious or incapacitated patients if it can be assumed that any reasonable patient would consent to care under the circumstances.

  - A patient's consent can be withdrawn at any time. If a patient withdraws their consent, then an EMT must stop treatment.

- Patients may lack **competency** or **capacity** to make medical decisions.

  - There are many reasons a person may have an altered mental state, including organic conditions (e.g., Alzheimer's disease), mood-altering substances, and medical conditions (e.g., concussion, lack of oxygen, stroke).

  - Patients with dementia or mental illness may have a designated guardian who can consent to treatment.

  - When the EMT determines that a patient does not have the capacity to make medical decisions, they should render care to the patient under implied consent.

HELPFUL HINT

Treating a patient without their consent can result in civil law-suits or criminal charges against the EMT for assault and battery.

- ○ Local protocols will regulate if and when law enforcement can give consent for people who have been arrested or who are not competent to give consent.
- ○ Care may be stopped if the patient returns to normal and declines care or if a person who has legal responsibility for the patient asks the EMT to stop care.

- For minor patients, the patient's guardian must provide consent.
  - ○ In most cases, the legal age of consent to treat is 18 years old.
  - ○ An **emancipated minor** has petitioned the court to be legally separated from their parents. They should be treated as an adult and asked for consent (if they can show the card verifying their emancipation).
  - ○ When a minor has a child, the minor is the guardian of that child and can make decisions about treatment for that child. However, the minor cannot make decisions about their own treatment.

- Patients who are competent may deny consent for treatment.
  - ○ The EMT may not force the patient to be treated or transported, even if their life is in danger.
  - ○ Every effort must be made to convince an individual to go to the hospital if the EMT believes that it is the right course of action for the patient.
  - ○ Law enforcement may be able to invoke their right to force a patient to seek help. However, this power usually only applies to people with mental illness or who are threatening self-harm.
  - ○ The EMT may contact medical control and discuss the situation with them. The patient may also talk directly to medical control.

- If a patient refuses care, the EMT should document the refusal.
  - ○ The EMT must have the patient (or guardian) sign a refusal-of-treatment form.
  - ○ The EMT should also thoroughly document the patient's mental status and the EMT's attempt to explain the need for care to the patient.

- An **advance directive** is a legal document that describes the medical treatment a person has consented to if they become unconscious.
  - ○ A **do-not-resuscitate (DNR)** order is written for patients who do not wish to be resuscitated in the event of cardiac or respiratory failure.
  - ○ EMTs should carefully examine advance directives to ensure they are valid (e.g., has patient and physician signatures).

- Some patients may have **health care proxies** who hold **durable power of attorney** and can make medical decisions on behalf of the patient.

HELPFUL HINT

If a patient is alert and competent, their medical decisions cannot be overridden by their health care proxy.

PRACTICE QUESTION

9. A call comes in for a sick child. Upon arrival, the EMT is met by a 16-year-old girl who says her child is sick and she wants him taken to the hospital. Another woman steps in and identifies herself as the mother of the 16-year-old. She says she will not allow the child to be taken to the hospital as he is not that sick. How should the EMT respond?

CONFIDENTIALITY

- In 1996, the United States federal government enacted the **Health Insurance Portability and Accountability Act (HIPAA)**. This act details how private health information (PHI) and electronic medical records (EMR) can be shared.

- All efforts must be taken to ensure the **confidentiality** of the patient's PHI.

  - Information describing who they are, where they live, their social security number, and their diagnosis must not be shared with anyone other than personnel involved in treating the patient.

  - Any paperwork that has the patient's information shall be secured at all times.

  - In most cases, an authorization form signed by the patient is required before releasing any PHI to anyone other than personnel directly involved in the patient's care.

  - The passing of information between dispatchers, field crews, medical control, and emergency departments must be HIPAA compliant to ensure the privacy of patients (e.g., never use the patient's name over the air waves).

- Violating HIPAA by sharing PHI can result in job loss or civil liability.

- Confidentiality also covers conversations between the EMT and patients or bystanders.

  - EMTs should not disclose information shared by patients to anyone other than relevant medical personnel.

  - During calls, EMTs should work to ensure that patients can share information with the EMT without being overheard by bystanders.

- EMTs should not discuss calls (personally or professionally) such that listeners can determine the patient's identity.

- EMTs may not access information about patients they did not directly care for. This is a violation of patient privacy and can lead to legal action and job loss.

PRACTICE QUESTION

10. An EMS crew recently transported a celebrity from their home to a hospital. The EMT who provided care later recounts to a coworker the reason for the treatment but does not mention the celebrity by name. Did the EMT commit a HIPAA violation?

1. EMTs cannot provide any medications for pain. They are only able to administer aspirin and nitroglycerin for possible ischemic chest pain and oral glucose.

2. The EMT should start by asking the parent if she can speak directly with the child. She should then crouch down to the patient's level, introduce herself, and explain that she is there to help the child. Because the child is frightened, she should use a non-threatening tone and not pressure the child to speak until he is ready.

3. The EMT has not included the patient's vital signs or any information about his response to treatment.

4. Vehicles can be driven for large amounts of time and long distances during a shift. Making sure fluids are topped off ensures that the vehicle can operate properly and safely and decreases the likelihood of a component failure at a critical time.

5. The driver should come to a stop at the intersection to make sure no traffic will be in the intersection when she passes through. Even though she has the right of way, drivers with a green light may not see her or stop in time. Going through the red light without stopping puts other drivers at risk.

6. Cleaning reduces the spread of disease and germs that might be present after a call.

7. The EMT may be legally liable. The EMT should have known that an altered mental state and a headache are symptoms of intracranial hemorrhage. He should have transported the patient to the ED for a full assessment or contacted medical control before releasing him.

8. Yes, the EMT will be protected under Good Samaritan laws. The EMT provided treatment within the scope of his training and committed no acts of negligence, so he is not liable for any injury the man suffered.

9. The 16-year-old mother is the guardian of the child and has the legal right to make decisions about her child's care. The grandmother has no legal right to determine the boy's care, so the EMT should prepare to transport the child.

10. Yes, the EMT most likely committed a HIPAA violation. The coworker may be able to identify the patient through gossip or news reports, meaning the EMT has now shared a patient's PHI and will be legally liable if the patient sues.

THIRTEEN: THE PSYCHOMOTOR EXAM

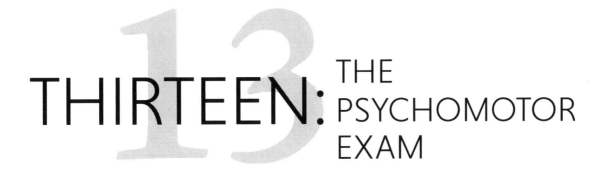

What is the Psychomotor Exam?

- The psychomotor examination is a standardized, hands-on test in which the EMT candidate must perform specific emergency medical skills.

  - The psychomotor exam is conducted in a proctored environment in which the EMT candidate may not reference notes or course material.

  - The examiners are typically EMT instructors and are not allowed to assist the EMT candidate.

  - The EMT candidate is graded using standard **NREMT performance checklists**, often referred to as "skill sheets."

- The psychomotor exam consists of seven skills:

  - Patient Assessment/Management – Trauma

  - Patient Assessment/Management – Medical

  - Bag-Valve Mask (BVM) Ventilation of an Apneic Adult Patient

  - Oxygen Administration by Non-Rebreather Mask

  - Cardiac Arrest Management/AED

  - Spinal Immobilization (Supine Patient)

  - Random EMT Skill

- The random EMT skill will consist of one of the following:

  - Spinal Immobilization (Seated Patient)

  - Bleeding Control/Shock Management

  - Long Bone Immobilization

  - Joint Immobilization

- All skills are scenario based, with the examiner relaying a synopsis of the simulated emergency after reading the instructions.

  - Scenario-based skills will require the EMT candidate to maintain dialogue with the examiner. For example, "I am palpating all four abdominal

HELPFUL HINT

The information in this chapter is meant to supplement the skill sheets, not replace them. You should reference the NREMT checklists as you read. They can be found at https://www.nremt.org/rwd/public/document/emt.

HELPFUL HINT

You will not be informed what the random skill is until that section of the test is about to begin.

quadrants for distension and tenderness" or "Your patient states he is prescribed nitroglycerine for chest pain."

- Each skill has **critical criteria**, which is a list of items that will lead to automatic failure.
  - In this chapter, critical criteria are shown in **bold**.
  - Although not listed under critical criteria, inability to complete an examination within the set time limit will also result in failure.
- This chapter will focus only on the NREMT-recommended psychomotor examination criteria. Some states or individual agencies may deviate from or modify the NREMT curriculum.

Patient Assessment/Management – Trauma

- This skill is designed to evaluate the EMT candidate's ability to effectively assess and treat an adult patient with multi-system trauma.
  - The simulated patient will have moulage (makeup or prosthetics imitating injuries), some of which may not be immediately visible during scene size-up.
  - The patient's injuries will vary in severity.
  - There will be two EMT assistants available.
  - **This skill must be completed within 10 minutes.**
- The NREMT checklist for this skill is divided into five areas: scene size-up, primary survey/resuscitation, history taking, secondary assessment, and reassessment.

Scene Size-Up

- **Use appropriate PPE or verbalize use of PPE to examiner.**
- **Determine if the scene is safe.**
  - During the exam, the EMT candidate determines scene safety by asking the examiner, "Is the scene safe?"
- Determine mechanism of injury. (The mechanism of injury will be inferred by the scenario description as read by the examiner but will still need to be verbalized by the EMT candidate.)
- Request additional resources if the patient could benefit from advanced life support (ALS) care.
- **Assess whether spinal immobilization would be performed based on mechanism of injury.**

HELPFUL HINT

During this skill, an EMT assistant can be used to hold manual in-line stabilization.

Primary Survey/Resuscitation

- Verbalize a general impression (a brief statement of the patient's stability based upon the size-up and mechanism of injury).

- Determine level of consciousness and expose patient (remove clothing) to determine chief complaint or life threats.

- **Manage airway, breathing, and circulation (ABCs), including hemorrhage and shock.**
  - **Provide high concentration oxygen and adequate ventilation.**
  - **Assess and treat ABCs before addressing other injuries.**

- **Determine patient priority and make a transport decision within 10 minutes of the start of the scenario.**

History Taking

- Gather vital signs.
  - Baseline vital signs are given verbally by the examiner once asked.
  - Each vital sign must be asked for individually.
  - The EMT candidate should be prepared to explain how he or she would obtain each vital sign (e.g., "I will obtain a heart rate by palpating the carotid artery with my index and middle fingers.")
  - Some examiners may require the EMT candidate to take actual vital signs.
  - If allowed by the examiner, obtaining vital signs may be delegated to an EMT assistant earlier in the scenario.

- Obtain SAMPLE history.
  - If a SAMPLE history cannot be obtained due to the patient's level of consciousness, the EMT candidate should verbalize this.

Secondary Assessment

- Inspect, palpate, and assess the patient head-to-toe for injury and function.

- Use the mnemonic DCAP-BTLS. (See chapter 2 for detailed information on secondary assessment of trauma patients.)

- The most successful method for completing the secondary assessment is to integrate portions of it into the Primary Survey/Resuscitation during ABCs (check the mouth and nose when checking the airway, or the chest when checking breathing).
  - If this method is used, it must be communicated to the examiner (e.g., "As I open the airway using the jaw thrust maneuver, I am performing an assessment of the mouth and nose.")

- Verbalize treatment for any injuries encountered during the secondary assessment.

Reassessment

- Reassess the patient every 5 or 15 minutes based on the patient's condition.

HELPFUL HINT

Not all items on the performance checklists have to be conducted in the order they are listed.

- If the patient's vital signs trend negatively, this is an indication the EMT candidate improperly performed an intervention or missed an injury.

PRACTICE QUESTION

1. How long does the EMT have to make a transport decision for the patient during the Patient Assessment/Management – Trauma skills exam?

Patient Assessment/Management – Medical

- This skill will measure the EMT candidate's ability to manage and treat an adult patient with a medical-related chief complaint.
  - The patient may ultimately be suffering from multiple illnesses of varying severity.
  - The examiner will verbally role-play most or all of the patient's responses.
  - There will be two EMT assistants (real or imaginary) to help as needed.
  - The time limit for this skill is 15 minutes.
- The NREMT checklist for this skill is divided into six areas: scene size-up, primary survey/resuscitation, history taking, secondary assessment, vital signs, and reassessment.

Scene Size-Up

- The same scene size-up procedures can be used for Patient Assessment/Management – Trauma and Medical skills exams.

Primary Survey/Resuscitation

- Verbalize a general impression (a brief statement of the patient's stability based upon the size-up and nature of illness).
  - The medical patient will often state their own chief complaint. However, there may be other life threats besides the chief complaint.
- Assess responsiveness and level of consciousness using the acronym AVPU. (See chapter 2 for detailed information on assessment of medical patients.)
- **Manage airway, breathing, and circulation (ABCs), including hemorrhage and shock.**
  - **Provide high concentration oxygen and adequate ventilation.**
  - **Assess and treat ABCs before performing secondary assessment.**
- **Determine patient priority and make a transport decision within 15 minutes of the start of the scenario.**

History Taking

- Take patient's history using the acronyms OPQRST and SAMPLE. (See chapter 2 for detailed information on assessment of medical patients.)

- OPQRST and SAMPLE do not have to be performed in order.

- The EMT candidate is encouraged to ask any necessary clarifying questions in addition to OPQRST and SAMPLE.

Secondary Assessment

- Perform a physical examination of the affected area and ask further clarifying questions specific to the body part or system involved.

- The secondary assessment does not need to be completed prior to patient transport.

HELPFUL HINT

Unacceptable affect with patients or personnel (e.g., aggression, impatience) is critical criteria that will result in failure.

Vital Signs

- Physically obtain vital signs from the simulated patient.

  ○ The examiner will compare the vital signs obtained by the EMT candidate with their own findings. The EMT must be within 10 mm Hg (BP), 10 beats per minute (HR), and 5 breaths per minute (RR) of the examiner.

  ○ After the actual vital signs are obtained, the examiner may adjust the figures to more accurately represent the scenario.

- The field impression of the patient is the EMT candidate's verbal opinion of what the patient's illnesses are.

- Verbalize treatment and interventions to the examiner.

  ○ If online medical direction is required, the examiner will play the role of the physician.

  ○ Explain the dosage, route, indications, and contraindications of any medications that are to be given.

Reassessment

- Reassess patient every 5 or 15 minutes based on the patient's condition.

  ○ If the patient's vital signs trend negatively, this is an indication the EMT candidate improperly performed an intervention or missed an illness.

- **Give accurate verbal transfer-of-care report.**

  ○ The transfer-of-care report is typically a brief statement of the patient's age, sex, chief complaint, illnesses/injuries, pertinent medical history, interventions, and vital sign trends.

PRACTICE QUESTION

2. The EMT candidate has completed the primary survey during the Assessment/ Management – Medical skills exam and determined the patient does not require immediate transport. What should the EMT do next?

BVM Ventilation of an Apneic Adult Patient

HELPFUL HINT

The BVM Ventilation skill exam is often done in conjunction with the Oxygen Administration by Non-Rebreather Mask examination.

- This skill is designed to measure the EMT candidate's ability to successfully provide artificial ventilations to an adult patient who has a pulse but is not breathing.
  - The EMT candidate will be required to use a bag-valve mask, supplemental oxygen, suction device, and an oropharyngeal airway adjunct.
  - The EMT candidate will need to assemble the bag-valve mask, oxygen components, and suction device during the examination.
- **Verbalize PPE precautions.**
- **Assess responsiveness.**
- **Assess pulse and breathing simultaneously for no more than 10 seconds.**
- **Open airway and suction the mouth and oropharynx.**
  - **Suction for no more than 15 seconds.**
- Insert oropharyngeal airway and begin BVM ventilation.
  - **After suctioning is complete, artificial ventilations must begin within 30 seconds.**
  - **Maintain appropriate ventilation rate (10 – 12 breaths per minute) and volume.**
  - **Do not stop ventilations for more than 30 seconds.**
- **Attach BVM to oxygen.**
  - Supplemental oxygen can be used immediately, or the oxygen can be postponed until after the first pulse check (about 2 minutes).
  - If the EMT candidate elects to wait until after the first pulse check to connect supplemental oxygen to the BVM, the examiner or an assistant will take over ventilations while the EMT candidate prepares the oxygen delivery system.

PRACTICE QUESTION

3. What is the maximum length of time the EMT candidate should spend suctioning an adult patient?

Oxygen Administration by Non-Rebreather Mask

- This skill is designed to measure the EMT candidate's ability to assemble the components of a supplemental oxygen system and provide oxygen therapy to a patient using a non-rebreather mask.
  - The patient will have no other injuries or illnesses.
  - The regulator and mask will be disconnected from the oxygen cylinder when the examination begins.
- **Verbalize PPE precautions.**

- Gather appropriate equipment.
  - Check to ensure the proper washer or O-ring is present on the regulator to prevent leaks.
- "Crack" the valve on the oxygen cylinder by opening it slightly for a brief moment to clear out any dust or debris in the port.
- Line up the pins on the regulator to the holes on the oxygen cylinder for proper assembly.
- After opening the cylinder valve, check the gauge and verbally state the pressure.
  - The pressure is measured in pounds per square inch, or psi (e.g., "The gauge reads approximately 2100 psi.").
- **After looking, listening, and feeling, verbalize the absence of leaks.**
- **Set flow rate to at least 10 liters per minute after the non-rebreather mask is attached.**
- **Prefill the reservoir bag on the non-rebreather mask.**
  - To prefill the reservoir bag, place a finger over the exhaust port on the inside of the mask.
- **Ensure the mask has a tight seal on the patient's face.**

PRACTICE QUESTION

4. Oxygen should be given at what flow rate during the Oxygen Administration by Non-Rebreather Mask skill exam?

Cardiac Arrest Management/AED

- This skill measures the EMT candidate's ability to use CPR and an AED to manage an adult patient in cardiac arrest. (See chapter 4, "Cardiovascular Emergencies," for detailed information on how to perform CPR and use the AED.)
  - No bystanders will be present.
  - After 2 minutes (5 cycles) of CPR, a second rescuer will arrive with an AED.
  - The EMT candidate will then use the AED while the second rescuer continues CPR.
  - The maximum time for this skill is 10 minutes.
  - Use the time allotted before the beginning of the examination to become familiar with the AED trainer and ensure all components are present and ready for use.
- **Take or verbalize appropriate PPE precautions and evaluate the scene for safety.**
- Upon determining the patient is unresponsive, request an AED and additional EMS assistance.

HELPFUL HINT

Interrupting CPR for more than 10 seconds is a critical criteria and will result in failure.

- **Check for pulse and breathing simultaneously for no more than 10 seconds.**

- **Immediately begin 1-rescuer CPR when the examiner states that the patient is apneic and pulseless.**

- After 2 minutes (5 cycles) of CPR, simultaneously reassess pulse and breathing for no longer than 10 seconds.

  o   During reassessment, the examiner will state that the patient is still apneic and pulseless, and a second rescuer has arrived with an AED.

- After directing the second rescuer to take over CPR (with less than 10 seconds of interruption), turn on the AED and follow the prompts.

HELPFUL HINT

Inform the second rescuer not to stop compression as you expose the chest and apply AED pads.

- Expose the patient's chest and apply AED pads while CPR is still in progress.

- Direct the second rescuer to stop CPR and stay clear of the patient as the AED analyzes the heart rhythm.

- **Once shock is advised by the AED, direct all individuals not to touch the patient; announce "All clear" before delivering shock.**

- **Resume CPR immediately after delivery of the shock.**

PRACTICE QUESTION

5.   An EMT candidate is taking the Cardiac Arrest Management/AED skill exam. She approaches the patient to perform a primary survey. The examiner tells her that the patient is unresponsive. The EMT candidate then simultaneously assesses airway and breathing, and the examiner then tells her the patient is apneic and pulseless. The EMT candidate immediately begins chest compressions.

What step did the EMT candidate not perform?

Spinal Immobilization (Supine Patient)

- The Supine Patient Spinal Immobilization exercise will test the EMT candidate's ability to secure a supine (lying flat on the back) patient to a long spine board.

  o   The patient will not have any illnesses or injuries apart from a suspected unstable cervical spine.

  o   Any approved spine board, straps, and padding may be used.

  o   The EMT candidate will be allowed one trained assistant to maintain manual in-line stabilization as directed.

  o   The EMT assistant and skill examiner will assist with moving the patient from the ground onto the spine board at the candidate's direction.

  o   The examination must be completed in 10 minutes or less.

HELPFUL HINT

The spinal immobilization (supine) examination is often combined with the random skill.

- **Take or verbalize PPE precautions.**

- **Direct the EMT assistant to apply and maintain in-line spinal immobilization.**

- **Apply properly sized cervical collar.**
  - ○ Check pulse, motor function, and sensory perception in all four extremities prior to applying cervical collar.
  - ○ **Ensure EMT assistant does not release manual stabilization after collar is applied.**
- Move patient onto long spine board.
  - ○ Provide instructions to the EMT assistant and skill examiner for their assistance in moving the patient onto the spine board.
  - ○ The EMT assistant maintaining manual stabilization of the head is responsible for initiating movement of the patient.

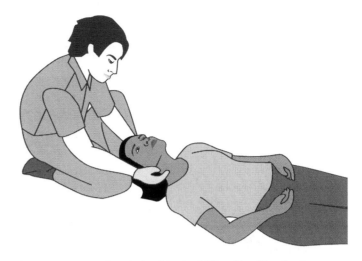

Figure 12.1. In-Line Spinal Immobilization (Supine)

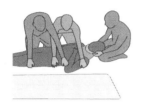 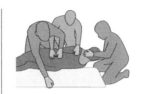 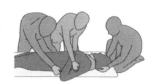

1. Maintain in-line stabilization with patient in supine position.

2. Grasp patient on far side and roll patient onto their side. Slide spine board under patient.

3. Roll patient onto the spine board.

Figure 12.2. Moving Patient to Long Spine Board

- Pad the voids between the patient and spine board as needed using appropriate padding.
  - ○ Padding any voids behind the patient's head can be completed here or immediately prior to securing the patient's head to the board.
  - ○ If padding voids is unnecessary due to the patient's body type, verbalize this to the examiner.
- **Secure patient's torso to spine board prior to securing the head.**
  - ○ **Secure patient's head in a neutral position.**
  - ○ **Prevent excessive movement of the patient or patient's head.**
- Secure the patient's legs and then the arms.
- **Reassess pulse, motor function, and sensory perception in all four extremities after securing the patient to the spine board.**

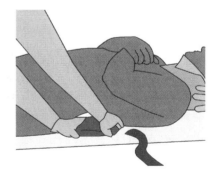

Figure 12.3. Padding Voids on Long Spine Board

PRACTICE QUESTION

6. The EMT candidate, the EMT assistant, and the examiner are in position to move the patient onto a spine board. Which person should initiate movement of the patient?

Spinal Immobilization (Seated Patient)

- The Seated Patient Spinal Immobilization tests the EMT candidate's ability to provide spinal immobilization of a seated patient to a long spine board.

  ○ The patient will be stable in a seated position with no illnesses or injuries apart from a suspected unstable cervical spine.

  ○ Any approved half-spine immobilization device may be used.

  ○ The EMT candidate will be allowed one trained assistant to maintain manual in-line stabilization as directed.

  ○ The examination must be completed in 10 minutes or less.

- **Take or verbalize PPE precautions.**

- **Direct the EMT assistant to apply and maintain in-line spinal immobilization.**

- **Apply properly sized cervical collar.**

  ○ Check pulse, motor function, and sensory perception in all four extremities prior to applying cervical collar.

  ○ **Ensure EMT assistant does not release manual stabilization after collar is applied.**

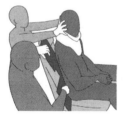

Figure 12.4. In-Line Spinal Immobilization (Seated)

- Position immobilization device and secure patient.

  ○ **Secure the patient's torso before securing the head.**

  ○ **Secure patient's head in a neutral position.**

  ○ **Prevent excessive movement of patient or patient's head.**

  ○ **Do not tighten the device to the torso such that it inhibits adequate chest rise and fall.**

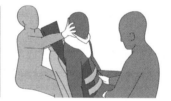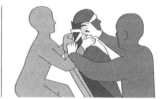

1. Slide half spine board behind patient.

2. Secure patient torso to board.

3. Secure patient head to board.

Figure 12.5. Securing Patient to Half-Spine Immobilization Device

- Verbalize the process of transitioning the patient from a seated position to a long backboard.

- **Check pulse, motor function, and sensory perception after verbalizing the process of securing the patient to a long backboard.**

PRACTICE QUESTION

7.   Which part of the body is attached first to the half-spine board?

Bleeding Control/Shock Management

- The Bleeding Control/Shock Management exercise tests the EMT candidate's ability to effectively treat an adult patient with arterial hemorrhage and hypoperfusion (shock).
  - The bleeding site will be at one of the four extremities.
  - Available equipment will include bandages, dressings, a tourniquet, a blanket, and a system for delivering supplemental oxygen.
  - The maximum time limit for this skill is 10 minutes.
  - Before the exercise begins, use the available time to become familiar with the equipment, particularly the tourniquet and oxygen delivery system, to avoid time delays later.
- **Take or verbalize PPE precautions.**
- Apply direct pressure to the wound using the available dressings and bandages.
  - The examiner will inform the EMT candidate that the wound continues to bleed.
- Immediately apply tourniquet proximal (closer to the torso) to the wound.
  - **Do not attempt other interventions (such as elevating the extremity or applying additional dressings) before applying the tourniquet.**

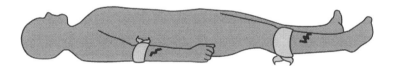

Figure 12.6. Tourniquet Placement for Arterial Bleeding in Extremities

  - The examiner will inform the EMT candidate that the patient is now exhibiting signs of hypoperfusion.
- Reposition the patient to a supine position if they will tolerate it, or place in a position of comfort.
- **Administer supplemental oxygen.**
- Prevent heat loss by covering the patient with a blanket.
- **Declare to the examiner that this is a priority patient requiring immediate transport.**

HELPFUL HINT

Placing the patient in the Trendelenburg position (legs elevated 8 – 12 inches above the level of the head) is no longer recommended.

8. An EMT candidate is performing the Bleeding Control/Shock Management skill exam. At what point should she expect to apply the tourniquet?

Long Bone Immobilization

- The Long Bone Immobilization exercise measures the EMT candidate's ability to effectively splint one of the following long bones in an adult patient: radius, ulna, tibia, or fibula.
  - This examination will not require the EMT candidate to perform a primary assessment or monitor the patient's ABCs.
  - There will be one EMT assistant available.
  - The use of traction, pneumatic, and vacuum splints is not allowed.
  - This skill must be completed within 5 minutes.
- **Take or verbalize PPE precautions.**
- **Direct the EMT assistant to apply manual stabilization of the injury by supporting the proximal and distal joints.**
- **Check pulse, motor function, and sensory perception distal to the injury.**
- Measure and apply the splint.
  - **Immobilize the joints above and below the injury.**
  - Methods for measuring and applying the splint will vary based on the devices available.
- Secure splinted extremity to the patient's body to restrict unnecessary movement.
  - Upper extremities can be secured to the torso using a swathe.
  - Lower extremities can be secured to each other with a rigid splint between, or to a long backboard.
- **Secure the hand or foot in a position of function.**
  - Extend the wrist slightly upward and allow the fingers to be flexed in a comfortable position. Do not extend the palm or fingers into a flat position.
  - The foot should be in a naturally upright position with no forced flexion.

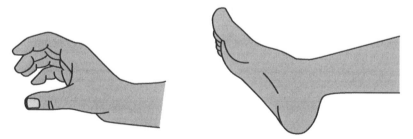

Figure 12.7. Position of Function for Hand and Foot

- Reassess pulse, motor function, and sensory perception distal to the injury.

PRACTICE QUESTION

9. After immobilizing a fractured tibia, how should the entire extremity be secured?

Joint Immobilization

- The NREMT Joint Immobilization exercise tests the EMT candidate's ability to effectively splint a shoulder injury using a sling and swathe on an adult patient.
  - The EMT candidate will not be required to perform a primary survey or monitor the patient's ABCs.
  - One EMT assistant will be provided.
  - This skill must be completed within 5 minutes.
- **Take or verbalize PPE precautions.**
- **Direct the EMT assistant to apply manual stabilization of the injury by restricting movement of the entire arm and providing support to the elbow and forearm area.**
- **Check pulse, motor function, and sensory perception distal to the injury.**
- Use a large triangle bandage (cravat) to apply the sling to the injured arm.
  - If available, use padding (such as additional bandages) between the knot and the neck.
  - Avoid tying the knot directly over the spine or carotid artery.
  - Form a pocket using the extra bandage material at the elbow to prevent the arm from slipping out of the sling. (The pocket can be formed by folding and pinning the excess material or tying a knot.)
- Apply the swathe over the injured arm and the torso, but do not include the uninjured arm.
  - A swathe is like a strap or belt and is used to restrict movement of the injured extremity.
  - A swathe is typically made by folding a triangle bandage into a strip approximately 2 inches wide, which is then wrapped over the injured arm and tied around the torso.
- **Reassess pulse, motor function, and sensory perception distal to the injury.**
  - Some states or agencies require distal circulation, motor function, and sensory perception to be checked after application of the sling and again after application of the swathe.

PRACTICE QUESTION

10. What is the difference between a sling and swathe?

HELPFUL HINT

The certifying state or testing agency may elect to have the EMT candidate immobilize a joint other than the shoulder.

HELPFUL HINT

The most appropriate distal pulse to check for an adult patient with a shoulder injury is the radial artery.

HELPFUL HINT

The only equipment available for immobilization during this skill exam will be large triangle bandages.

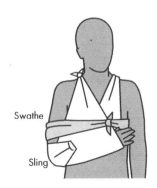

Swathe

Sling

Figure 12.8. Sling and Swathe

ANSWER KEY

1. Transport must be initiated or called for within 10 minutes.

2. The EMT candidate should tell the examiner that he has determined immediate transport is not necessary and that he will continue assessment and treatment on the scene. He may then begin the patient history and secondary assessment.

3. An adult patient should not be suctioned for more than 15 seconds at a time. Prolonged suction is a critical failure point.

4. The oxygen flow rate should be at least 10 L/min.

5. After determining that the patient was unresponsive, the EMT candidate should have sent the assistant to get the AED and requested additional EMS assistance.

6. Movement must only be initiated by the person holding manual in-line stabilization of the head (in this case, the EMT assistant). The EMT candidate should provide instructions to the EMT assistant and skill examiner for moving the patient and direct the EMT assistant to initiate movement.

7. The patient's torso should be secured first. Failing to secure the torso before the head will result in failure of the examination.

8. A tourniquet should be applied immediately after the examiner notifies the EMT candidate that the wound continues to bleed after direct pressure application. Additional bandages, elevation of the extremity, and using pressure points are not required before tourniquet application and could result in critical failure.

9. To entirely secure an injured lower extremity, the legs can be secured together with a rigid splint in between or the legs can be secured to a long spine board.

10. A sling is designed to support the weight of the injured extremity. A swathe is a narrow strap or bandage intended to keep the injured appendage from excessively moving.

FOURTEEN 14: PRACTICE TEST

DIRECTIONS: READ THE QUESTION, AND THEN CHOOSE THE MOST CORRECT ANSWER.

1. To select the proper size nasopharyngeal airway, measure
   A. from the nostril opening to the earlobe.
   B. the diameter of the selected nostril.
   C. the circumference of the cranium.
   D. from the corner of the mouth to the earlobe.

2. You are treating a 73-year-old patient complaining of chest pain. Which of the following vital signs is a contraindication for nitroglycerin administration?
   A. respiratory rate of 22 breaths per minute
   B. blood pressure of 90/50 mm Hg
   C. resting heart rate of 130 bpm
   D. skin that is hot and dry

3. You are called to a 61-year-old unconscious female. Upon arrival, you find her lying motionless in bed. After opening the airway and observing no pulse or breathing, your next step is to
   A. immediately begin CPR.
   B. check for signs of trauma.
   C. move the patient to the floor or other hard surface.
   D. insert a nasopharyngeal airway.

4. An 84-year-old woman called 911 after accidentally setting her hand down on her stovetop. Upon arrival, you note an obvious burn injury to her entire palm. You should describe the burn as covering what percent of her body surface area?
   A. 1%
   B. 5%
   C. 9%
   D. 18%

5. A patient was struck in the upper right abdomen with a baseball and has substantial bruising. The patient may have injured his
   A. spleen.
   B. appendix.
   C. urinary bladder.
   D. liver.

6. A patient who responds to a physical stimulation but not to EMTs calling their name would be considered
   A. unresponsive.
   B. alert.
   C. responsive to verbal stimuli.
   D. responsive to painful stimuli.

7. A 45-year-old male with a history of diabetes is complaining of abdominal pain and nausea. The assessment reveals a blood sugar of 385. The patient's symptoms are MOST likely being caused by

   A. hypoglycemia.

   B. alcohol withdrawal.

   C. diabetic ketoacidosis.

   D. pancreatitis.

8. A 75-year-old male has left-sided weakness and slurred speech that resolves while you are evaluating him. This patient MOST likely had a

   A. myocardial infarction.

   B. transient ischemic attack.

   C. hemorrhagic stroke.

   D. migraine headache.

9. A patient with cardiogenic shock is expected to have

   A. hypertension and trouble breathing.

   B. decreased urine output and warm, pink skin.

   C. increased urine output and cool, clammy skin.

   D. hypotension, weak pulse, and cool, clammy skin.

10. The incident commander at a motor vehicle collision assigns you to treat a motorcyclist who was hit by a moving car. The patient is awake and talking with a chief complaint of severe pain to the waist and leg. You find an obvious deformity to the right femur, and his pelvis is unstable. While your EMT partner holds manual traction, your next step is to

    A. secure the patient to a long spine board.

    B. tightly wrap the pelvis with bandages.

    C. elevate the injured leg above the head.

    D. apply a traction splint.

11. You are assessing a 6-year-old child with an acute asthma attack. You find a pulse oximetry reading of 91%. You should first

    A. request an ALS intercept.

    B. provide supplemental oxygen.

    C. begin rescue breathing.

    D. administer a nebulized albuterol treatment.

12. You are providing CPR to a 54-year-old male in cardiac arrest as your EMT partner assembles and operates the AED. You stop compressions, and your partner delivers a shock from the AED. Your next step is to

    A. immediately resume chest compressions.

    B. wait for the AED to provide instructions.

    C. check pulse and breathing for no longer than 10 seconds.

    D. place the patient in recovery position.

13. Which of the following terms defines chest pain resulting from the coronary arteries being unable to supply an appropriate amount of oxygenated blood to meet the needs of the heart?

    A. angina pectoris

    B. congestive heart failure

    C. cerebrovascular accident

    D. coronary vein distension

14. A 73-year-old female with a history of smoking and chronic cough is complaining of shortness of breath after a recent lung infection. Knowing these symptoms, you suspect that she has

    A. sepsis.

    B. valley fever.

    C. tuberculosis.

    D. COPD.

15. You are treating a patient who accidentally amputated his finger while attempting to clean a large packaging machine. Suddenly, the patient's coworker yells that she found the finger in a puddle of blood on the factory floor. Your next step is to

   A. leave the finger in place and call the police.

   B. photograph the finger as evidence.

   C. place the finger in a clean bag in the freezer.

   D. wrap the finger in moist, sterile gauze.

16. You locate an adult patient who has a penetrative neck wound from sharp-force trauma. You notice bubbles forming at the site of the wound. Law enforcement has already secured the scene. Your priority treatment should include

   A. applying a C-collar.

   B. palpating the cervical spine.

   C. applying an occlusive dressing.

   D. checking the pupils for size and reactivity.

17. You arrive on scene and are about to enter a house when you hear gunshots from inside. You should

   A. enter the home to investigate.

   B. sound the siren to alert bystanders.

   C. leave the home and contact law enforcement.

   D. remain in front of the home and wait for someone to come out.

18. For a patient to successfully sue an EMT for malpractice, they must prove that the EMT

   A. purposefully caused the injury.

   B. was the cause of the injury.

   C. knew the injury occurred.

   D. felt no remorse for the injury.

19. A 19-year-old male is complaining of abdominal pain in the right lower quadrant. Detailed examination reveals rebound tenderness and fever. The patient MOST likely has

   A. pancreatitis.

   B. endometriosis.

   C. kidney stones.

   D. appendicitis.

20. You are called to care for a patient who was floating for 30 minutes in water at a temperature of 39.9°F (4.4°C) after his boat capsized. The patient is alert but confused. What should you do first?

   A. administer 100% oxygen

   B. move the patient to a warm area and then remove his clothing

   C. apply an AED

   D. apply heat packs to the patient's hands

21. You are evaluating an infant immediately after birth and find a pulse of 40 bpm. You stimulate the infant and provide oxygen with a non-rebreathing mask. You should next

   A. start compressions.

   B. attach the infant to an AED.

   C. administer epinephrine.

   D. allow the mother to hold the infant.

22. When communicating with a patient you should

   A. use medical terms to demonstrate competence.

   B. always remove bystanders to make the patient more comfortable.

   C. speak loudly to establish authority.

   D. ask open-ended questions to gather as much information as possible.

23. A patient found unconscious outside a bar wakes during assessment and states that he does not want to be transported. He knows the month and year, but he does not know where he is or how he got there. You may provide care for the patient because

   A. he is intoxicated.

   B. implied consent was given while he was unconscious.

   C. he is not competent.

   D. you cannot cease care once you have contact with the patient.

24. You are assessing a 72-year-old male patient with trouble breathing and pink, frothy sputum. The patient reports that he was treated for a myocardial infarction 2 weeks earlier. You should suspect the patient has developed

   A. pneumonia.

   B. pulmonary embolism.

   C. pulmonary edema.

   D. hemorrhagic stroke.

25. A patient with upper GI bleeding should be expected to have

   A. increased heart rate.

   B. decreased heart rate.

   C. warm, dry skin.

   D. bounding peripheral pulses.

26. After receiving online instruction from medical direction to help your asthmatic patient with their metered-dose inhaler, you should prepare the device by

   A. warming it for 10 seconds in the microwave.

   B. holding it upright and flicking the canister.

   C. shaking it vigorously.

   D. cooling it for 5 minutes in the refrigerator.

27. Online medical direction authorizes you to administer up to 3 doses of nitroglycerin to your patient, who has a chief complaint of chest pain. You know that you must wait at least how long between doses?

   A. 30 seconds

   B. 5 minutes

   C. 30 minutes

   D. 1 hour

28. Which of the following is NOT a reason to terminate CPR?

   A. The patient regains a pulse.

   B. Patient care is transferred to ALS providers.

   C. The patient is transported to a hospital.

   D. The patient's spouse asks you to stop.

29. During your secondary assessment of a 12-year-old boy who fell off his bike, you find an abrasion on his knee with slow and oozing bleeding that seems to be clotting itself. This bleeding would be categorized as

   A. venous.

   B. severe.

   C. capillary.

   D. profuse.

30. Your ambulance is dispatched to a middle school for a seventh-grade student who tripped and fell with a pencil in her hand. Upon arrival to the health office, you observe the patient in severe pain with the pencil impaled in her eye. Your intervention primarily consists of

   A. quickly removing the object.

   B. surrounding the object with gauze and stabilizing with a cup.

   C. irrigating the eye with saline solution.

   D. securing the patient to a long spine board.

31. After applying water-based lubricant to a nasopharyngeal airway, insert it

   A. as quickly as possible.

   B. by placing the bevel toward the septum.

   C. into one nostril while plugging the other.

   D. by placing the bevel toward the cheek.

32. A patient with partial thickness burns on 30 percent of his body is at risk for complications related to

   A. rhabdomyolysis.

   B. hyperglycemia.

   C. hypothermia.

   D. hemorrhagic stroke.

33. You arrive on a scene and discover an overturned semi hauling hazardous materials. Where should you park the ambulance?

   A. downwind from the accident

   B. as close to the semi as possible

   C. uphill from the accident

   D. on the road to block traffic

34. A 15-year-old female developed hives, difficulty breathing, and stridor after eating a peanut butter cookie. The definitive treatment for this patient is

   A. epinephrine.

   B. beta agonist.

   C. nitroglycerin.

   D. oxygen.

35. An abdominal stab wound to which organ is MOST likely to result in acute hemorrhage?

   A. stomach

   B. liver

   C. small intestine

   D. colon

36. A patient has pain and redness on her left forearm right after swimming in the ocean. She says that she saw a jellyfish and then her arm began to hurt. Her vital signs are stable, and she is not having any respiratory problems. You should

   A. wash with salt water and bandage the wound.

   B. remove the stinger with a credit card.

   C. immediately give the patient epinephrine.

   D. evacuate all swimmers from the beach and call animal control.

37. You apply a splint too tightly on a patient's lower leg and cut off circulation to the patient's foot. You do not notice and transport the patient to the hospital. You have most likely committed

   A. abandonment.

   B. assault and battery.

   C. negligence.

   D. false imprisonment.

38. To relieve chest discomfort in a patient with pericarditis, you should

   A. apply a heating pad to the patient's chest.

   B. apply cool compresses to the patient's chest.

   C. have the patient sit up and lean forward.

   D. administer sublingual nitroglycerin.

39. A contraindication for the insertion of an oropharyngeal airway is

   A. blockage from the tongue.

   B. bleeding within the mouth.

   C. an intact gag reflex.

   D. jugular vein distention.

40. What is the proper method for opening the airway of an unconscious patient who fell from the top of a 16-foot ladder?

A. jaw-thrust maneuver

B. head tilt–chin lift maneuver

C. Heimlich maneuver

D. Sellick maneuver

41. You respond to assist ocean lifeguards with an 18-year-old female who dove into a shallow sandbar and is now complaining of severe neck pain. Your assessment reveals a blood pressure of 88/66 mm Hg and a heart rate of 48 bpm. You believe this patient is exhibiting signs of

A. concussion.

B. neurogenic shock.

C. hypothermia.

D. septic shock.

42. You and your EMT partner are performing two-rescuer CPR on a pulseless and apneic adult patient. You are currently providing compressions and your partner is providing ventilation. You should plan to switch roles

A. every 2 minutes.

B. once the EMT performing compressions is too tired to continue.

C. never, as this will waste critical time.

D. after 2 cycles.

43. After being unable to rouse a 4-month-old child from an unresponsive state, you listen and feel for breathing while simultaneously palpating which pulse for 10 seconds?

A. femoral

B. vena cava

C. ankle

D. brachial

44. Aspirin is given to patients with chest pain because it

A. dilates blood vessels

B. slows blood clot formation

C. relieves pain

D. fights infections

45. You are treating a patient with a penetrating wound just above the clavicle. After applying a pressure dressing to the wound, you notice the blood begins to soak through the bandages. Your next step is to

A. apply additional dressing.

B. instruct the patient to lean back and let gravity control the bleeding.

C. use a liquid bandage or glue to seal the wound.

D. remove the dressing and apply a new one.

46. You arrive at a scene to find an adult male home alone with an open fracture of the ulna. The patient is speaking to you in a language you do not understand. You should

A. use gestures to get nonverbal consent for treatment.

B. not treat the patient until a translator can be found.

C. ask the patient in loud, clear English if he consents to treatment.

D. wait for the patient to lose consciousness and treat under implied consent.

47. A sunken fontanel on an infant is associated with

A. dehydration.

B. traumatic brain injury.

C. hypotension.

D. congenital defects.

48. You respond to a nursing home for a patient in cardiac arrest. The staff produces a do-not-resuscitate (DNR) order for the patient stating that the patient does not want medication during cardiac arrest. You should

A. start CPR immediately.

B. contact medical direction for pronouncement of death per protocols.

C. call for ALS intercept to administer epinephrine.

D. contact the patient's family and ask if they want CPR started.

49. What vital sign is taken to assess perfusion in patients under 3 years old?

A. systolic blood pressure

B. capillary refill

C. brachial pulse

D. rectal temperature

50. You are assessing a patient with chest pain who begins to act violently and throw items at you. What should you do?

A. ask bystanders for help restraining the patient

B. grab the patient and subdue him

C. leave the scene

D. retreat and call for law enforcement assistance

51. You are called to a high school for a 16-year-old football player who experienced a hard collision to the body. His chief complaint is difficulty breathing accompanied by one-sided chest pain. You palpate a deformity of the rib cage. This patient is likely experiencing

A. traumatic pneumothorax.

B. diaphragm spasm.

C. renal failure.

D. pulmonary edema.

52. Which of the following is NOT an indication for supplemental oxygen administration?

A. altered level of consciousness

B. abdominal pain

C. shock

D. cardiac arrest

53. A psychological emergency patient being transported to the hospital points at the back door of the ambulance and states she sees spiders. You should

A. call for a different ambulance to transport the patient.

B. tell her the spiders are real but are not dangerous.

C. tell her there are no spiders.

D. change the topic to distract the patient.

54. Which of the following can be applied to counteract neck flexion when opening the airway of a supine pediatric patient?

A. manual in-line stabilization

B. cervical collar

C. padding under the shoulders

D. pressure to the forehead

55. Many patients experiencing an aortic aneurysm present with

A. jugular vein distention.

B. low blood sugar.

C. no symptoms.

D. swelling in the lower extremities.

56. A fracture located at the base of the skull is known as which kind of fracture?

A. linear

B. crown

C. basilar

D. cervical

57. Upon your arrival for a patient complaining of intense shoulder pain after falling down a flight of stairs, you notice an obvious deformity at the joint, and you cannot palpate a distal pulse. You suspect this patient has experienced

   A. a compound fracture.

   B. a dislocation.

   C. sciatica.

   D. hyperextension.

58. You are preparing to take over chest compressions on a 44-year-old apneic patient in cardiac arrest. The depth of your compressions should be

   A. 1 – 6 inches.

   B. 2.0 – 2.4 inches.

   C. 25% of the depth of the chest.

   D. as deep as you can go.

59. During an initial assessment, you discover that the patient is not breathing. You should first

   A. check a pedal pulse.

   B. provide rescue breaths.

   C. request an ALS intercept.

   D. get the AED from the vehicle.

60. Blood pooling within the brain tissue is known as

   A. intracerebral hemorrhage.

   B. epidural hematoma.

   C. Battle's sign.

   D. compartment syndrome.

61. A 44-year-old male was involved in a motor vehicle crash (MVC), and you have determined the patient is unstable. You should immediately

   A. request police assistance.

   B. take the patient's vital signs.

   C. immediately splint any broken bones.

   D. perform a rapid head-to-toe assessment.

62. You are assessing an 11-month-old infant with a barking cough, a respiratory rate of 66, and a very runny nose. To help the patient's breathing, you should place the child

   A. sitting upright in a parent's lap.

   B. on a stretcher in a prone position.

   C. in reverse Trendelenburg.

   D. in semi-Fowler's.

63. A 35-year-old woman is confused and acting irrationally according to her friends. Her skin is cool and clammy, and her blood glucose level is 32. You should

   A. provide 100% oxygen via a non-rebreathing mask.

   B. provide the patient with oral glucose or sugar.

   C. provide immediate transport in left lateral recumbent position.

   D. restrain the patient and request an ALS unit.

64. A 17-year-old male presents with sudden-onset sharp chest pain. You note that he is tall and thin and that the pain is worse on deep inspiration. You should suspect

   A. spontaneous pneumothorax.

   B. esophageal rupture.

   C. diabetic ketoacidosis.

   D. ascending aortic rupture.

65. An electrician was wiring a circuit panel when he was shocked. He fell away from the panel, and another electrician shut off the power. You find the patient to be pulseless and apneic. You should

   A. treat the electrical burns and transport.

   B. begin CPR and apply the AED.

   C. move the patient away from the scene.

   D. provide rescue breathing and AED without compressions.

66. You arrive at the home of a patient who is suicidal. She is on a couch in the middle of a large room and appears to be agitated. Police are on scene as well. You should

   A. remain in the doorway.

   B. kneel in front of the patient.

   C. stand directly over the patient.

   D. make sure she has access to an exit.

67. A 25-year-old pregnant female calls 911 because she has started to have contractions. You evaluate the patient and find the infant is crowning and the mother is feeling the urge to push. You should

   A. immediately load-and-go to the hospital.

   B. instruct the mother not to push and prepare for transport.

   C. instruct the mother not to push until an ALS unit arrives.

   D. call for ALS and prepare to deliver the infant.

68. An 84-year-old male patient was found lying in a back bedroom. He is wearing a soiled diaper, and you observe animal feces in the room. The caregiver on scene is a 15-year-old girl who states that the man does not need any care. What should you do?

   A. assess the patient and allow the 15-year-old to sign a refusal form

   B. contact social services and file an adult neglect report

   C. move the patient to the shower and clean him before transport

   D. call for an ALS intercept to assist with care

69. Which of the following is NOT a symptom of hypertensive crisis?

   A. blurred vision

   B. ear ringing

   C. flushed skin

   D. nausea and vomiting

70. An 83-year-old male has a sudden onset of right-sided weakness with a splitting headache and slurred speech. The patient's symptoms are MOST likely being caused by

   A. stroke.

   B. myocardial infarction.

   C. diabetic ketoacidosis.

   D. hypoglycemia.

71. As you prepare to administer nitroglycerin to a patient experiencing chest pain, you must verify

   A. the expiration date of the medication.

   B. the patient's blood type.

   C. that you have the antidote to the nitroglycerin.

   D. that the patient has food to eat with it.

72. Cardiac arrest in children and infants is MOST often caused by

   A. respiratory arrest.

   B. accidental overdose.

   C. electrocution.

   D. acute coronary syndrome.

73. The AED pad placement for a 4-month-old patient is

   A. only one pad on the center of the chest.

   B. one pad directly on top of the other.

   C. one pad on the center of the chest and one on the center of the back.

   D. one pad on the upper right and one on the lower left chest.

74. Which of the following is NOT a common symptom of myocardial infarction?

   A. chest pressure or tightness

   B. diaphoresis

   C. nausea or vomiting

   D. wheezing or crackles

75. A hiker fell through ice while crossing a river and then hiked 2 hours to a vehicle access trail. At the trail, you note that the patient's feet are white, waxy, and hard to the touch. You should

   A. rub both feet to warm them.

   B. immerse both feet in warm water.

   C. splint both feet and give the patient oxygen.

   D. apply pressure dressing to both feet.

76. You are called to care for a roofer who has passed out on a hot day. The patient was acting confused before he passed out. He is now unconscious, hot, and dry. He MOST likely has

   A. heat cramps.

   B. heat exhaustion.

   C. heat stroke.

   D. heat rash.

77. During one-rescuer BVM ventilation, which technique is preferred to maintain a patent airway and proper mask seal?

   A. cricoid pressure

   B. vagal maneuvers

   C. "EC" clamp

   D. palm wrap

78. You receive a call for a 3-year-old who is having difficulty breathing. On assessment, you find the patient is in tripod position, wheezing on exhalation, and using accessory muscles. You should suspect

   A. pneumonia.

   B. pulmonary embolism.

   C. foreign body aspiration.

   D. asthma.

79. Your unconscious patient has excess secretions, including vomitus, in his mouth. After attaching the rigid catheter to the suction unit, your next step is to

   A. begin suctioning while inserting the catheter into the patient's oral airway.

   B. blindly swab the patient's mouth while applying suction.

   C. insert an airway adjunct and begin suctioning around it.

   D. position the tip of the catheter where it can be seen prior to applying suction.

80. Inadequate blood flow to the tissues and organs as the result of problems with the circulatory system is known as

   A. shock.

   B. hemorrhage.

   C. dyspnea.

   D. hypotension.

81. You respond to an adult patient bleeding significantly from blunt-force trauma to the head. The patient's heart rate is 130 bpm with a blood pressure of 102/68 mm Hg. The patient's skin is cool, pale, and diaphoretic. You suspect this patient is experiencing which of the following conditions secondary to the head trauma?

   A. neuropathy

   B. hemorrhagic shock

   C. anemia

   D. gastroenteritis

82. An EMS unit is dispatched to a residential address for a 58-year-old male with chest pain. You should report to dispatch when you

   A. arrive at the scene.

   B. enter the patient's home.

   C. begin assessing the patient.

   D. determine the nature of illness.

83. A 95-year-old woman is having severe abdominal pain and has been vomiting blood. The patient is confused and does not want to go to the hospital. Her son tells you that he wants her transported. You must transport the patient if

   A. the son has durable power of attorney.

   B. the son gives informed consent.

   C. the patient has a do-not-resuscitate order.

   D. the patient is competent.

84. You are caring for an 85-year-old man who has fallen down the stairs. When placing the patient on a backboard, what precaution should be implemented due to the patient's age?

   A. insert an airway adjunct after the patient has been secured on the backboard

   B. ensure the voids between the patient and backboard are padded

   C. check carotid pulse every 5 minutes

   D. restrain the patient before placing him on the backboard

85. You are preparing to deliver an infant. You notice that when the water breaks the fluid is light green. You know that the fluid is

   A. a normal color.

   B. stained with meconium.

   C. mixed with blood.

   D. infected with bacteria.

86. A 17-year-old patient has explained to you that she does not want to be transported. Her parents are not on scene. The patient can refuse care if she is

   A. competent.

   B. an emancipated minor.

   C. pregnant.

   D. accompanied by a grandparent.

87. A college student dove into a shallow lake and struck his head on the bottom, hyperextending his neck. He is floating facedown in 2 feet of water. You should

   A. pull the patient from the water by his arms.

   B. slide a backboard under the patient and pull him out prone.

   C. lift the patient's head out of the water and check for breathing.

   D. move the patient's arms above his head and grasp his biceps while rotating him face up.

88. While the AED is analyzing the patient's heart rhythm, the EMT should

   A. briefly discontinue CPR.

   B. check pulse and breathing for no longer than 10 seconds.

   C. insert an airway adjunct.

   D. raise the patient's legs above heart level.

89. A patient has just delivered an infant. You should first

   A. check the infant for a brachial pulse.

   B. suction the infant's mouth and nose.

   C. lift the infant and slap its feet.

   D. rub the infant vigorously.

90. Which of the following is a life-threatening source of chest pain?

   A. indigestion

   B. rib fracture

   C. pneumothorax

   D. sternum contusion

91. You are assessing an infant immediately after birth. Findings are as follows:

pink trunk with blue extremities

pulse of 120 bpm

strong vigorous cry

moving spontaneously

breathing well

What is the infant's APGAR score?

A. 7

B. 8

C. 9

D. 10

92. You respond to a 6-month-old patient with a weak brachial pulse and no respirations. After opening the airway, you provide artificial ventilation at a rate of

A. 1 – 6 breaths per minute.

B. 10 breaths per minute.

C. 12 – 20 breaths per minute.

D. 60 breaths per minute.

93. Which of the following is true for the mouth-to-mouth form of artificial ventilation?

A. It should never be used.

B. It is recommended only for patients whose medical history is known.

C. It should be used only on immediate family members.

D. It is not recommended unless no other methods are available.

94. You are triaging patients at the scene of a multi-car motor vehicle crash. Which patient is at highest risk for a crush injury?

A. an unrestrained passenger

B. one who was ambulatory at the scene

C. one who was ejected from the vehicle

D. one with a prolonged extraction

95. Which dressing would be MOST appropriate for a patient with a partial thickness wound to the epidermis?

A. transparent dressing

B. occlusive dressing

C. nonstick adherent dressing

D. bulky dressing

96. You are assessing a 14-year-old patient with delirium, respiratory distress, and headache. Upon examination of the airway, you note a burn to the roof of the patient's mouth. You should suspect

A. ingestion of a hot beverage.

B. inhalation of chemicals from a compressed gas can.

C. ingestion of dry ice.

D. marijuana use.

97. Which appearance is MOST consistent with an avulsion?

A. open wound with presence of sloughing and eschar tissue

B. skin tear with approximated edges

C. shearing of the top epidermal layers

D. separation of skin from the underlying structures that cannot be approximated

98. Approximately 90 minutes after a catastrophic earthquake, you are dispatched to the treatment area of a partial building collapse. Rescue workers bring you a 34-year-old female with an obvious and significant leg deformity who has just been extricated from underneath the rubble. You suspect your patient has

A. syncope.

B. deviated septum.

C. rhabdomyolysis.

D. hemorrhagic stroke.

99. A patient with emphysema tells you that he feels like he can't breathe. You should help the patient so he is

    A. lying flat on his back.

    B. in a prone position.

    C. sitting up and leaning forward.

    D. lying on his side with feet elevated.

100. A patient with a history of deep vein thrombosis who is complaining of sudden difficulty breathing along with chest pain that worsens with deep breaths is possibly experiencing

    A. appendicitis.

    B. kidney stones.

    C. pulmonary embolism.

    D. congestive heart failure.

101. Which of the following is NOT a symptom included in Cushing's triad?

    A. altered respiratory pattern

    B. pinpoint pupils

    C. hypertension

    D. bradycardia

102. Hyperventilation syndrome is MOST often caused by

    A. air pollution.

    B. allergic reaction.

    C. psychological reasons.

    D. painful stimuli.

103. An unresponsive patient in ventricular fibrillation requires

    A. epinephrine.

    B. nitroglycerin

    C. low-flow oxygen.

    D. defibrillation.

104. As an EMT in a mountainous region, you come across a patient from out of town who recently hiked quickly to the top of a tall peak and is now experiencing dyspnea, fatigue, and a worsening cough. You suspect this patient has

    A. high-altitude pulmonary edema.

    B. decompression sickness.

    C. respiratory failure

    D. pneumonia.

105. The hardening and narrowing of the arteries due to plaque buildup is known as

    A. aneurysm.

    B. atherosclerosis.

    C. thrombosis.

    D. melanoma.

106. While completing the SAMPLE history of your hypertensive patient, she tells you her ears are ringing. Which of the following terms do you use to note this symptom in your patient care report?

    A. photophobia

    B. tinnitus

    C. audiography

    D. migraine

107. You respond to the laboratory of a local university for a 19-year-old research assistant who inadvertently spilled a chemical on her torso. After treating the patient, your EMT partner is preparing to load her in the ambulance. Before leaving the scene, you should

    A. attempt to neutralize the residual chemical.

    B. obtain a sample of the chemical and bring it to the hospital.

    C. test the chemical for acidity.

    D. document the chemical name and its properties.

108. A patient with an oxygen saturation of 84% would be considered

    A. normal.

    B. mildly hypoxic.

    C. moderately hypoxic.

    D. severely hypoxic.

109. Which of the following is a psychological disorder characterized by severe mood swings between mania and depression?

    A. anxiety

    B. bipolar disorder

    C. schizophrenia

    D. clinical depression

110. During a history, a patient states that they have recently started taking Adderall for attention-deficit/hyperactivity disorder. The EMT knows that this drug places the patient at a higher risk for

    A. seizures

    B. renal failure

    C. stroke

    D. bradycardia

111. You arrive at a scene to find a woman clutching her throat. When you ask if she is choking, she is unable to speak but nods yes. You should first

    A. establish an airway by tilting the chin back

    B. administer five quick chest compressions

    C. administer two rescue breaths

    D. perform the abdominal-thrust maneuver

112. Oxygen cylinders should always be stored

    A. in a heated room.

    B. in an approved flammable gas cabinet.

    C. on their side.

    D. upright.

113. The use of standard precautions is required for contact with all of the following EXCEPT

    A. blood

    B. urine

    C. sweat

    D. vomit

114. Which of the following medications is prescribed to patients at high risk for deep vein thrombosis?

    A. Celebrex (celecoxib)

    B. Ambien (zolpidem)

    C. Topamax (topiramate)

    D. Xarelto (rivaroxaban)

115. Breathing that does not support life due to insufficient oxygen intake is known as

    A. asystole.

    B. respiratory arrest.

    C. respiratory failure.

    D. pulmonary shock.

116. You are treating an apneic patient with a tracheostomy. What are the proper steps for ventilation?

    A. wait for ALS to intubate the patient

    B. cover the tracheal opening and ventilate through the mouth and nose

    C. provide high-flow supplemental oxygen blow-by

    D. attach the one-way valve of a pocket mask or BVM directly to the trach tube

117. Septic shock results from

    A. head trauma.

    B. significant infection.

    C. traumatic blood loss.

    D. prolonged exposure to cold temperatures.

118. Your 12-year-old female patient plays multiple types of contact sports. After a sporting event, she complains of chest pain at the point where her ribs meet her breastbone. While palpating this area you notice it is inflamed. You suspect she most likely has

   A. costochondritis.

   B. flail segment.

   C. heartburn.

   D. floating ribs.

119. Which of the following types of blast injuries is caused by the human body being thrown against a hard surface after an explosion?

   A. secondary

   B. shockwave

   C. tertiary

   D. ferrous

120. A patient has acknowledged your arrival on scene and is asking for help. The patient has given

   A. direct consent.

   B. written consent.

   C. implied consent.

   D. expressed consent.

ANSWER KEY

1. A.

For nasopharyngeal airway placement, measure from the opening of the nostril to the tip of the earlobe.

2. B.

Nitroglycerin is contraindicated in the presence of a systolic blood pressure of less than 100 mm Hg.

3. C.

Patients requiring CPR must be moved onto a hard surface before starting compressions.

4. A.

Using the rule of palm, also known as the rule of one, the size of the patient's palm is approximately 1% of their body surface area.

5. D.

The right upper quadrant contains the liver, pancreas, gallbladder, small intestine, and colon. The liver is a vascular organ, and significant bruising may result if it is injured.

6. D.

When checking a patient's level of consciousness, use the acronym AVPU (Alert, Verbal, Pain, Unresponsive). An **A**lert patient answers questions. In response to **V**erbal prompting, the patient moans or moves when being called. In this scenario, the patient responds to a physical or **P**ainful stimulus. An **U**nresponsive patient does not respond at all.

7. C.

This patient is experiencing diabetic ketoacidosis, which is determined by the blood glucose reading. A blood glucose of less than 70 is hypoglycemia, above 200 is hyperglycemia, from 350 to 800 is diabetic ketoacidosis, and above 800 is hyperglycemic hyperosmolar syndrome.

8. B.

The patient had a transient ischemic attack (TIA). The symptoms of TIA resolve themselves with no permanent effects.

9. D.

Classic signs of cardiogenic shock include hypotension; a rapid pulse that weakens; cool, clammy skin; and decreased urine output.

10. A.

Since a traction splint cannot be applied due to a suspected pelvic fracture, the next best choice is to secure the patient to a long spine board.

11. B.

The priority intervention for a patient with SpO_2 below 94% is supplemental oxygen. If the patient has an albuterol nebulizer, it may be administered after supplemental oxygen has been started.

12. A.

CPR should resume immediately after delivering a shock from an AED.

13. A.

Angina pectoris, or simply angina, is the term describing chest pain resulting from poor blood flow to the heart.

14. D.

COPD (chronic obstructive pulmonary disease) is most commonly caused by smoking. The chronic cough associated with COPD is often exacerbated by lung infection.

15. D.

Amputated appendages should be wrapped in sterile gauze moistened with saline before being placed on ice. They should never be frozen.

16. C.

An occlusive dressing should be applied to any open neck wound to prevent an air embolus from entering the blood vessels.

17. C.

If the scene is not safe, you should not enter the scene. You should contact the appropriate agency to mitigate the hazard (in this case, the police).

18. **B.**

   To sue for malpractice the patient needs to prove four things: the EMT had a duty to act; the EMT acted improperly; the EMT was the cause of the injury; and there was an injury or harm caused by the action.

19. **D.**

   Appendicitis typically presents with a fever, right lower quadrant pain, and rebound tenderness. Occasionally the patient will have referred pain around the umbilicus.

20. **B.**

   Move the patient to a warm area like the back of the ambulance or a building. Remove wet clothes to facilitate rewarming.

21. **A.**

   You should start CPR if the pulse of a newborn infant is less than 60 bpm. You should also request ALS intercept.

22. **D.**

   Asking patients open-ended questions (as opposed to yes/no questions) will help you gather more information about the patient and scene.

23. **C.**

   This patient would not be considered competent to deny care because he is unable to demonstrate that he knows where he is or the history of present illness.

24. **C.**

   The patient is experiencing symptoms of pulmonary edema, a complication of left-sided heart failure.

25. **A.**

   Upper GI bleeding causes signs and symptoms of hypovolemia, including tachycardia; cold, clammy skin; and weak peripheral pulses.

26. **C.**

   Inhalers contain a propellant in addition to medication. Shaking the inhaler prior to administration ensures a proper mixture of medication and propellant.

27. **B.**

   Multiple doses of nitroglycerin should be separated by at least 5 minutes.

28. **D.**

   CPR should continue unless the patient regains a pulse or patient care is transferred to someone of equal or higher training, such as an ALS provider or emergency room physician.

29. **C.**

   Capillary bleeding is slow and oozing. It is usually a result of minor abrasions and can sometimes clot itself.

30. **B.**

   Objects impaled in the eye should first be stabilized with soft material such as folded or rolled gauze, then protected with rigid stabilization such as a paper cup.

31. **B.**

   To insert a nasopharyngeal airway, place the bevel (angled portion) toward the septum and smoothly slide it in.

32. **C.**

   Damage to the skin caused by burns with large body surface area affects the body's ability to thermoregulate and puts patients at risk for hypothermia.

33. **C.**

   As part of scene size-up, you should determine the best location to park the ambulance. At a HazMat incident, be sure to park uphill, upwind, and upstream to prevent the hazardous materials from contaminating the ambulance.

34. **A.**

   The symptoms described indicate anaphylactic shock. The definitive treatment for this is epinephrine (often in the form of an EpiPen).

35. **B.**

   Solid organ (e.g., liver) injury usually results in hemorrhage, while hollow organ (e.g., stomach, small intestine, colon) injuries lead to spillage of gastrointestinal contents.

36. **A.**

   As with other animal bites or insect stings, if there is no concern of an anaphylactic reaction, you should clean and bandage the wound. Jellyfish stings should be washed with salt water.

37. C.

Providing improper care for a patient may be negligence.

38. C.

Sitting up and leaning forward will pull the inflamed cardiac sac away from the muscle and relieve the chest discomfort.

39. C.

An oropharyngeal airway should not be inserted when the patient has an intact gag reflex, as this may cause vomiting and aspiration.

40. A.

The jaw-thrust maneuver is used to open the airway of trauma patients with suspected head, neck, or back injury.

41. B.

Key findings for neurogenic shock include spinal trauma combined with significantly low blood pressure and bradycardia.

42. A.

When two EMTs are performing CPR, they should switch roles every 5 cycles to avoid fatigue. Five cycles should take approximately 2 minutes.

43. D.

The brachial artery of the upper arm is used to check the pulse of infants.

44. B.

The mechanism of action of aspirin includes antiplatelet properties that reduce the likelihood of blood clots forming.

45. A.

If the wound continues to bleed through and a tourniquet is not an option, apply additional dressing. Never remove a pressure dressing once it has been applied.

46. A.

When a patient does not speak English, you may use gestures to get implied consent (e.g., you may gesture at the patient's arm, and the patient may nod or lift the arm in response).

47. A.

If the fontanel is sunken the infant could be dehydrated.

48. A.

DNR orders may indicate specific treatments that should be withheld. You should read the DNR order and follow the patient's wishes documented on it. Because the DNR only addresses medication, you should initiate CPR.

49. B.

Capillary refill is used to assess perfusion in children less than 3 years old.

50. D.

When faced with a patient who suddenly becomes violent, retreat from the scene and call for help to protect the safety of the patient, bystanders, and yourself.

51. A.

Traumatic pneumothorax is the result of thoracic trauma and often presents with unilateral chest pain and dyspnea.

52. B.

Altered level of consciousness, shock, and cardiac arrest are all indications for prehospital supplemental oxygen.

53. D.

When caring for a patient having delusions, do not confirm or deny the delusion. Confirming plays into the delusion, and denying may cause an altercation. Change the subject or distract the patient by reassessing vital signs or with conversation.

54. C.

Placing padding under the shoulders of a pediatric patient can counter neck flexion and reduce the risk of injury while opening the airway.

55. C.

Aortic aneurysms can develop slowly over time, with no obvious symptoms among many patients.

56. C.

Basilar fractures are those that occur at the base of the skull.

57. **B.**

Dislocations occur at the joint and are caused by sudden significant force, such as falls. The shoulder is a common joint for dislocation, and the symptoms will likely include a deformity along with intense, localized pain. Severe dislocations can cause vascular disruption.

58. **B.**

Current guidelines for adult CPR indicate a chest compression depth of 2.0 – 2.4 inches.

59. **B.**

When you find a problem during the initial assessment, correct the problem before moving to the next step. Here, the EMT finds during the initial assessment that the patient is not breathing, so the EMT should provide rescue breaths immediately.

60. **A.**

Intracerebral hemorrhage is the pooling of blood within the brain tissue.

61. **D.**

In trauma situations, perform a rapid head-to-toe assessment in unstable patients. You should also transport immediately.

62. **A.**

The child should remain with the parent in an upright position. Taking the child from the parent could cause anxiety and crying and worsen the respiratory distress.

63. **B.**

This patient has hypoglycemia. She should be given sugar orally if she is conscious.

64. **A.**

Tall, thin teenage males are the most likely population to experience a spontaneous pneumothorax. Symptoms typically arise suddenly with pain worsening on inspiration.

65. **B.**

Pulseless patients who have been electrocuted respond well to CPR and AED use.

66. **D.**

The patient is agitated. Do not put yourself in a position where you could be injured if the patient becomes combative. Always look for an exit route before needing it.

67. **D.**

If birth is imminent, call for ALS and prepare to deliver the infant on scene. Signs of imminent birth include contractions less than 2 minutes apart, crowning, and feeling the urge to push. If the mother has had multiple births and says she is about to give birth, that is also a sign of imminent birth.

68. **B.**

EMTs who observe adult abuse or neglect have a responsibility to file a complaint with the appropriate social service government agency.

69. **C.**

Flushed skin is not a symptom of hypertensive crisis.

70. **A.**

The patient is most likely having a stroke. Strokes can present with one-sided weakness or numbness, facial droop, headache, slurred speech, confusion, or altered mental status.

71. **A.**

The expiration date of medication should always be verified early to ensure it can be used.

72. **A.**

Respiratory arrest is the most common cause of cardiac arrest in infants and children.

73. **C.**

For infants and small children, it will likely be necessary to apply one pad to the center of the chest and the second pad to the center of the back.

74. **D.**

Wheezing and crackles are not symptoms of myocardial infarction.

75. **C.**

The patient has frostbite. Handle the feet gently and splint them. Administer oxygen to the patient.

76. **C.**

A patient with heat stroke may be found unconscious; confused; and with hot, dry skin. The patient will no longer be sweating.

77. **C.**

The "EC" clamp, achieved by placing the fingers in the shape of an "E" and "C," is the preferred method for achieving an effective face seal during one-rescuer BVM ventilation.

78. **D.**

The child is presenting with signs of asthma exacerbation, including trouble breathing, tripod positioning, wheezing on exhalation, and use of accessory muscles.

79. **D.**

The tip of the catheter should be positioned before applying suction and only in places where it can be seen.

80. **A.**

Shock, or hypoperfusion, is a state of inadequate blood flow to the tissues and organs.

81. **B.**

Tachycardia and hypotension are symptoms of hemorrhagic shock along with cool, pale, and moist skin. Hemorrhagic shock, a form of hypovolemic shock, is most often caused by trauma.

82. **A.**

The EMS unit should report to the dispatcher when they have arrived at the scene.

83. **A.**

Durable power of attorney gives an individual the power to make medical decisions for another person.

84. **B.**

Patients over 65 have a loss in fatty tissue and joints that do not move as well as those of a younger patient. Padding the voids will make the backboard much more comfortable for the patient.

85. **B.**

The fluid is stained with meconium (the infant's feces).

86. **B.**

An emancipated minor can make choices regarding their medical care as long as they are competent.

87. **D.**

Use care in removing the patient from the water due to the likelihood of a spinal cord injury. Maintain in-line stabilization and rotate the patient face up to clear the airway.

88. **A.**

CPR should be momentarily halted, and nobody should touch the patient while the AED is analyzing the patient's heart rhythm.

89. **B.**

To stimulate breathing after the infant is born, suction the mouth and nose.

90. **C.**

Pneumothorax is a life-threatening source of chest pain.

91. **C.**

The APGAR score is 9.

pink trunk with blue extremities: 1

pulse of 120 bpm: 2

strong vigorous cry: 2

moving spontaneously: 2

breathing well: 2

92. **C.**

The rate of artificial ventilations for infants and children is 12 – 20 breaths per minute.

93. **D.**

Mouth-to-mouth is recommended only if there are no other means available for artificial ventilation.

94. **D.**

A patient in a motor vehicle crash with a prolonged extraction will likely have sustained compressing or crushing force or pressure damaging underlying vascular and musculoskeletal structures.

95. **C.**

Nonstick adherent dressing such as a Telfa pad is the appropriate choice.

96. **B.**

Adolescent patients presenting with frostbite burns to the roof of the mouth are most likely abusing inhalants, typically in the form of aerosols, glues, paints, and solvents.

97. D.

An avulsion is characterized by the separation of skin from the underlying structures that cannot be approximated.

98. C.

Crush pressure that is sustained for a long period (> 60 minutes) can lead to a rapid breakdown of muscle tissue known as rhabdomyolysis. Sometimes shortened to "rhabdo," this condition is the second leading cause of death following earthquakes.

99. C.

A patient with emphysema can improve their breathing by sitting up and leaning forward.

100. C.

The most common form of pulmonary embolism (PE) is a blood clot due to deep vein thrombosis. A key symptom of PE is pleuritic chest pain that worsens upon inhalation and exhalation.

101. B.

Cushing's triad, a sign of increased intracranial pressure and/or herniation syndrome, does not include pinpoint pupils.

102. C.

While hyperventilation can be caused by an underlying medical condition, it is most often a result of a psychological concern.

103. D.

Ventricular fibrillation is a shockable dysrhythmia that requires defibrillation to return the heart to a sinus rhythm.

104. A.

High-altitude pulmonary edema occurs after a rapid ascent to altitudes greater than 8,200 feet.

105. B.

Atherosclerosis occurs when arteries are hardened and/or narrowed due to the deposition of fatty plaques on the inner walls.

106. B.

Tinnitus is the medical term for the perception of ringing in the ears.

107. D.

If possible, you should document the chemical name and its properties and provide this information to the receiving hospital. Never bring chemicals into the ambulance or hospital.

108. D.

A patient with a pulse oxygenation of less than 85% is considered severely hypoxic.

109. B.

Bipolar disorder is characterized by extreme shifts between mania and depression.

110. A.

Seizures are a serious, adverse drug effect that may occur when taking Adderall.

111. D.

In responsive patients with airway obstruction, the first intervention should be the abdominal-thrust (Heimlich) maneuver.

112. C.

To prevent damage to the regulator and valve, oxygen cylinders should be stored on their side so they cannot fall or be knocked over.

113. C.

Standard precautions are recommended whenever the nurse comes in contact with blood or body fluids that could transmit blood-borne pathogens.

114. D.

Xarelto (rivaroxaban) is an anticoagulant that helps prevent clots and DVT.

115. C.

A patient in respiratory failure is still breathing, but the breaths are not sufficient to support life.

116. D.

The universal fitting on the one-way valve of pocket masks and BVMs will attach directly to a tracheostomy tube.

117. B.

Septic shock is the result of a massive infection, typically of the urinary or respiratory tract, damaging the blood vessels.

118. A.

Costochondritis is an inflammation of the junction where the ribs and sternum meet. This condition can be caused by repeated minor chest trauma.

119. C.

Tertiary blast injuries are those caused by the human body being thrown into a hard surface, such as a wall, by the blast force of the explosion.

120. D.

A patient verbally asking for help is giving expressed consent.

Follow the link for your second EMT practice test: **ascenciatestprep.com/emt-online-resources**

" " " BEYOND " " "
ARCHITECTURE

MARION MAHONY AND
WALTER BURLEY GRIFFIN

AMERICA " AUSTRALIA " INDIA

EDITED BY ANNE WATSON

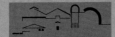

POWERHOUSE PUBLISHING
PART OF THE MUSEUM OF APPLIED ARTS AND SCIENCES

First published 1998.
Powerhouse Publishing, Sydney

Powerhouse Publishing
part of the Museum of Applied Arts and Sciences
PO Box K346 Haymarket NSW 1238 Australia.
The Museum of Applied Arts and Sciences incorporates the Powerhouse Museum and Sydney Observatory.

Project management: Julie Donaldson*
Editing: Bernadette Foley
Design: Colin Rowan* and Rhys Butler
Picture research: Anat Meiri* and Melanie Cariss*
Rights & permissions: Gara Baldwin*, Anat Meiri and Melanie Cariss
Proofreading: Karen Ward
Index: Caroline Colton
Printing: Inprint Pty Ltd, Brisbane
Produced in Stone Serif and Gill Sans Light. Title and chapter heads hand lettered
based on Griffin's letterhead.
* Powerhouse Museum

National Library of Australia Cataloguing-in-Publication

Beyond architecture: Marion Mahony and Walter Burley Griffin in America, Australia
and India
Bibliography.
Includes index.
ISBN 1 8317 068 5

1. Griffin, Marion Mahony, 1871–1961. 2. Griffin, Walter Burley, 1876–1937. 3.
Architecture, Modern — 20th century. 4. Architects — Biography. I. Watson, Anne
(Anne Jeanette). II Powerhouse Museum. 720.92

Published in conjunction with the exhibition *Beyond architecture: Marion Mahony and
Walter Burley Griffin in America, Australia and India* at the Powerhouse Museum
22 July 1998 — May 1999.

Major sponsor

Sponsors HBO + EMTB architecture   QANTAS

Supporters
Crone Associates, The E.G.O. Group, Multiplex and Peddle Thorp & Walker.

The museum gratefully acknowledges the generous assistance of the Walter Burley
Griffin Society and the contribution to the first printing of the book by Griffin Press.

Cover image: Facade of the Pyrmont Incinerator, courtesy of Fairfax Photo Library.
Inside cover: Detail drawing of Pyrmont incinerator tiles by Trevor Waters, 1988.

CONTENTS

GRIFFIN CHRONOLOGY

1871, 14 Feb	Marion Lucy Mahony (MLM) born, Chicago, Illinois.
1876, 24 Nov	Walter Burley Griffin (WBG) born, Maywood, Illinois.
1893	World's Columbian Exposition, Chicago.
1894	MLM graduates in architecture from Massachusetts Institute of Technology, Boston.
1894	MLM works for Dwight H Perkins on Steinway Hall.
1895–1909	MLM works for Frank Lloyd Wright at Oak Park, Chicago, the last four years on an occasional contract basis.
1899	WBG graduates in architecture from the University of Illinois at Urbana–Champaign.
1899–1901	WBG works at Steinway Hall, Chicago, successively for architects Dwight H Perkins, Robert C Spencer Jr and Henry Webster Tomlinson.
1901–06	WBG works for Frank Lloyd Wright at Oak Park.
1903	MLM designs Unitarian Church of All Souls, Evanston, Illinois. Her first major independent project.
1903–04	WBG designs W H Emery house, Elmhurst, Illinois. First major domestic commission and first substantial house in Walter's early style.
1906	WBG sets up his own practice at Steinway Hall.
1909–11	MLM works for Hermann Von Holst at Steinway Hall on Frank Lloyd Wright's uncompleted projects and new projects including the David Amberg house, Grand Rapids and Adolph and Robert Mueller houses, Decatur.
1911	WBG designs 'Solid Rock' house for William F Tempel, Winnetka, Illinois. The first house erected in Walter's mature style and his first house of reinforced concrete.
1911	MLM joins WBG's practice.
1911, 29 June	WBG and MLM marry in Michigan City.
1912	WBG designs J G Melson house, Rock Crest–Rock Glen, Mason City, Iowa: WBG's first major expression of 'organic' architecture and anticipates later projects in Castlecrag, Sydney.
1912	Griffins win international competition for the design of Australia's new capital, Canberra.
1913, Aug	WBG is invited to Australia by the Commonwealth Government and in October is appointed Federal Capital Director of Design and Construction. He returns to the US for six months to settle his American practice.

1914, Feb	WBG and MMG visit Europe for three weeks to appoint adjudicators for Parliament House competition.
1914, May	WBG and MMG leave America for Australia accompanied by architects Roy Lippincott and George Elgh. Of approximately 125 architectural projects in America since 1900, about 65 were constructed.
1914–20	WBG works on the implementation of the Canberra plan and on other urban planning projects such as Griffith and Leeton in New South Wales and Eaglemont in Victoria.
1914–37	Practice established in Melbourne. Of approximately 72 projects for private residences and major buildings, 48 were completed.
1914–37	Practice established in Sydney. Of approximately 100 projects for private residences and major buildings, 33 were completed.
1915–18	WBG/MMG design Newman College, University of Melbourne, in association with A A Fritsch Architects.
1916	WBG/MMG design Cafe Australia, Collins Street, Melbourne.
1917, May	Knitlock construction system patented by WBG and David C Jenkins. A system of interlocking, precast concrete tiles used to construct roofs, interior and exterior walls.
1919	WBG forms the Greater Sydney Development Association Ltd (GSDA), with the aim of purchasing land and developing a residential estate on the shores of Sydney Harbour.
1920	WBG's position as Federal Capital Director of Construction and Design terminated. Walter's refusal to join the newly formed Federal Capital Advisory Committee effectively ended his role in Canberra.
1921–24	WBG/MMG design Capitol House–Capitol Theatre, Swanston Street, Melbourne, in association with Peck & Kemter Architects.
1921	WBG, with shareholders, purchases 650 acres (263 hectares) of land on the foreshores of Sydney Harbour in the areas now known as Castlecrag, Castle Cove and Middle Cove.
1922	WBG designs Leonard House, 46 Elizabeth Street, Melbourne.
1924, Nov	The Griffins return to the US for three months.
1925	MMG moves to Castlecrag from Melbourne, and WBG joins her a few months later. Over the next decade, they live at various addresses in Castlecrag and design more than 50 houses, of which sixteen are built.
1929–37	The Reverberatory Incinerator & Engineering Company (RIECo) incorporated by Nisson Leonard–Kanevsky, John Boadle and Vasilie Trunoff. WBG in partnership with Eric Milton Nicholls completes thirteen incinerators throughout Australia.
1930	WBG and Eric Nicholls partnership established; the firm, Griffin and Nicholls, continues after WBG's death in 1937.
1930	WBG/MMG design Haven Scenic Theatre (open–air theatre), Castlecrag.
1930	MMG joins the Sydney Anthroposophical Society
1930, Nov	MMG returns to Chicago.
1931	WBG joins the Sydney Anthroposophical Society.
1932, Sept	MMG returns to Castlecrag.
1935	WBG/MMG design Pyrmont incinerator, Sydney.
1935, Oct	WBG travels to Lucknow, India, having received a commission to design Lucknow University Library.
1936, May	MMG joins WBG in India.
1936–37	WBG designs approximately 100 projects in India, about half of which are individual buildings for the United Provinces Industrial and Agricultural Exhibition. Those built include the Pioneer Press building and pavilions for the United Provinces Exhibition, both in Lucknow.
1937, 11 Feb	WBG dies in Lucknow, aged 60, after developing peritonitis following a gall bladder operation.
1938	MMG returns to Chicago.
1949	MMG completes her memoirs 'The magic of America'.
1961, 10 Aug	MMG dies in Chicago of heart failure, aged 90.
1987	WBG's unmarked grave in Lucknow is provided with a memorial slab and enclosure.
1997	MMG's ashes re–interred with a new memorial plaque at Graceland Cemetery, Chicago.

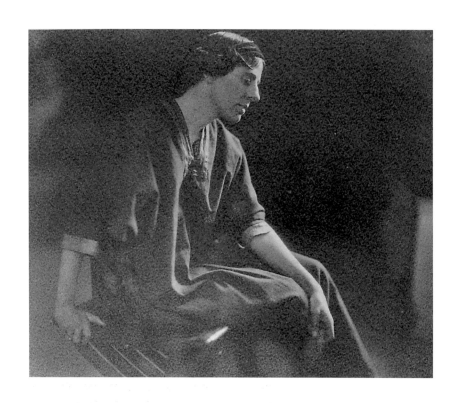

Marion Mahony Griffin and Walter Burley Griffin, about 1915.
Photographs courtesy Nicholls collection, Sydney.

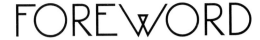

FOREWORD

The impetus for this book, and the exhibition which it accompanies, was driven by the demolition in 1992 of one of Sydney's landmark Griffin buildings — the Pyrmont incinerator. By way of memorialising this striking building, Sydney City Council allocated funding to a number of Griffin projects, including an exhibition and the conservation of architectural materials salvaged from the incinerator. As the repository for the patterned wall tiles and other elements from the incinerator, the Powerhouse Museum demonstrated its early commitment to preserving and interpreting the Griffin legacy.

The publication of this collection of essays on aspects of the lives and careers of Marion Mahony and Walter Burley Griffin demonstrates the museum's dedication to scholarly research and to bringing the remarkable achievements of these two important architects to a wider audience.

The essays by American and Australian Griffin scholars address the Griffins' architectural contribution — which encompasses the disciplines of town planning, landscape architecture and interior design as well as the design of buildings — and also the philosophical, aesthetic and ideological contexts that directed and informed their vision. Ultimately, they strove to find architectural solutions which expressed a balance between society and the environment, an affinity between the human spirit and the natural world. It is the intention of both the exhibition and this book to present a holistic view of the Griffins' lives through an analysis of the tangible legacy of their architectural and design work and the intellectual background to its creation.

In doing so the essays traverse many new areas of research and present fresh ideas and interpretation as well as newly discovered source material and hitherto unknown projects and objects. The museum has been given privileged access to several institutional and private collections and many images which are published here for the first time. This is the first book on the Griffins that reproduces Marion's splendid satin architectural renderings and tree studies in colour and pays long overdue attention to the Griffins' designs for furniture and lighting.

Finally, *Beyond architecture* provides a lasting record of the diversity of the Griffins' creativity and the extensiveness of their legacy. Its penetrating essays and the richness of its images underscore the importance of the Griffins in Australian architectural and social history and the significance of their contribution in India and early twentieth-century America. If, by the example of their own uncompromising vision and the legacy of their architecture, they can be said to have influenced the course of modern Australian architecture, then this comprehensive record of their achievement will consolidate their status as two of our most important architects.

Terence Measham
Director, Powerhouse Museum

INTRODUCTION

When Nancy Price wrote her Sydney University undergraduate thesis on and in consultation with Walter Burley Griffin in 1933, she could not have foreseen the extensive body of Griffin-related research and writing that would accumulate in the years to come. Since then there have been many theses — most notably that of respected Griffin authority Peter Harrison in 1970 — innumerable articles, several books, television documentaries, plays and compositions for music and dance relating to the Griffins. They have been the subject of conferences and symposia and Walter Burley Griffin's name, like Utzon and the Opera House, is still regularly coupled with Canberra, in spite of his and Marion's singular lack of success in realising their grand democratic vision for the new capital.

Despite all this attention we are still awaiting the 'definitive' Griffin biography. And despite the regular invocation of the Griffins' names in association with places such as Canberra and Castlecrag in Australia, most non-architects are only partially aware of the nature and extent of their extraordinarily productive careers, or indeed of the grand drama of their lives.

Architecture was central to the Griffins' lives; they lived and breathed it. Witness the large number of projects — over 350 built and unbuilt — in the 30 or so years of their joint architectural practice in three countries. But their creativity and their contribution extended well beyond architecture. As well as specific architectural and urban design projects the Griffins designed interior schemes, furniture, floor coverings, tableware and lighting, and were responsible for a number of technological innovations, most notably the Knitlock precast concrete block building system patented in 1917. They wrote and lectured extensively on a range of subjects from social economics to architecture to Australian flora. Marion's superb tree drawings and paintings survive as an enduring record of the Griffins' passionate concern for the Australian landscape and its preservation, decades before such concerns received widespread currency.

As the Griffins' creativity ranged beyond architecture, so any analysis of their extremely prolific creative output would be incomplete without consideration of the ideological, philosophical and spiritual beliefs that informed their work. Both Walter and Marion grew up and worked in progressive circles in Chicago where issues of social and urban reform encouraged debate and experimentation in many areas of design and community life. Indeed, the Griffins' decision to settle in Australia was inspired by their idealistic perception of the opportunity Canberra offered for the expression of the great 'democratic civic ideal'.

In Australia the Griffins moved in non-conformist circles, befriending members of minority ethnic communities, pacifists, suffragists and political activists. In Sydney they became members of the Anthroposophical Society, as did a number of other Castlecrag residents. The society's focus on creativity and spirituality as the core of individual endeavour held great appeal for the Griffins, both in their architecture and their lifestyle.

This collection of essays by Griffin scholars in North America and Australia, while not intended as a definitive coverage of Walter and Marion's lives, does aim to convey the extensiveness and diversity of their careers and to 'bring them to life', both professionally and personally. Thus Paul Kruty's opening essay examines the unique social and creative climate of turn-of-the-century Chicago and emphasises the seminal importance of this energetic intellectual environment in the formation of the Griffins' attitudes and philosophies. Marion and Walter's contribution to architecture, particularly in America, has always been somewhat eclipsed by the towering reputation of Frank Lloyd Wright, for whom they both worked in Chicago. This essay and that of Paul Sprague should dispel the popular misconception that they merely plagiarised Wright. On the contrary, there is much evidence to suggest that they introduced a number of ideas into the Oak Park studio that Wright was to adopt as his own.

Paul Sprague ranks Walter Burley Griffin as a 'leader', with Louis Sullivan and Wright, rather than a follower of the midwest architectural movement, and draws our attention to the significance of several projects that depart radically from Wright and signal the arrival of a mature, original style anticipating many of the later preoccupations of modernism.

Both Paul Sprague and Anna Rubbo examine, from very different angles, the nature and extent of Marion Mahony's collaborative and independent role as a designer and extraordinarily gifted artist. Anna Rubbo's extensive research into Marion's long life indeed reveals her to be a 'larger than life' character whose remarkable talents and achievements in an almost entirely male profession have hitherto been undervalued or ignored. Passionate, energetic and a dedicated architect and wife, her story is now being accorded the attention it deserves.

Long overdue for analysis too is a detailed account of the spiritual and ideological bases of the Griffins' work. James Weirick's extended essay reveals many new facts and insights into the role of spirituality in Marion and Walter's lives and challenges theories suggesting that esoteric or occult symbolism directed and shaped their work. This essay traces the Griffins' 'spiritual journey' from Emersonian beginnings in Chicago to a testing of their social and political idealism during the Canberra years — an experience that in turn led to their interest in theosophy and then, more keenly, their association with anthroposophy in the Castlecrag community. Inseparable from this spiritual journey, their architecture developed a new design vocabulary that found its first and most profound expression in the building details for the Canberra plan.

Just as Marion's role in her partnership with Walter is being reassessed so too are Walter's activities as a landscape architect, a profession he studied for and then practised throughout his adult life. Christopher Vernon evaluates the significance of Walter's landscape work in the United States and Australia, and emphasises Walter and Marion's lifelong regard for nature and their concern for the preservation of the natural environment. Both became extremely knowledgeable about Australian flora and were dedicated to advocating its inclusion in local planting schemes.

Jeffrey Turnbull examines the Griffins' ideologies and philosophies, not through the lens of their architecture, but through the often radical literary, philosophical and political influences that shaped their lives. Such beliefs, in turn, acted as an important conduit through which their network of remarkable clients, friends and acquaintances was developed in Australia and India.

Both Marion and Walter stressed the importance of integrating exterior architecture and interior schemes, and my essay on their designs for furniture and lighting is the first survey of this important component of their creative output. It reveals the nature and extent of their design of interior elements and its significance in any consideration of the Griffins' architectural careers.

Sydney's 1935 Pyrmont incinerator — or more accurately its demolition — provided the raison d'être for the exhibition that inspired this publication. Peter Navaretti's essay establishes the incinerator's important position in the Griffins' work and its crucial role as an expression of their architectural ideas and philosophical and spiritual beliefs. Such beliefs predisposed them to respond enthusiastically to the very different spiritual and physical environment of India — to which Walter and Marion travelled in 1935 and 1936 respectively. As Paul Kruty's essay elucidates, the Indian work, known only today through Marion's superb drawings and photographs of the few completed buildings, represents the creation of a new modernist aesthetic as well as the culmination of their architectural practice, for it was in India that Walter met his untimely death early in 1937.

David Dolan's concluding reflection draws together the diverse threads of the essays presented in this book and examines the speculation and misinterpretation that has both fuelled the Griffin 'enigma' and ensured the longevity of scholarly debate and enquiry. But will there ever be a last word on the Griffins? Will we ever feel confident that the disentangling of their complex, sometimes puzzling, lives and careers is complete and that they, as personalities, are fully explained and deciphered?

Quite possibly not, for theirs were many layered lives, often unorthodox, certainly peripatetic and decades ahead of their time. Their contribution was not simply one of introducing new architectural and planning concepts. By challenging accepted opinion, by their uncompromising vision of a democratic society living in sympathy with the natural environment, they also articulated and anticipated many social and environmental issues of today. It is the continuing relevance and universality of their humanism that will ensure the endurance of their ability to intrigue, provoke and inspire.

Anne Watson

CHICAGO 1900:
THE GRIFFINS
COME OF AGE

PAUL KRUTY

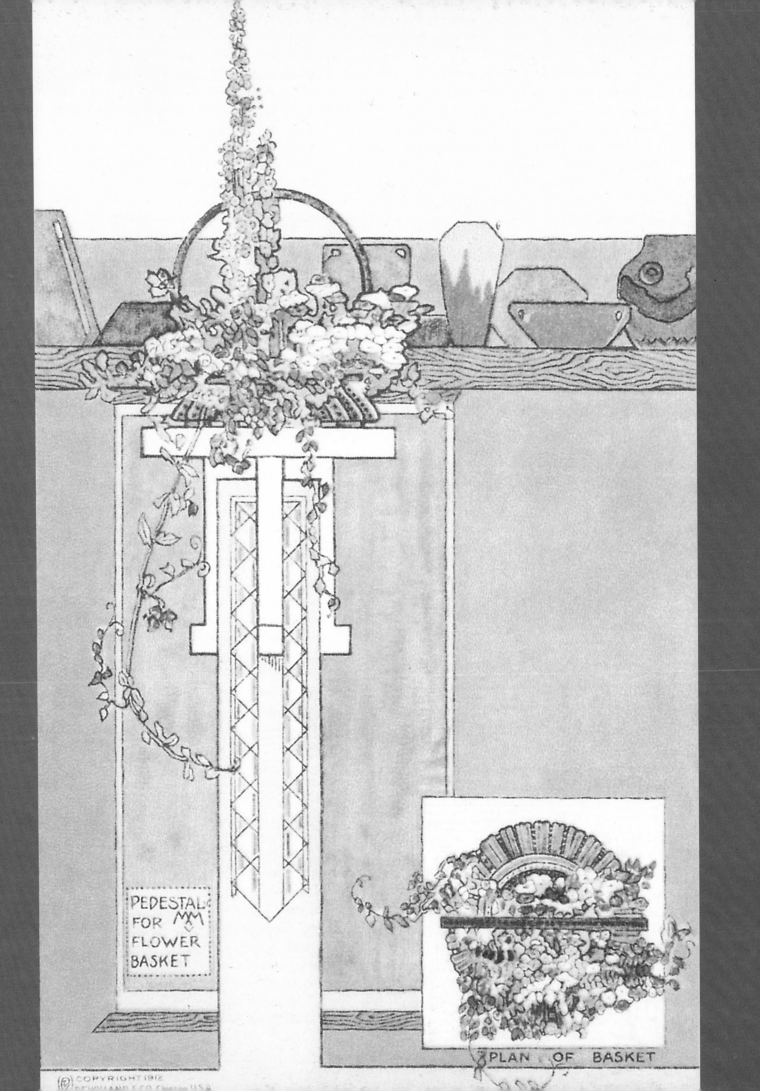

PEDESTAL
FOR
FLOWER
BASKET

PLAN OF BASKET

In June 1899, Walter Burley Griffin, armed with a degree in architecture from the University of Illinois and a passion for landscape gardening, arrived at Steinway Hall on East Van Buren Street in downtown Chicago. Exiting the elevator on the eleventh floor, he was greeted by Dwight Perkins, his new employer, who introduced him to two other architects who had offices on this floor, Robert C Spencer Jr and Myron Hunt.[1] Ascending the spiral stairs to the twelfth floor drafting room that the three shared, Griffin began his first day's work as a draftsman. Until late the previous year, Frank Lloyd Wright and his chief assistant, Marion Lucy Mahony, had also occupied the space. After leaving Steinway Hall they first moved a few blocks west to the Rookery building, then several miles west to the studio adjoining Wright's house in suburban Oak Park. These two architects were soon to become intimately tied to Griffin's life and art.

Constructed in 1895 to a design by Dwight Perkins, Steinway Hall almost from its inception was home to many Chicago architects. The group that Griffin worked for in the loft formed what the *Chicago Inter-Ocean* newspaper called a new 'community in architecture' whose members believed 'in the principles of cooperation rather than the idea of competition'.[2] Although the reporter appeared to be less clear about where 'this experiment' would lead, he believed that it was somehow important as 'evidence of a progressive spirit and is along general lines of social evolution'. This 'evolution' was based on the search for a new kind of architecture. 'Convinced that the time has come when Chicago is ready to demand more artistic work as well as buildings which will meet every demand of utility, they have set themselves high standards, which by mutual criticism and encouragement they strive to maintain.'

Perkins, Spencer, Hunt, and Wright, the newspaper report expanded, were sharing expenses, architectural ideas and drafting staff in the Steinway Hall loft. Thus following his stint with Perkins, Griffin drafted for Spencer. He was also 'lent' to a variety of Steinway Hall architects, including Adamo Boari, who was friendly with the group but less committed to their artistic vision. Finally, in January 1901, Griffin was drafting for another tenant in the loft, Henry Webster Tomlinson, when Tomlinson entered into partnership with Frank Lloyd Wright.[3] Six months later, Walter Burley Griffin was working side by side with Marion Mahony in Wright's suburban office.

In the vast city of Chicago, with its dense commercial core, growth and change were a way of life. The village of Chicago had been incorporated in 1833 with a mere 550 inhabitants; less than four decades later its metropolitan population had reached 350,000.[4] The city paid a price for this unregulated expansion, coupled with drought and bad luck, when in 1871 its business centre and much of its housing were destroyed by fire. Within twenty years, however, Chicago was ready to host the World's Columbian Exposition, a fair of such gigantic proportions that Europe took notice and American culture was changed forever. Both events affected the lives of Chicagoans. While the fire forced the Mahonys to move far out of the city into the suburbs,[5]

Right: Marion Lucy Mahony (left) and Catherine Tobin Wright in a photograph probably taken by Frank Lloyd Wright, about 1895, in Oak Park, Illinois.
Photograph courtesy The Frank Lloyd Wright Home and Studio Foundation, Oak Park (cat no H+S H213).

Previous page: Postcard designed by Marion, 1912, for the P F Volland Company, Chicago. The card bears the 'MMG' monogram. The Griffins also designed the company's offices in 1912.
Courtesy Nicholls collection, Sydney.

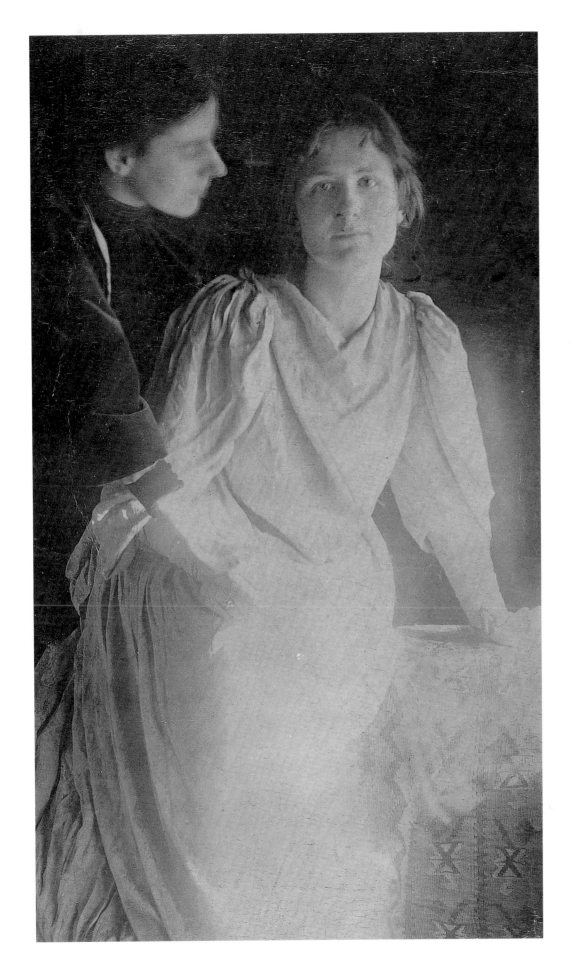

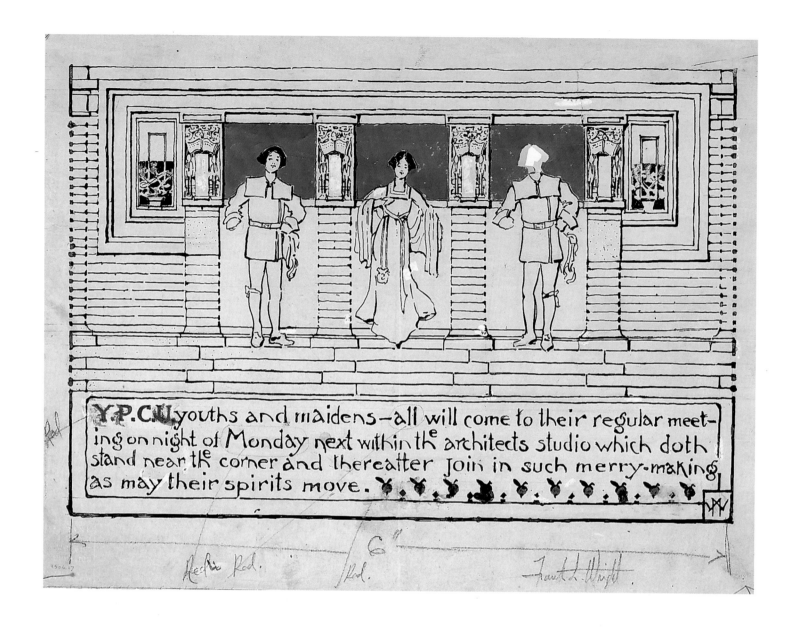

Above: Maginel Wright, invitation, ink and watercolour, about 1900, 30 × 40.5 cm. For this invitation to a party at her brother's Oak Park studio, Maginel placed three costumed figures between the four columns of the Chicago Avenue entrance. Marion Mahony later claimed that the composition of the column capitals — foliage, open book, plans and two secretary birds — was created by the sculptor Richard Bock from a sketch of hers.
Courtesy of the Frank Lloyd Wright Foundation, Scottsdale, Arizona (9506.017).

the Columbian Exposition converted young Griffin into an ardent believer in the possibilities of urban planning enhanced by landscape gardening, that is, a practitioner in the emerging field of landscape architecture, as it came to be called.

The landscape of the Chicago region was also new, changed from what it had been for thousands of years as rapidly as the city itself grew. The endless prairies, the indigenous people who camped in the prairie groves that had stood like islands in the sea of grass, and the extraordinary abundance of wildlife, all were long gone by the 1890s. In their place stood the great modern American city, with its collar of expanding suburbs and its vast territories of farms and villages, linked by a network of rail lines and interdependencies like a great spider's web.[6]

Chicago's cultural pretensions had risen with its population. In the wake of the World's Fair, the city could boast a new public library and an art institute, both fitted in the garb of European classicism.[7] It had its own grand opera house in the gigantic Auditorium building, whose neighbour, the Fine Arts building, housed galleries and studios for musicians and artists.[8] A school of tonalist landscape painters attempted to capture the new midwestern landscape, while all but ignoring Chicago, the economic magnet that had produced it. In the 1890s, the egalitarian ideals of the English arts and crafts movement found ready acceptance, with the Chicago Arts and Crafts Society founded on 22 October 1897 at Jane Addams' famous settlement house, Hull House.[9] The book arts began to flourish, as graphic artists including Will Bradley and W W Denslow worked with publishers such as Stone & Kimball and Way & Williams to match good design with trade editions of modern fiction.[10] Technological developments allowed the construction of a new kind of building — the skyscraper — that had begun to fill Chicago's tightly bordered downtown. And an architect had emerged who attempted to tie all of this together, to produce a kind of architecture that was inspired by, that grew naturally from, the life of this energetic, brash young city, which seemed to represent the very future of America itself. This was Louis H Sullivan (1856–1924).[11]

Chicago's architects were in a peculiar position in the western world's age of architectural revivalism. The nineteenth-century dialogue between past and present might have a certain visceral significance in Europe, where Roman temples, gothic churches and renaissance palaces were part of daily life. In America there could only be half of the conversation; without the physical facts of a cultural heritage, there were only the consciously reproduced copies. In the midwest, this situation was more heartfelt: it extended even to the American colonial revival, which had become so popular on the east coast since the 1880s. Chicago had no colonial buildings; the 'historic' structures of the Potawatomi Indians or the French Voyageurs disappeared along with those who had built them. Thus, while a generation of European architects in the 1890s, including Otto Wagner, Victor Horta and Charles Rennie Mackintosh,

wished to create a new architecture that would stand alongside the historical styles as a valid architecture for a modern age, their American counterparts had the even more elementary goal of creating what they saw as the very first style for the new country. The new architecture in Chicago was to be as much an American or a democratic architecture as it was a modern architecture.

Arguments about the need for a new American style of architecture did not hold much interest for most architects, who continued to find the meaning of a contemporary building to be validated by its relationship with methods of design associated with past monuments of western architecture. For Louis Sullivan, however, this was the great issue of the age, and his ideas transformed Walter Burley Griffin. In June 1900, the Architectural League of America held its second annual convention in Chicago, in the Auditorium theatre a block away from Steinway Hall.[12] Sullivan addressed the convention on the subject of 'The young man in architecture'.[13] Attacking American architecture as being composed of 'ninety parts aberration, eight parts indifference, one part poverty, and one part Little Lord Fauntleroy', he enjoined his young listeners to follow not their history books but 'Inspiration', which he defined as 'the intermediary between God and man, the pure fruition of the soul at one with immaculate nature'. And he specifically charged them with joining him in the search for modern architecture. 'If any one tells you that it is impossible within a lifetime to develop and perfect a complete individuality of expression, a well-ripened and perfected personal style, tell him that you know better, and that you will prove it by your lives.' Sullivan's words came to Griffin at the perfect moment; he later admitted that they completely changed his life.[14]

Yet Griffin was already on the path that would eventually lead to the Melson house in the USA, Newman College in Melbourne, Castlecrag in Sydney, and the library and museum for the Raja of Mahmudabad in India. Even before he heard Sullivan speak, Griffin was responding to Sullivan's ideas. Sullivan's influence was everywhere around him. For example, in a lecture published in June 1898, Robert Spencer attempted to answer the question, 'Is there an American style of domestic architecture?', and praised the more original aspects of what we would call the Shingle style as opposed to the academic recreations of eighteenth-century American buildings.[15] In fact, the Steinway Hall group was attempting to put into practice Sullivan's mystical call for an American architecture. By the time of Griffin's arrival, a larger group was gathering informally to discuss modern architecture over steaks at the Bismarck restaurant.[16]

The local public forum for the discussion of architecture was the Chicago Architectural Club, which held monthly meetings in club rooms at the Art Institute and mounted an annual exhibition in the spring. The club, begun in 1885 as a sketching club for young draftsmen, grew rapidly in size and stature, organising its first exhibition in 1888 and publishing its first illustrated catalogue in 1894. Griffin was already a member when in November 1900 the

English architect C R Ashbee was the guest of honour.[17] In the next catalogue following this visit the club published Wright's famous response to Ashbee, 'The art and craft of the machine'. At the monthly meeting of March 1901, the topic was formal abstraction and the geometric basis of architecture — what was termed 'pure design'. The question was, 'Should architectural design and the study of historic styles follow and be based upon a knowledge of pure design?' Spencer and Wright, among a host of others, argued about the answer.[18]

By the late 1890s, the Steinway Hall group came to dominate the activities of the Chicago Architectural Club and had taken control of the jury of admissions for the annual exhibition. This *coup d'état* culminated in the landmark 1902 exhibition. With Spencer serving as president, and the jury of admissions consisting of Spencer and two other members of the Bismarck dinner group, George Dean and Richard Schmidt, an entire room was given over to Wright's work (although he was never a dues-paying member), and designs by Sullivan and his followers dominated the remaining spaces. One reviewer could only grumble, 'To glance at the catalogue one would think that this "L'art nouveau" of ours was the only manner of existence in architecture here'.[19]

Griffin began to formulate his own goal to create an architecture which responded to specific needs of clients and the capabilities of new materials, and that was as thoroughly 'designed' as any architecture, but whose style was personal to the architect and not dictated by fashion or tradition — as new as the landscape and culture from which it sprang. These ideas were first realised in Chicago (and America itself) by Louis Sullivan and were shared by Griffin's elder colleague, Frank Lloyd Wright. But they did not come to Griffin through Wright; rather, Griffin's sympathies with Sullivan's ideals attracted him to Wright and conversely made him an appealing asset to Wright.

Despite changing fortunes, Griffin remained committed throughout his life to creating a personal modern architecture that was rationally derived and enriched with the unified decoration called for by Sullivan. In 1913 he attempted to explain to the president of the University of Illinois, his alma mater, 'the principles I am trying to help work out in practice toward an architecture which will be disassociated from literary cults and have better possibilities of becoming democratic and American than an architecture loaded down with non-functional, superimposed and really irrelevant features'.[20] He always acknowledged Sullivan's role in his development, admitting in 1913 to the Royal Victorian Institute of Architects, 'I would probably have followed the lines others had if I had not the advantage of contact with an independent thinker in Chicago, Mr. Louis H. Sullivan ... one who has had opportunity not only to exercise his independence in his own work, and in his own way, but through his pupils to express the validity of his ideas'.[21] One month before he died in 1937, Griffin reiterated his view of Sullivan: 'This century, while still young, was shown the way by architectural

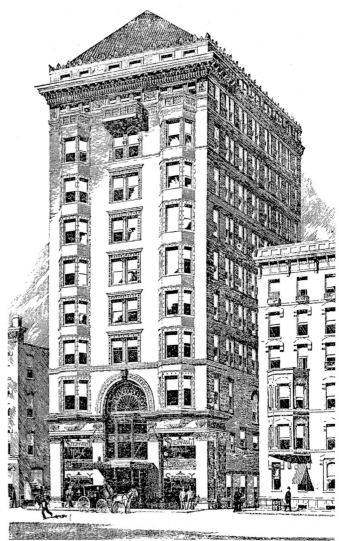

STEINWAY HALL, VAN BUREN STREET, CHICAGO.
Dwight & Perkins, Architect; Prof. Lewis J. Johnson, Designer of Steel Work.

Above: Steinway Hall, 64 East Van Buren Street, Chicago. Dwight Heald Perkins moved into the eleventh floor, whose windows are visible above the projecting cornice, and shared the attic space under the hipped roof with a changing group of progressive architects. Steinway Hall was demolished in the early 1970s.
From *Engineering News*, 34, 17 October 1895, p 251.

Right: Walter Burley Griffin, about 1899. In his graduation portrait from the University of Illinois, Griffin sports a starched collar and bow tie. In addition, he proudly displays his university affiliation by the pin on his lapel, an eight-pointed star surrounding the letters 'UI'.
Photograph courtesy National Library of Australia, gift of Dr Hermann Pundt.

forerunners at the end of the last, among whom Louis H. Sullivan was the first'.[22]

Marion Mahony understood Sullivan's polemical stance as practised by his followers, including her employer, Frank Lloyd Wright, and was a champion in her own way for a modern American architecture. However, she apparently did not wish to create a personal style of architecture herself, or to build an independent practice. The dozen buildings, spanning an equal number of years, that can be attributed solely to her do not form a consistent body of work.[23] Her talents lay elsewhere. Following her graduation from the Massachusetts Institute of Technology in 1894,[24] Mahony drafted for Dwight Perkins, her first cousin (himself an MIT graduate and just beginning independent practice), before joining Wright's modest office in Sullivan's Schiller building the following year. Just when Mahony's immense gift for architectural rendering first appeared is not clear, but in addition to spending long hours producing working drawings for Wright, she made original designs for ornamental details which Wright used in his architecture. For example, she later asserted that the stork capitals on Wright's studio addition, physically created by the sculptor Richard Bock, were taken from a design of hers.[25]

In January 1898, Mahony was among twelve would-be architects who took the first licensing examination in the history of the profession, administered in Chicago's City Hall.[26] The Illinois General Assembly had passed the world's first licensing law the previous June. While practising architects like Wright were given licences under a 'grandfather' clause, drafting staff who wished to become architects were now required to be tested during a three-day examination. In her fourth year of drafting for other architects, Mahony wished to be certified as a professional architect. She garnered 74 out of a possible 100, the third highest grade, and became the first woman anywhere in the world to receive a licence to practise architecture. A number of journals reported this fact, including the *Architect* of London, which noted that, of these first candidates, 'one was a lady, but the majority were graduates of scientific and architectural schools', apparently assuming that these were mutually exclusive.[27]

In a similar way, Griffin, after graduation from the University of Illinois and two years drafting, and newly inspired by Louis Sullivan's call to such young men in architecture as himself, took the licensing examination at Chicago's Armour Institute on the three days beginning 19 June 1901. He earned some of the highest marks awarded up to that time, receiving a final grade of 90. Griffin then joined Wright's studio in Oak Park. This marked a turning point in his career. While his professional introduction to Wright presumably came through his employment by Webster Tomlinson, Griffin clearly entered the suburban office with different aspirations and new qualifications. He was now a fully licensed architect, able to practise under his own name if he chose. His later claim that he was virtually a partner of Wright appears to be much nearer the truth than Wright's assertion to the Australian architect and historian,

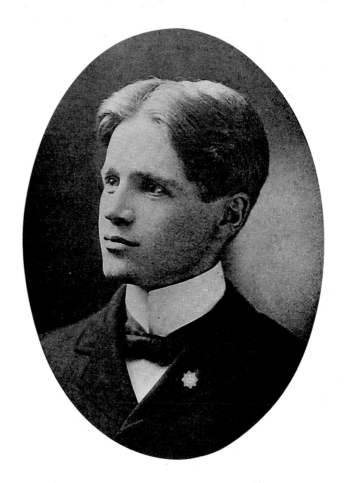

Robin Boyd, that Griffin was a 'novice' when he entered the Oak Park studio.[28] Beginning in the summer of 1901 three licensed architects were working in Wright's studio: the firm's namesake, who had been granted a licence without examination, and his remarkable associates, Mahony and Griffin, both of whom had distinguished themselves at the state's rigorous three-day licensing ordeal — and who, unlike their employer, had professional degrees from the two leading architectural schools in the country at the time.

They were joined at the studio by a changing handful of others in one of the most exciting creative adventures in the history of modern architecture. For example, in May 1904 the staff consisted of: Mahony and Griffin, William E Drummond, Charles E White Jr, Francis Barry Byrne and Isabel Roberts.[29] Griffin served as project manager on some of the larger office commissions, including the Hillside Home School near Spring Green, Wisconsin, and the Larkin building in Buffalo, New York. He also contributed landscape plans as they were occasionally needed, a subject about which Wright had little knowledge and, at this stage of his career, little interest.

In some ways the work day at the Oak Park studio echoed the free exchange of ideas at the Steinway Hall loft. Although there was a single architect under whose name they all worked, Wright was generous about allowing his more ambitious employees to maintain separate private practices as long as this did not interfere with studio work. Thus in 1902 Griffin accepted the commission to design a house for his highschool friend, William Emery, and Mahony designed a church for her family friend, the Reverend James Vila Blake. In fact, Griffin tried to juggle two separate practices outside of office hours, embarking on his second independent career as a landscape architect. On 3 September 1901 (some two months after he began to work for Wright), Griffin signed a contract to provide plans for the 'Improvement of Grounds' at the Eastern Illinois State Normal School, which proved to be a complex and time-consuming project.[30]

Griffin's and Wright's ideas began to intertwine in ways that Mahony's and Wright's never had. Mahony certainly made original contributions, mostly of an ornamental nature, to Wright's buildings; and she later claimed that on several occasions he had improperly used her independent architectural sketches for his own work. But almost from the beginning Griffin and Wright began to spar over fundamental issues of design, construction and management. Ever the empirical architect, Wright never hesitated to change details of a design even during construction in order to achieve the visual effect he desired. Griffin's penchant for rational systems and typologies led him in different directions. The basic idea of the module — a repeated unit in plan that regulated the size of rooms and the placement of walls, doorways and windows — is as 'un-Wrightian' as it is 'Griffinesque'. It cannot be a coincidence that it first occurs in Wright's work in 1902, after his mature style has fully appeared, and within a year of Griffin's entry into the office. In a similar manner, the square plan, centred

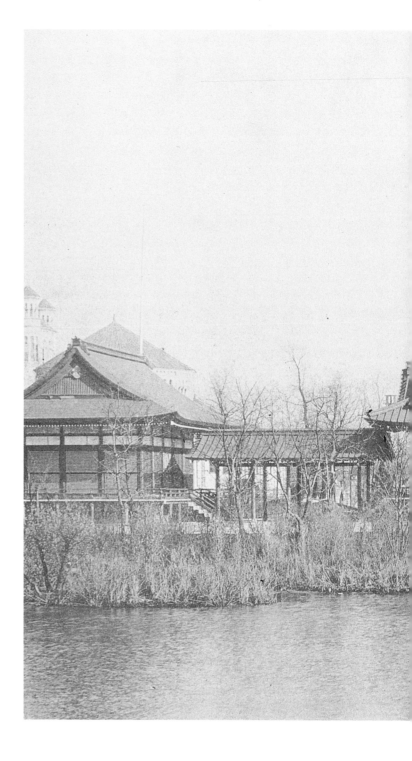

The Japanese pavilion, known as the Ho-o-den or the Phoenix Palace, at the World's Columbian Exposition, Chicago, Illinois, 1893. Designed by the government architect, Masamichi Kuru, and based on the Ho-o-do erected near Kyoto in 1053, it was located on an island in the middle of the fairgrounds.
Photograph by C D Arnold, as published in *American Architect and Building News*, 28 April 1894.

BEYOND ARCHITECTURE

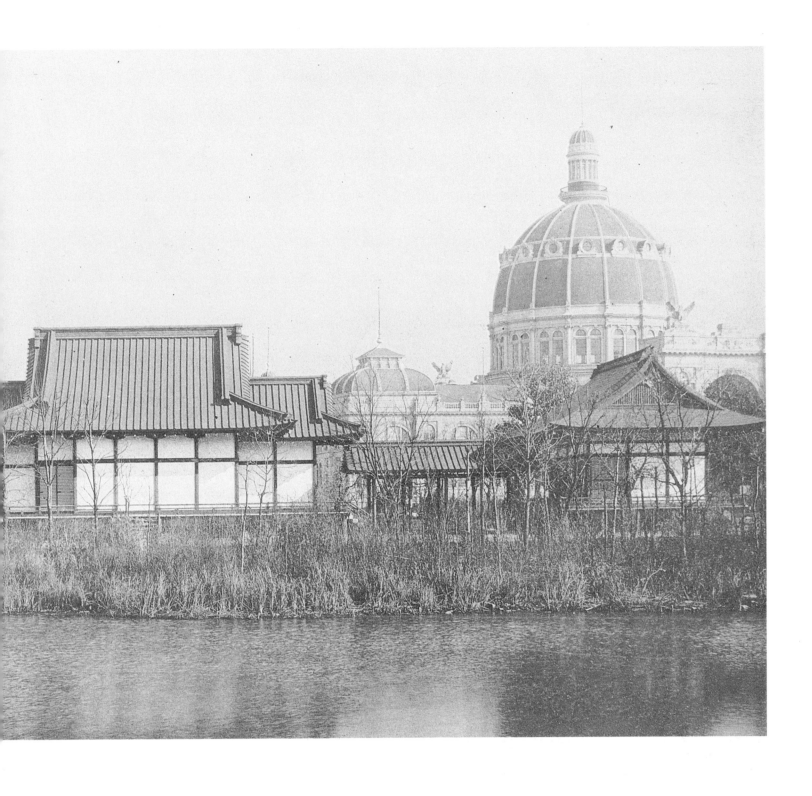

on a fireplace, around which the living and dining areas form a continuous L-shaped open space, is Griffin's formal simplification of the spatial revolution of Wright's Prairie houses. Although this project (*right*) is one of Wright's most famous, it is in fact a collaboration between Griffin, who created the original plan borrowed here by Wright, and Mahony, who did the rendering.[31]

Griffin's personal career also began to cross paths with Wright's — he fell in love with Wright's sister Maginel, a capable graphic artist a year younger than Griffin, and asked her to marry him.[32] In October 1904, however, Maginel married Chicago artist Walter J 'Pat' Enright. In the next decade, Maginel worked as a designer for the P F Volland Company (*see p 14*), whose offices in the Monroe building Griffin designed in 1912, and for whom Mahony, now Mrs Griffin, designed 'art postcards'.

Mahony's personal feelings toward Griffin during the five years when they both worked for Wright are not recorded; Griffin for his part was deeply hurt by Maginel's rejection and took no personal notice of Mahony. While she admired Wright at this time, Mahony held real affection for Wright's wife Kitty; Mahony later devoted many hours during 1909 and 1910 trying to help the abandoned Oak Park family, after Wright travelled to Europe in the company of Mamah Cheney, the wife of one of his clients.[33]

In 1904 Griffin visited the World's Fair in St Louis and again discovered, as he had at Chicago's World's Fair, the tremendous power of monumental buildings as coordinated in a geometric landscape.[34] If he was in a better position to dismiss the formal qualities of the buildings, he now saw them as an ensemble and observed their setting with the eye of a 27-year-old practising architect rather than as a sixteen-year-old highschool student. He also made contact at the fair with the vice-commissioner of the Imperial Chinese Commission, Wong Kai Kah (1860–1906), and through him received his first commission for the design of a city, an addition to the Chinese port of Shanghai. Alas, the project came to naught and the drawings were lost when Mr Wong died in Nagasaki, Japan, in January 1906 while returning to China.[35]

In mid February 1905, Wright felt sufficiently secure to entrust his office in Griffin's care as he travelled to Japan for the first time. Griffin managed the office well enough — perhaps too well, for on Wright's return a tension developed between the two architects which lasted throughout the year. Wright was particularly alarmed by the amount of artistic licence Griffin had taken with several of the projects, while Griffin was disappointed that Wright insisted on reimbursing him for salary owed and money loaned with Japanese prints. Early in 1906, on the strength of the contract to landscape the campus of the Northern Illinois State Normal School, Griffin decided to establish his own practice. This difficult decision was further aided by work sent his way by former employers Robert Spencer and Henry Webster Tomlinson. The catalyst was undoubtedly Griffin's discovery that Dwight Perkins had finally vacated his space in the Steinway Hall loft for larger quarters.[36] Griffin promptly moved into Perkins' old office to work alone.

Right: Frank Lloyd Wright, 'A Fireproof House for $5000'. Although published as a work by Wright, this design is actually a collaboration between Wright, Mahony and Griffin. The original idea of the floor plan is Griffin's. It is based on a square divided into quarters. The living and dining spaces comprise three of the quarters, wrapping around a central fireplace to form an L of continuous space. In the fourth quarter is the separated kitchen and stairway to the second floor. Because of the cramped space a small extension beyond the square is required to fit the necessary stairs. This is the arrangement of the Harry V Peters house, the first house Griffin designed after leaving Wright's office, which was constructed in October and November 1906. Wright created his version early in the following year and turned it over to Mahony, who drew the perspective and signed it in the lower right with 'MLM'.

From *The Ladies Home Journal*, April 1907, p 24.

A Fireproof House for $5000

Estimated to Cost That Amount in Chicago, and Designed Especially for The Journal

By Frank Lloyd Wright

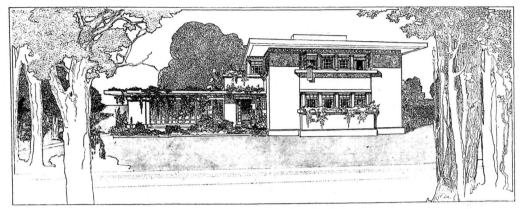

One Side of the House, Showing the Trellised Extension

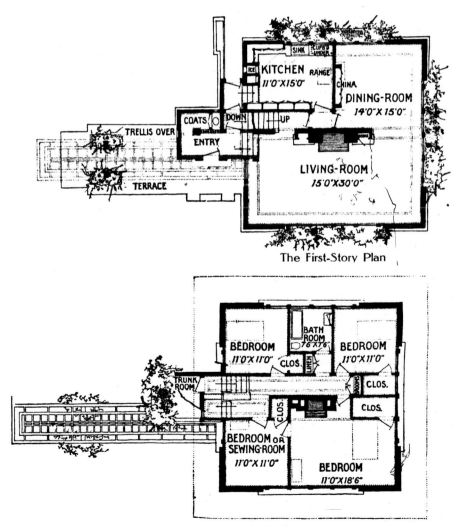

The First-Story Plan

The Second Story

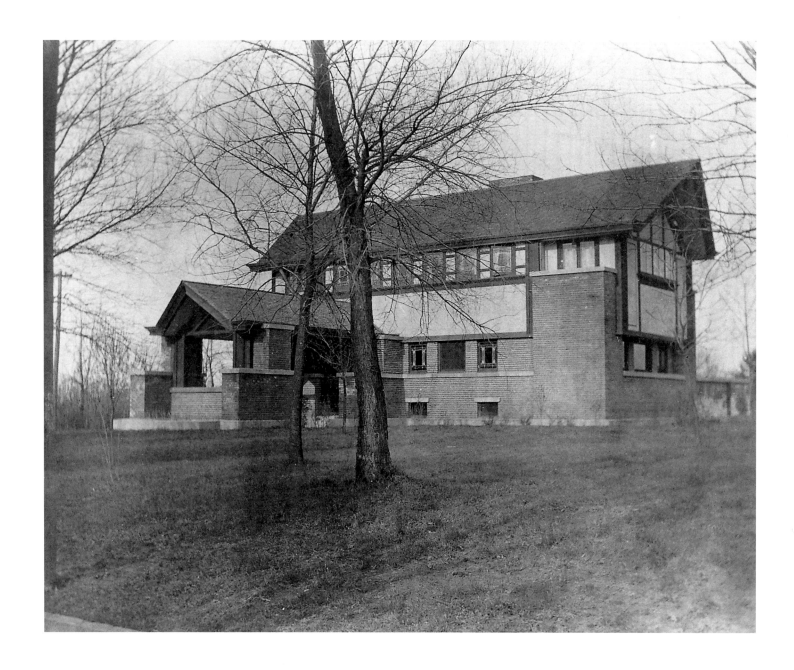

Above: William Emery house, designed by Walter Burley Griffin in 1903 and built in Elmhurst, Illinois. Conceived while Griffin worked for Frank Lloyd Wright, the Emery house borrows much from Wright's new Prairie style, but exhibits many of Griffin's personal aesthetic preferences, including overhanging gabled roofs and massive corner piers. However, precedent for the extraordinary interior, with its series of interlocking spatial levels, cannot be found in Wright's work. This photograph was taken in 1908 by William Gray Purcell, Griffin's friend, colleague and the architect to whom he had hoped to turn over his practice in 1914 when he travelled to Australia on his first three-year appointment.

Photograph courtesy the Northwest Architectural Archives, William Gray Purcell papers, University of Minnesota Libraries, St Paul, MN.

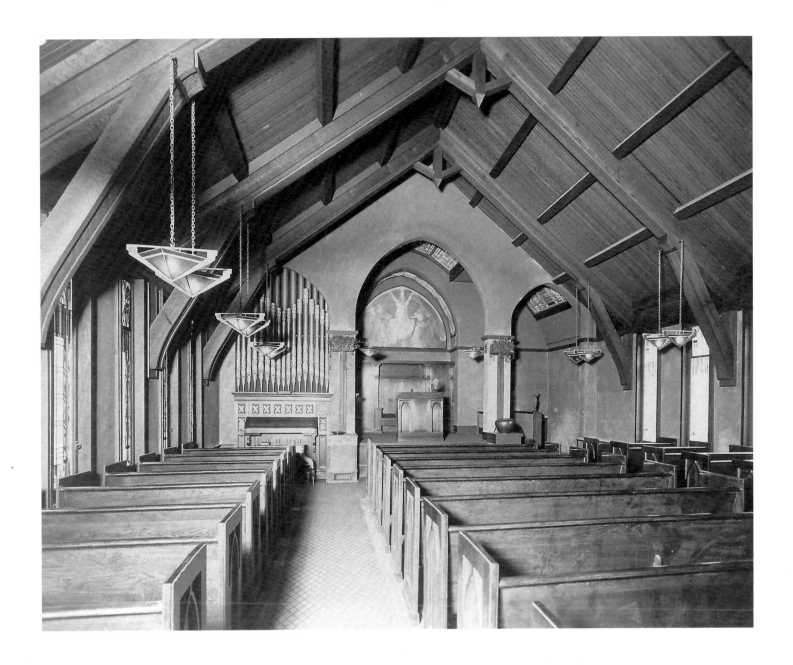

Above: The Church of All Souls, designed by Marion Lucy Mahony in 1903 and built in Evanston, Illinois. While employed by Frank Lloyd Wright, Mahony prepared two versions of the church for the Reverend James Vila Blake. The second was constructed. This undated view of the interior shows Mahony's hanging lamp fixtures, leaded stained-glass windows and skylights, and a mural painted by her. The arts and crafts interior mixes medieval forms with the simple abstracted shapes and surfaces typical of the work of the Chicago architects who followed Louis Sullivan's call for a modern American architecture, a group known today as the Prairie School. The building was demolished in the 1960s.

Photograph courtesy the Art Institute of Chicago.

Mahony, by this time, had also ceased working full time for Wright. Despite the literature which claims that she stayed with Wright continuously from 1895 to 1909, it is clear that by 1905 she worked for Wright only occasionally on an individual contract basis. Indeed, at the end of 1905, the office was forced to hire Louis Rasmussen to prepare a rendering of Wright's Smith Bank in Dwight, Illinois, as Mahony was not available.[37] Yet on 4 March 1906, Charles White reported, 'Marion Mahony has been doing great work (the Unity [Temple] perspectives are hers)'.[38] After 1906 Mahony signed perspectives with her monogram, 'MLM', a procedure that full-time drafting staff would never consider but that was routine for contract renderers, including Rasmussen.

By 1906, Walter Burley Griffin and Marion Mahony were seasoned professionals in their thirties. The world beckoned and it would be theirs. They had blossomed under the intellectual flowering of Chicago in the 1890s and had passed through trial-by-fire in Wright's office. Griffin now established himself as an independent architect with a practice that within five years would be thriving, while in 1906 Mahony invented a style of presentation drawing that would change the way the world saw Wright's architecture and, later, Griffin's architecture. Finally, in 1911 Walter and Marion would become partners in marriage and architecture, and soon embark on careers that would take them far away from the Chicago of their youth. But the intellectual, aesthetic and professional foundations to their lives had already been solidly set by their midwestern experiences. The ideas and inspiration that Griffin and Mahony received at the beginning of their careers in their hometown Chicago would carry them through a lifetime of architectural and personal exploration.

Notes

1. For Perkins, see E E Davis and K Indeck, *Dwight Heald Perkins: social consciousness and Prairie School architecture*, Gallery 400, Chicago, 1989. For Spencer, see Paul Kruty, 'Wright, Spencer and the casement window', *Winterthur Portfolio*, vol 30, Summer/Autumn 1995, pp 103–27; and for Hunt, see Jean Block, 'Myron Hunt in the midwest', pp 9–21, in *Myron Hunt, 1868–1952: the search for a regional architecture*, Baxter Art Gallery, Pasadena, 1984. The general background for much of this essay may be found in H Allen Brooks, *The Prairie School: Frank Lloyd Wright and his midwest contemporaries*, University of Toronto Press, Toronto, 1972.

2. 'Community in architecture', *Chicago Inter-Ocean*, 2 May 1897. The four were identified as 'R. C. Spencer, who took the Rotch traveling scholarship in 1888; Frank Wright, who was formerly with Adler & Sullivan; Myron Hunt, who came from the office of Shepley, Rutan & Coolidge; and Dwight Heald Perkins, from the office of D. H. Burnham'.

3. Announced, among many places, in *Brickbuilder*, vol 10, January 1901, p 20. According to the 1899 edition of the *Lakeside Directory of Chicago*, Tomlinson was in 1106 and Perkins, Spencer and Boari in 1107, Steinway Hall. The loft itself was number 1200.

4. According to the 1870 census, the population of Cook County was 349,966; William Cronon, *Nature's metropolis: Chicago and the great west*, W W Norton & Co, New York, 1991, p 301.

5. Marion Mahony recalled, 'I was born in Chicago, 1871, and was carried in a clothes basket with my older brother Jerome away from the Chicago fire out to Winnetka'; undated letter written in response to a letter dated 19 June 1951 from William Gray Purcell, Purcell collection, Northwest Architectural Archives, University of Minnesota. At the time of the fire, Griffin's parents were not yet married. In 1871 his father, George, was a twenty year old living on the city's north side.

6. The reconfigured aspect of the midwestern landscape is the central thesis of Cronon's *Nature's metropolis*.

7. Both designed by the Boston firm of Shepley, Rutan and Coolidge and under construction in 1892.

8. See Perry R Duis, '"Where is Athens now?" The Fine Arts Building 1898 to 1918', *Chicago History*, vol 6, Summer 1977, pp 66–78.

9. For Chicago's role in this movement, see Richard Guy Wilson, 'Chicago and the international arts and crafts movement: progressive and conservative tendencies', pp 209–27, in John Zukowsky, ed, *Chicago architecture, 1872–1922: birth of a metropolis*, Prestel-Verlag, Munich, 1987. See also, H Allen Brooks, 'Chicago architecture: its debt to the arts and crafts', *Journal of the Society of Architectural Historians*, vol 30, no 4, 1971, pp 312–17.

10. For an overview of Chicago's progressive movements, including literature and the book arts, see Perry Duis, *Chicago: creating new traditions*, Chicago Historical Society, Chicago, 1976.

11. For the most succinct statement of this reading of Sullivan, see Paul E Sprague, 'Louis H. Sullivan', entry in Adolf K Placzek, ed, *Macmillan encyclopedia of architects*, Collier Macmillan Publishers, London, 1982, vol 4, pp 152–63.

12. As James Weirick is fond of pointing out in conversation, Sullivan's office in the Auditorium tower looked down on the Steinway Hall loft, where the largest collection of his followers, including Griffin, were gathered.

13. The full text appears in *Brickbuilder*, vol 9, June 1900, pp 115–19.

14. Griffin's partner Eric M Nicholls told the American historian Mark Peisch, 'W.B.G. told me that hearing L.S. give his talk on "A Young Man in Architecture" completely changed his life'; letter, 5 November 1965, Peisch collection, Avery Architectural and Fine Arts Library, Columbia University. Nicholls further recalled Griffin telling him that 25 years after that speech, on his first return to the United States after settling in Australia, 'Sullivan was the one person he had wanted to see in America'. Alas, Sullivan had died the previous year.

15. R C Spencer Jr, 'Is there an American style of domestic architecture?', *Arts for America*, vol 7, June 1898, pp 569–72. Similar arguments by other members of the emerging Prairie School include George R Dean's 'A new

movement in American architecture', *Brush and Pencil*, vol 5, March 1900, pp 254–59; and Elmer Grey's 'Indigenous and inventive architecture for America', *Brickbuilder*, vol 9, June 1900, pp 121–23.

16. Recalled by Robert Spencer in 'Chicago School of Architecture', a paper delivered on 26 September 1939 to the Illinois Society of Architects, a transcript of which is in the Ricker Library of Architecture and Art, University of Illinois, Urbana-Champaign. Wright later claimed that the group called itself 'the Eighteen'; *A Testament*, Bramhall House, New York, 1957, p 34.

17. *Construction News*, vol 11, 1 December 1900, p 423. Griffin is first listed as a member of the Chicago Architectural Club in 1900. Marion Mahony was never active in the club.

18. 'Personal and club news', *Brickbuilder*, vol 10, March 1901, p 64. Spencer's text was published in *Brickbuilder*, vol 10, June 1901, pp 120–22. For a brief discussion of one aspect of 'pure design' see Narciso Menocal, 'Form and content in Frank Lloyd Wright's Tree of Life window', *Elvehjem Museum of Art Bulletin* (1983–84), vol 31, no 26.

19. 'Chicago: the exhibition of the Architectural Club and its catalogue', *American Architect*, vol 76, 26 April 1902, p 29.

20. W B Griffin to Edwin J James, 12 February 1913, University of Illinois archives.

21. W B Griffin, 'Architecture in American universities', *Journal of the Proceedings of the Royal Victorian Society of Architects*, September 1913, p 173.

22. Walter Birley [*sic*] Griffin, 'Architecture in India', *The Pioneer*, 9 January 1937, p 17.

23. For Mahony's role in Griffin's work, see Paul Sprague's essay in this book. See also, David T Van Zanten, 'The early work of Marion Mahony Griffin', *Prairie School Review*, vol 33, no 2, 1966, pp 5–23. The controversial subject will be examined in considerably greater detail in *Walter Burley Griffin: the complete American work*, a catalogue raisonné under preparation by Professor Sprague and myself.

24. See James Weirick, 'Marion Mahony at M.I.T.', *Transition*, Winter 1988, pp 49–54. Mahony's thesis is reprinted in the same issue, pp 47–48.

25. In her reply of 1951 to Purcell's queries noted above, Mahony recalled, 'I had also done the design Wright used for his colonnaded entrance to the Oak Park office extension of his house'.

26. See Paul Kruty, 'A new look at the beginnings of the Illinois Architects' Licensing Law', *Illinois Historical Journal*, vol 90, Autumn 1997, p 154.

27. *Architect*, vol 59, 18 February 1898, p 112.

28. To Boyd's letter to Wright of 27 May 1946 asking about Griffin, which ended, 'It would be of tremendous interest to us, and deeply appreciated, if you could send some information, if only a brief opinion of his work and ability as you remember it', Wright replied on 14 June, 'Walter came to me as a young man — a novice from the University of Illinois. He was a faithful apprentice for about four years'; correspondence in the Frank Lloyd Wright archives, Taliesin West, Scottsdale, Arizona.

29. As reported in a letter by Charles White, published in N K Morris Smith, ed, 'Letters, 1903–1906, by Charles E White, Jr, from the studio of Frank Lloyd Wright', *Journal of Architectural Education*, vol 25, Fall 1971, p 105.

30. University archives, Eastern Illinois University, Charleston, Illinois. In the surviving specifications, Griffin is listed as 'landscape gardener'. Not surprisingly, on 6 October he was forced to write an apology for the lateness of his plans and specifications.

31. For a full discussion of these issues, see Kruty and Sprague, *Walter Burley Griffin: the complete American work*.

32. Many years later Maginel Wright, then Mrs Barney, recalled that Griffin's marriage proposal 'came as a complete surprise'; notes to a conversation, 17 February 1958, Peisch papers, Avery Architectural and Fine Arts Library.

33. Roy Lippincott, who worked with Mahony in Von Holst's office trying to complete Wright's remaining projects, in recalling 'the days just before and just after Wright's departure for Europe with Mrs. Cheney' explained, 'Marion was a very close friend of Kitty Wright's and spent considerable time out there with her during that time'; letter to David Van Zanten, 17 February 1966. I am indebted to Professor Van Zanten for giving me access to his professional papers relating to Griffin.

34. Letter, Frank Lloyd Wright to Darwin Martin, 6 October 1904, published in Bruce Brooks Pfeiffer, ed, *Frank Lloyd Wright: letters to clients*, the Press at California State University, Fresno, 1986, pp 13–14. Explaining to Martin the status of Griffin's landscape plan for the Martin and Barton houses, Wright reported that Griffin 'went to the Exposition last night taking it with him to finish up on the way'.

35. See 'Wong Kai Kah' in *Obituary record of graduates of Yale, 1900–1906*, Yale University, New Haven CT; see also, John K Fairbank, ed, *The I.G. in Peking: letters of Robert Hart, Chinese Maritime Customs, 1868–1907*, Harvard University Press, Cambridge, 1975, vol II, pp 1338–39, 1401. Wong's name is also transliterated as Wang Kai Kiah and Huang K'ai-chia.

36. *American Contractor*, vol 27, 24 February 1906, p 43.

37. Letter, 22 February 1906, enclosing a cheque of US$25 to Mr Rasmussen for a watercolour of the building; First National Bank of Dwight collection, Burnham Library, Art Institute of Chicago. For Wright, Rasmussen also rendered the first version of the San Diego Cinema project. A decade before he had provided numerous perspectives for Louis Sullivan.

38. Smith, 'Letters', p 110.

MARION MAHONY AS ORIGINATOR OF GRIFFIN'S MATURE STYLE: FACT OR MYTH?

PAUL SPRAGUE

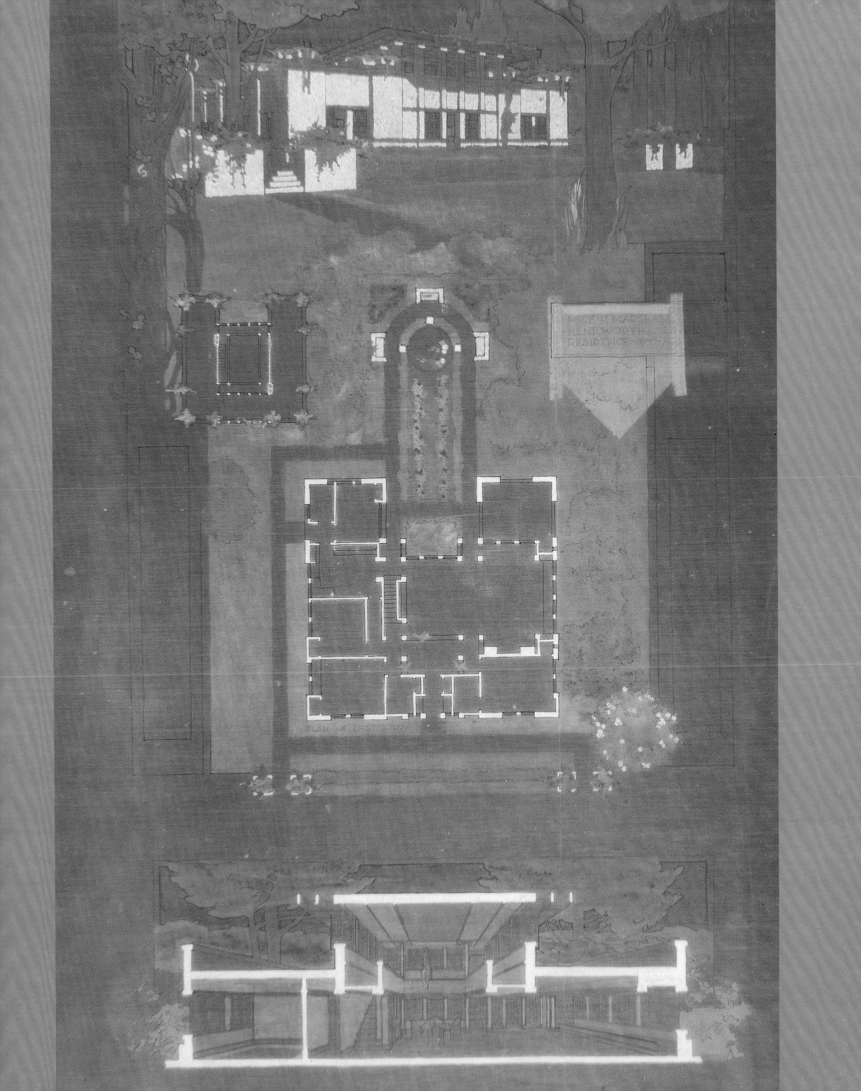

PLAN OF FIRST STORY

Had Walter Burley Griffin not outgrown his early dependence on the architecture of Frank Lloyd Wright, he would be remembered merely as another follower of that architectural giant.[1] Not content, however, to pursue so easy a path, and passionately devoted to the ideals of his intellectual mentor, Louis Sullivan, who promoted the creation of modern architectural styles not tied to the past, Griffin consciously sought independence from both the historic styles of architecture and from the architectural styles of Sullivan and Wright. He achieved this goal in mid 1910. In creating his new style, Griffin employed elementary geometric masses sometimes relieved by walls of broken stone and rough-surfaced wooden trellises. The dynamic primitivism thus attained is best studied in such seminal works as the F P Marshall house, 1910, the Frank Pallma house ('Solid Rock'), 1911, the William F Tempel house, 1912, (built in a slightly revised form for James Blythe in 1913), the Joshua Melson house, 1912 (*see pp 43 and 96*), the architect's own house, 1912, and the Stinson Memorial Library, 1912.

When these buildings and others like them by Griffin are compared with the work of the other American architects who, after the turn of the century, were intent upon developing new styles of architecture, there is no question that, in terms of imagination, originality and artistic prowess, Griffin ranked with the leaders. The only architects whose work embodied greater genius than Griffin's were Louis Sullivan, who initiated the movement that ought rightly to be known as the Sullivan School,[2] and Frank Lloyd Wright, who brought to a pitch of perfection one line of development leading away from the modern style Sullivan had originated.

Even though Griffin did not reach the lofty pinnacles attained by his mentors, his achievement stands well above that of any other American architect who sought modernity by abandoning the historic styles. He should not be seen merely as a follower but as a leader, together with Sullivan and Wright, of the movement in the midwest which sought to establish new architectural styles that would be personal and at the same time would give mystical expression to the cultural essence of twentieth-century Chicago.

Those scholars who have studied Griffin's work seriously have generally recognised and applauded his mature style. For example, H Allen Brooks, the first person to produce a relatively lengthy and serious study of Griffin's work in his 1957 PhD dissertation, 'The Prairie School: the American spirit in midwest residential architecture, 1893–1916', wrote that: 'By 1911 Griffin's own personal style began to emerge through the Wright inspired forms and soon there was no trace of the master's work in that of the pupil ... and although he was strongly influenced by Frank Lloyd Wright for several years, he was a talented enough designer to create an architectural expression of his own'.[3]

Had the evaluation of Griffin's American achievement remained as Brooks left it some forty years ago, it would be easy enough to argue that Griffin should be ranked along with Sullivan and Wright as one of the three distinguished originators of modern architecture in America.

However, time has not been so kind to Walter Burley Griffin. In a recent essay, 'The life and work of Marion Griffin', Janice Pregliasco writes that: 'as in the Wright studio, Marion was the design talent of Walter's office', and 'the first house Marion designed for herself was at the focal point of a thirty-home development Walter was planning called Trier Center ...'.[4] The house she speaks of at New Trier, which would have become the home of the Griffins had they not moved to Australia, is entirely typical of Walter's mature style. Pregliasco then suggests the next logical step by remarking that 'historians have noted the sudden maturity of Walter's architecture beginning in 1910. Walter's movement away from Wrightian-inspired idioms to a more personal style was directly related to his professional and romantic collaboration with Marion'.[5]

If we were to follow this line of reasoning to its apparent conclusion, we would be forced to admit that if Mahony was 'the design talent' in the Griffin office and the person who designed at least one building in Walter's mature style, then Walter's apparent maturity in 1910 must not have been his own doing, but that of his exceptionally artistic wife, acting for him. The next step would surely be to assert that it was not Walter, but Marion, who was the designing architect in the Griffin office, with Walter relegated to planning, landscaping and getting the business. Although Pregliasco does not go quite this far when discussing the American projects, she certainly seems to do so when speaking of the work in India. There she asserts that Marion, who was in charge of the drafting force of the Indian office, designed 'over one hundred buildings', while 'Walter represented the office to the outside world, and he was involved in the numerous introductory meetings required by Indian clients as well as contractors and government officials'.[6] If this is true, then Walter Burley Griffin ought to be assigned a minor position and Mahony moved to centre stage as the real architect behind the Griffin myth. In consequence, she must be elevated to partnership with the acknowledged leaders of the Sullivan School in a triumvirate consisting of Sullivan, Wright and herself.

But can this really be true? Not at all, as I intend to prove. Yet how was it that such a myth began? Given Pregliasco's assertions, it might appear that the origins of the myth should be sought in the writings of feminist authors intent upon correcting prejudicial evaluations by male writers. Generally, the female scholars who have examined Mahony's career have been remarkably temperate in their judgments, and none save Pregliasco have even hinted that Mahony might be the author of Griffin's mature architectural style.[7] Surprisingly, when the literature is searched, it turns out that the originator of the myth was none other than H Allen Brooks himself.

The idea that Walter may have derived his mature style from Mahony was set in motion by Brooks quite inadvertently in his PhD thesis, then continued in his distinguished book, *The Prairie School: Frank Lloyd Wright and his midwest contemporaries*, now the standard work on the subject.[8] That Brooks had no intention of demeaning

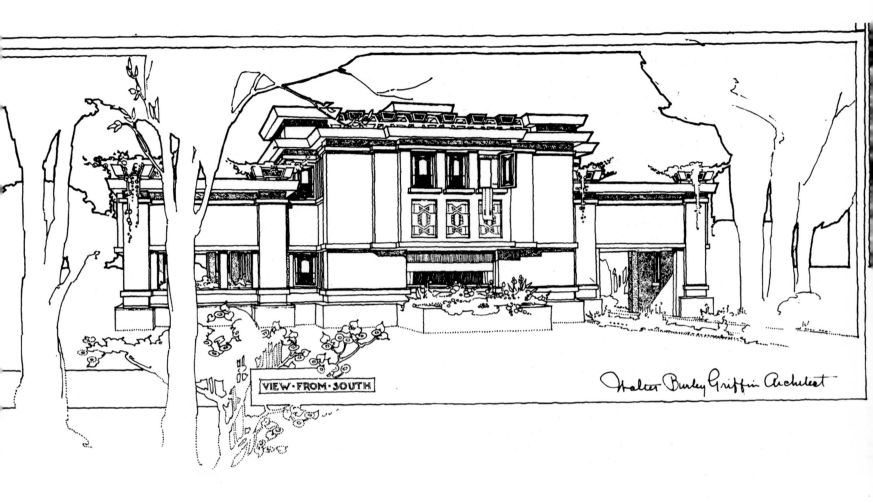

VIEW · FROM · SOUTH

Walter Burley Griffin Architect

Above: William F Tempel house, Winnetka, Illinois, designed late 1911 by Walter Burley Griffin, built in slightly revised form for James Blythe, Mason City, Iowa, 1913. Detail of ink on linen drawing by Marion Mahony Griffin.
Courtesy the Mary and Leigh Block Museum of Art, Northwestern University, Illinois, 1985.1.113.

Previous page: F P Marshall house, Winnetka or Kenilworth, Illinois, designed about May 1910 by Walter Burley Griffin, not built. Lithograph and watercolour on silk sateen, by Marion Mahony, dated 10 June 1910 with monogram 'MLM', 119.3 × 53.3 cm.
Courtesy Avery Architectural and Fine Arts Library, Columbia University, New York (1000.015.0021).

Following page: Frank Pallma house ('Solid Rock'), Winnetka, Illinois, designed late 1910 by Walter Burley Griffin, standing, roof altered. Ink on linen drawing by Marion Mahony Griffin, 107 × 58 cm.
Courtesy the Mary and Leigh Block Museum of Art, Northwestern University, Illinois, 1985.1.98.

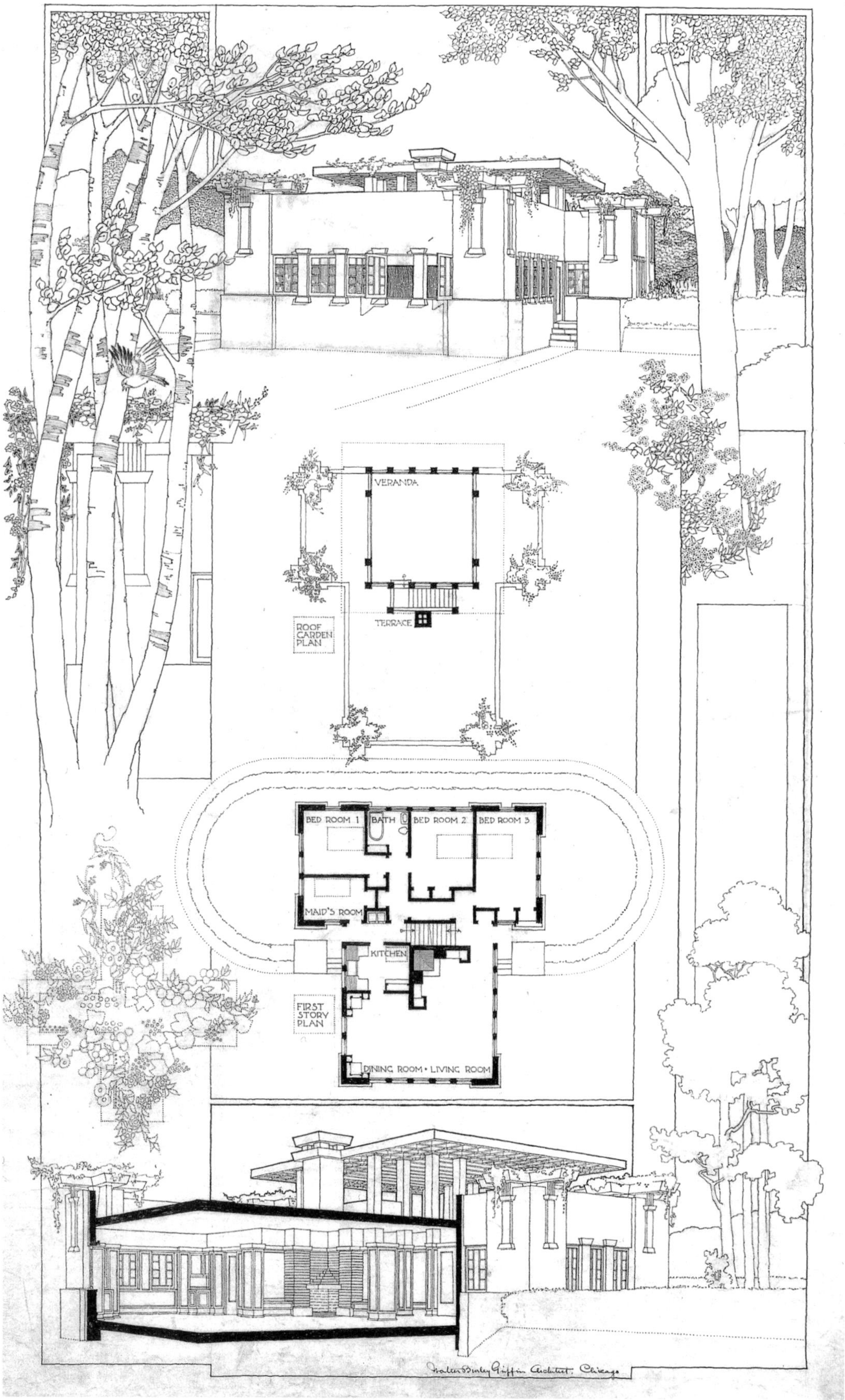
VERANDA
TERRACE
ROOF GARDEN PLAN
BED ROOM 1
BATH
BED ROOM 2
BED ROOM 3
MAID'S ROOM
KITCHEN
FIRST STORY PLAN
DINING ROOM • LIVING ROOM

Griffin's achievement is clear enough from his overall evaluation of Griffin, where he writes that the architect's

> achievement had been considerable, even when measured against his former teacher Wright. He had pioneered the development of vertical space in contrast to Wright's concern for horizontal flow. He had exploited the use of concrete and its structural expression in residential architecture at a time when Wright was still proposing, but not building, houses of concrete ... In terms of planning and urban design Griffin's work was more respectful of nature and has proved more realistic and enduring ... And not least significant is the fact that Griffin had achieved a viable architectural expression which, though initially based on that of his teacher, had continued to evolve and develop as the architect added his own ideas to those which he had learned.[9]

Even so, Brooks supposed that many of the essential features of Walter's mature style were the product of Marion's genius, not his. He came to this conclusion through an entirely credible analysis of both Walter's and Marion's architecture between 1909 and 1913, the main difficulty with his study of their work being that he reasoned forward from an incorrect assumption. This was his acceptance of erroneous dates for the design by Mahony of the Henry Ford house at Dearborn, Michigan.

In 1909, after helping close Wright's practice in Oak Park, when the architect went abroad for a year to work on several publications about his architecture, Mahony moved early that autumn to the office of Hermann Von Holst at Steinway Hall in Chicago. There she became head of a division which Von Holst set up to finish Wright's outstanding commissions, according to a contract Wright signed with Von Holst on 22 September 1909, and to carry out such work as might come to Von Holst's office by persons seeking plans in the style of Wright. While there Mahony designed four large houses: for C Harold Wills, Detroit, Michigan, 1909, not built; David Amberg, Grand Rapids, Michigan, 1909; and Robert Mueller and Adolph Mueller, both at Decatur, Illinois, 1910. Later, after marrying Griffin in June 1911 and transferring to his office, she returned briefly to work for Von Holst on two commissions whose clients wanted houses of a Wrightian type — but not by Wright. One was for Henry Ford; the other was for one of his lieutenants, Norval Hawkins. The first was partly erected to Mahony's design; the second did not progress beyond preliminary drawings.

In his thesis, Brooks supposed that the Henry Ford house 'actually reached the construction stage about 1910 or 1911'.[10] In fact, it is now certain that Mahony did not make any designs for the house before February 1913.[11] However, unaware of the correct dating of the Ford design, Brooks naturally assumed that any buildings by Walter dating after 1911 that exhibited architectural elements similar to those of the Ford house, must owe those features to Mahony's inventiveness. Even after David Van Zanten provided more accurate dates for the Ford house in his 1966 article 'The early work of Marion Mahony Griffin',[12] Brooks continued to believe that the house had been designed earlier than it

actually was, and accepted in his book, *The Prairie School*, the date of 1912 because that year is lightly pencilled on an ink drawing of the house.[13] Supposing that Griffin's Melson house and the Stinson Memorial Library, each of which have walls of rugged stone similar to those Mahony proposed to use in the Ford house, were designed after the Ford house, Brooks wrote about the Ford house that:

> the predominance of rather heavy rustic ashlar masonry can be ascribed to Marion Mahony's predilection for such materials and her appreciation of their intrinsic massive effect ... Similar window treatment and the use of masonry later appear in Walter Burley Griffin's work (Melson house, for example) and must be considered part of Marion's influence upon her husband. However, such design-elements are also in keeping with Griffin's own characteristics (liking for massiveness, etc.), making it readily understandable why this adoption would take place. One might say that Marion helped push Walter Burley Griffin in the direction he wanted to go, but the exact degree is difficult to calculate.[14]

As for the Melson house, Brooks wrote in his dissertation, that 'the manneristic keystones seem an unfortunate bid for novelty, and the ashlar, indicative of the cliff from which the house grows, creates an extremely busy wall surface. These characteristics, however, would appear as Marion's contribution to the design ...'[15] In his book, Brooks adopted a more cautious approach in evaluating the Melson house and said about it only that 'the rough limestone, embankment site, and diamond-shaped window mullions all recall her earlier work'.[16]

Curiously, by the time Brooks discusses the Stinson Library in his book,[17] he appears to have forgotten all about his belief that the origins of Walter's mature style lay in Marion's previous work, so overwhelmed does he seem to be by the visual impact of the library. In fact, were one to read only Brooks' praise of the library and his positive assessment of Walter's mature style, which follows directly after it, one would never suspect that previously in the same text he had attributed to Marion many of the library's essential characteristics, for here he says nothing about her contributions to Walter's mature style. It is almost as if he no longer believed what he had written earlier in the book. If that is what Brooks really believed when he wrote the book, he would be correct. Because Marion Mahony Griffin did not design the Ford house until February 1913,[18] its stylistic elements must be derived from Walter's Melson house, designed about April 1912 and the Stinson Library, designed about September 1912, not the reverse. The style of Walter Burley Griffin's maturity — first announced in mid 1910 with his design of the F P Marshall house, continued and expanded in his Melson house and Stinson Library — served Marion Mahony Griffin well when faced with the daunting task of designing a house for one of America's most wealthy industrialists in 1913.

It is not unexpected that Mahony should have drawn on Griffin's work for inspiration and motif. Her role in the Von Holst office was to finish Wright's outstanding work and to make designs for clients who wanted buildings in the style

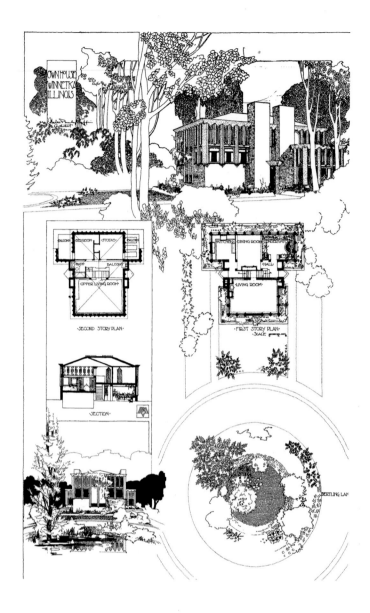

of Wright. She was not asked to develop and define a style of her own. Thus it was expected she would make new designs which mimicked Wright's. And this is what she did at first. Her house for C H Wills of 1909 certainly might be mistaken for a design by Wright as would her houses for David Amberg and Robert Mueller, both of 1910. Brooks believed that Wright actually left 'behind some elevational drawings that Mahony utilized', when designing the Robert Mueller house.[19]

By contrast, the Adolph Mueller house seems less Wrightian in character. Yet does it exemplify, as Brooks claims, 'all the characteristics thus far associated with Mahony...', or is it 'most purely hers', as Pregliasco declares?[20] The answer as I see it is decidedly in the negative, for what the Adolph Mueller house resembles most closely are houses in Walter Burley Griffin's early style, especially his design for the Irving Payne house of 1907 and for the Gilbert Cooley house of 1908.[21] It would seem, therefore, that beginning in the autumn of 1910 Marion Mahony, then attracted to Walter Burley Griffin and drawn to his architecture, switched aesthetic role models from Wright to Griffin.

As our examination of Mahony's work indicates, she seemed unable to develop an independent style of her own. Instead she preferred to base her architectural designs on the work of architects she admired. Up to the autumn of 1910, she followed Wright's example. Then with her design for the Adolph Mueller house, made in October 1910, she drew sustenance from Griffin's work of his early period. By 1913, however, when she designed the Henry Ford house, her inspiration was her husband's mature architecture, specifically that of the Melson house and the Stinson Library.

That Mahony preferred to design by referring for guidance to the work of architects whom she respected is also supported by the recently discovered design by her for the house of Norval Hawkins, sales manager of the Ford Motor Company from 1907 to 1919.[22] Both in plan and elevation it is based on Griffin's 1906 design for the house of his brother Ralph, not built until 1909–10.[23] Unlike her designs for the houses of Adolph Mueller and Henry Ford, made in 1910 and 1913 respectively and done at times when Griffin might actually have assisted or advised her as she developed the design of each, he could not have helped her with the Hawkins drawings. These are dated 10 November 1913, and in that month he was in Australia and had been there for some time.

This does not mean that the Hawkins design is flawed because it was reminiscent of the earlier house by Griffin, for in many ways it is better than the original. It does suggest, however, that Marion Mahony Griffin lacked the architectural imagination necessary to invent original concepts of her own. We have seen this to be so beginning with her designs in the manner of Wright when first working for Von Holst, then her switch to Griffin as a model beginning with the Adolph Mueller house which refers to his early style, then to Griffin's late style when confronted by the Ford commission, then back to his early style for the Hawkins house. Apparently she recognised this deficiency for once she transferred to Griffin's office, she evidently was

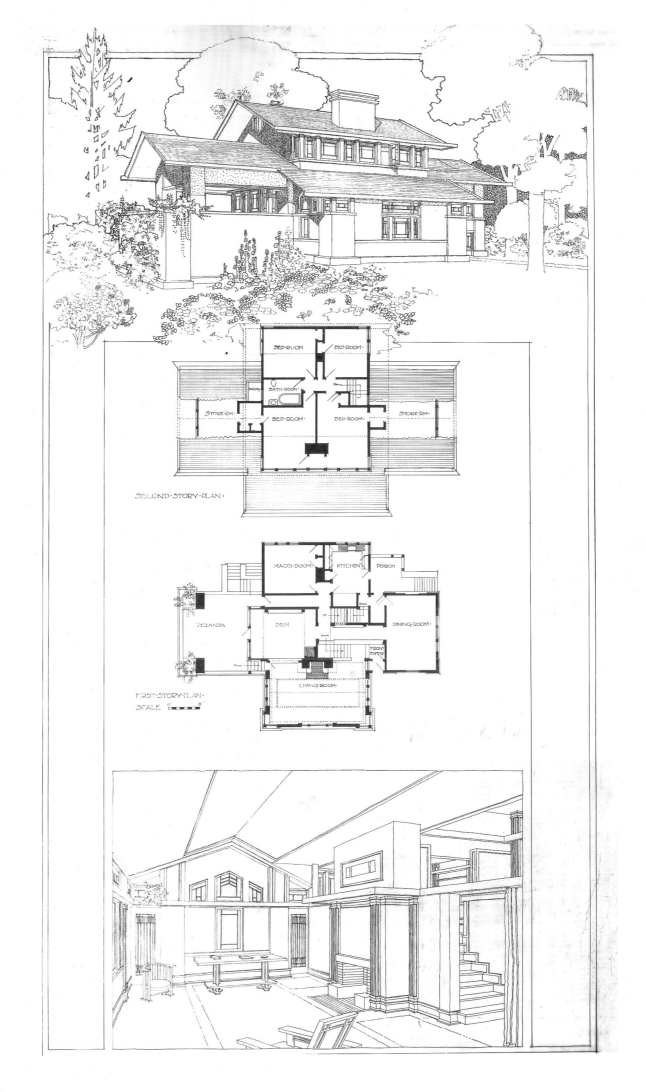

SECOND·STORY·PLAN·

BED·ROOM·   BED·ROOM·

BATH·ROOM·

STORE·RM·   BED·ROOM·   BED·ROOM·   STORE·RM·

MAIDS·ROOM·   KITCHEN·   PORCH·

VERANDA   DEN   DINING·ROOM·

FRONT·
ENTRY·

LIVING·ROOM·

FIRST·STORY·PLAN·
SCALE·

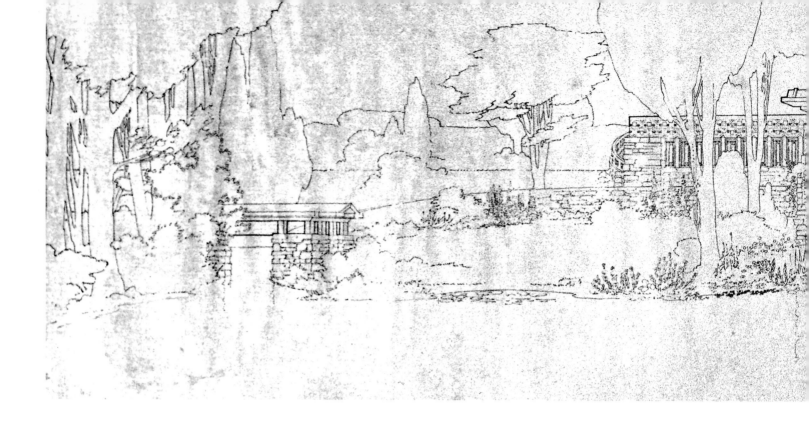

satisfied to leave to Walter the task of making the initial sketches for commissions while she worked on later phases of the design. At least this appears to be the case if we can trust her own occasional remarks and those of others to that effect. According to Mahony, after joining the Griffin office, 'she had thrill after thrill. Problems which she had seen struggled over in office after office and never solved were being solved one after another. Inspiration, the source of information, had been tapped and she watched [Walter] with awe and amazement and understanding'.[24]

Elsewhere she wrote that: 'I presently became deeply centered in the task of lending a hand in all the emergencies that arose. Truly I lost my self in him and found it completely satisfying'.[25]

Roy Lippincott, her brother-in-law, who first worked for Mahony in the Von Holst office, and who moved to the Griffin office with her in 1911, believed that: 'It would be very hard to discover any effect that she might have had on Walt's work before the Australian days. She had an almost worshipful regard for his genius, and repeatedly expressed to me the opinion that it was far greater in basic elements than Wright's'.[26]

What then was Marion's role in the Griffin office after transferring there in 1911? She saw it as assisting Walter in realising his visions of architecture. This she did by managing the drafting room, supervising the drafting force, making the required drawings for presentation and construction, and convincing clients to approve Walter's designs by making the wonderful perspectives and elevations for which she is rightly known and acclaimed. This does not mean that Mahony was not an architect, for certainly she was, not only because she possessed the proper credentials — a degree from the Massachusetts Institute of Technology, and

a licence to practise architecture granted by the state of Illinois — but also because she personally designed at least eleven buildings and saw five of them built. In addition, she was a female architect when few existed, and among them, she was one of the very few to practise. If she had done nothing else, this should be enough to secure her a distinctive place in history. But she did more; she immersed herself in the early modern movement in Chicago and worked for and with two of its outstanding leaders, Frank Lloyd Wright and Walter Burley Griffin. Moreover, her gifts for rendering, drafting and detailing helped to further the reputations of both architects.

What is less clear, however, is just how gifted she was as a designing architect. Had she not made any independent designs there would be no way to appraise her architectural ability except through her rendering and drafting, but she did and it is on the basis of those designs, especially the ones done while working in the office of Hermann Von Holst that this evaluation must rest. Unfortunately, even when her work is approached with the greatest sympathy, it must be admitted that much of its interest lies in the rejection of historical precedent. Had she come up with a distinctive approach to design free of the trammels of the historic styles, this might well have been enough to propel her to high status, even without regard to the innate aesthetic character of her designs. But she did not reach this plateau, partly because she was asked to make designs in the style of Wright, and partly because she was unable to elude the overpowering forcefulness, first of Wright's conceptions, then of Griffin's.

In fact, when one thinks of superior artistic qualities, the image is not of Mahony's architecture, satisfactory as it may be in the parochial sense, but of her work in the two-dimensional arts. As renderer, muralist and designer of

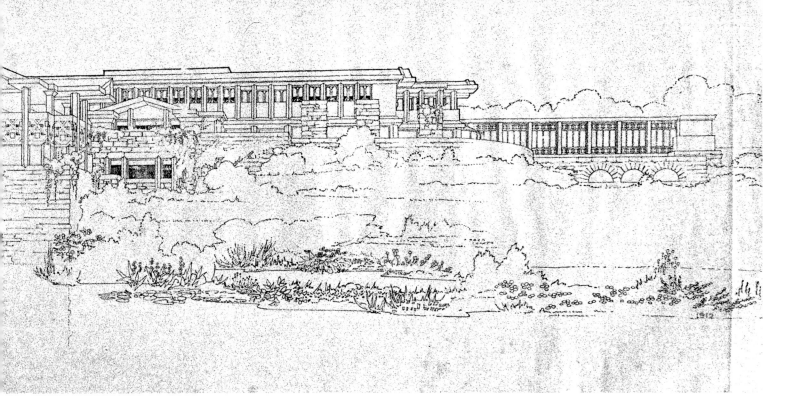

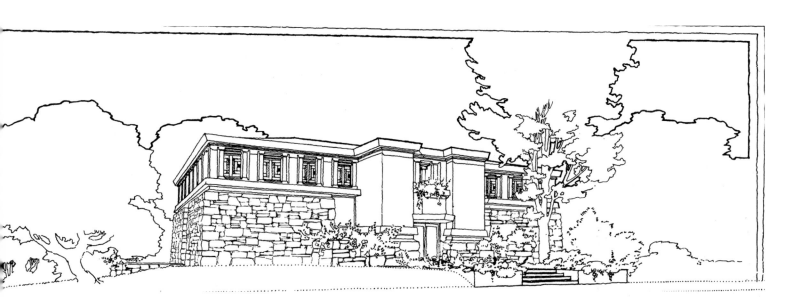

Top: Henry Ford house, Dearborn, Michigan, designed about February 1913, only foundations built. Ink on linen drawing by Marion Mahony Griffin, 41 × 142 cm.

Above: Stinson Memorial Library, Anna, Illinois, designed about September 1912 by Walter Burley Griffin, standing. Detail of ink on linen drawing by Marion Mahony Griffin.

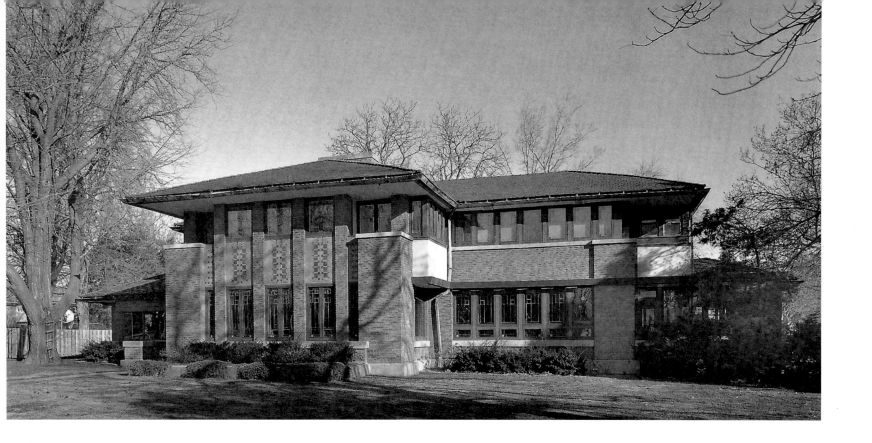

patterns, fireplace fronts, inlaid tile panels, art glass windows, doors, sconces, furniture, and other essentially two-dimensional accoutrements associated with architecture, Marion was supreme. Reluctantly perhaps we come back full circle to Marion as artist rather than Marion as architect, when we search for her true intrinsic excellence. Indeed, there is some likelihood that had she never known either Wright or Griffin, she might well have touched fame through her artistic renderings, architectural drawings and designs for architectural ornamentation in two dimensions. Perhaps it is time we stopped trying to measure her work by the architectural yardstick, recognise her abilities for what they were, and applaud her for the renown she actually achieved in her specialised branch of art.

Having examined the origins of the myth that threatens to continue to cast doubt on Walter Burley Griffin as originator of his mature architectural style, let us now survey, however briefly, the evolution of Walter Burley Griffin's American architecture. While it is generally supposed that Griffin's early style is largely based on the work of Frank Lloyd Wright, there is much about it which, almost from the beginning, shows independence. The very idea of designing prairie-hugging houses in the manner of Wright was not something in which Griffin often indulged as is suggested by his earliest important works, the stables for Thomas Wilder of 1902 and the 1903 house for William Emery, both of which stood tall above the prairie of Elmhurst, Illinois.[27] Also, as these examples demonstrate, Griffin preferred Japanese gables to Wright's hip roofs and placed a much greater emphasis on cubic geometry in the massing of his buildings. In subdividing his windows, Griffin favoured simple muntins of wood arranged in geometric

patterns, which generally echoed the basic massing of the building, over Wright's delicate and ornate art glass windows. There is no building by Griffin for which an obvious module, used to regulate its layout, cannot be discovered, so enamoured was he of this planning device. In fact, there is evidence that it was from Griffin that Wright learned about the module, or 'unit system' as Wright would call it, which Wright used only sparingly in his own work before 1919. Like Wright, Griffin also embraced open plans, though his were more simple and compact than those of his mentor. In fact, it is likely that Wright borrowed from Griffin the rudimentary L-shaped open plan which so fascinated Griffin after 1903, when in 1906 or 1907, Wright designed for *The Ladies Home Journal* a small cubic house of concrete. Finally, Griffin seemed to favour vertically integrated space, split-level planning and cathedral ceilings, none of which much interested Wright but all of which Griffin exploited from the beginning as is evident in his Emery house of 1903 (*see p 22*) and in two early houses of 1906, the one for Harry Peters and the other for his brother, Ralph Griffin (*see p 69*).

During the evolution of Griffin's early style, it is possible to detect hints of the severe geometry that would characterise his later work. This is especially evident in the two-flat residence that he designed in 1907 for Mrs Bovee, the store he did in 1908 for the Paul Cornell estate, and his house for Harry Gunn of 1909.

Once Griffin announced his mature style in the form of the F P Marshall house in 1910, he reserved its use for his more important commissions, or at least for those clients whom he thought willing to accept something new and radical, while continuing to offer designs in his early style to those who were more timid. The buildings he designed in his

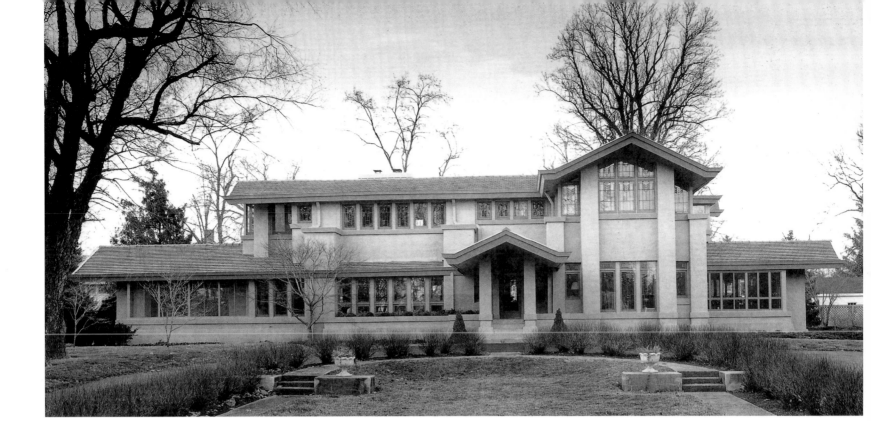

new cubic manner have a family resemblance, though the innovative variations from one to the next are considerable. Any attempt to describe these buildings must begin by calling attention to Griffin's characteristic simplified massing of his buildings accomplished by reducing their cubic forms to a kind of primitive geometry. Everywhere smooth surfaces serve to articulate and dramatise the elementary geometry which makes up the basic strata of his buildings.

These are generally rectilinear in form, though for contrast and effect Griffin introduced sharp-edged bases, cornices and piers between windows, the keen edges produced by rotating the bases, cornices and piers through 45 degrees from the wall surfaces above and below them. Angular bases and cornices of this kind are especially evident in the Clark Memorial Fountain of 1910 and in the Portland Cement Exhibition building of 1911; angular piers may be seen in Griffin's design of 1912 for his own house.

Ornamental panels, also consisting of simple geometric shapes, were used sparingly by Griffin for surface ornament, as in the Clark Fountain or in his house of 1912 for William Tempel, though in general Griffin avoided ornamenting his cubic masses. Instead he preferred to decorate his buildings by subdividing their windows with wooden muntins forming patterns which echo the overall geometric characteristics of the building. In a few cases, he translated his ornamental vision into stained glass as he did when designing the Stinson Memorial Library and the Koehne villa and studio of 1913, though this was rare.

Generally Griffin subdivided the massive surfaces of his buildings into piers and panels, all of them largely rectilinear in shape. Even in the few, seemingly different buildings, where Griffin specified walls of broken, uncoursed

Above: Adolph Mueller house, Decatur, Illinois, designed as built about September 1910 by Marion Mahony assisted by Walter Burley Griffin.
Photograph by Mati Maldre, 1991.

Above left: Robert Mueller house, Decatur, Illinois, designed about June 1910 by Marion Mahony.
Photograph by Mati Maldre, 1991.

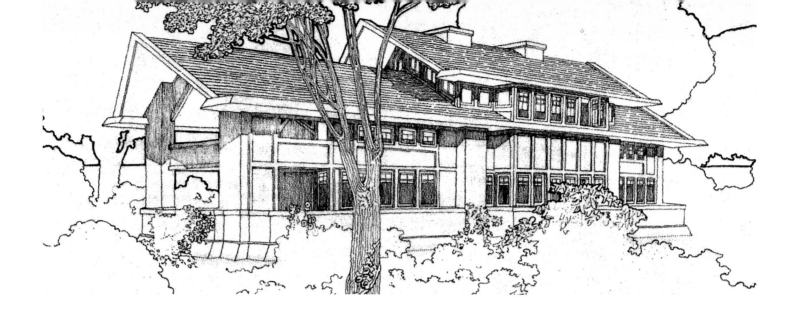

stone, projecting and receding from an unseen surface, the overall character of each is very much like his smooth-surfaced designs, at least whenever the observer mentally transforms the ragged stonework into smooth surfaces. Buildings of this type include the Melson house and the Stinson Library, though the over-scaled concrete keystones which break the skyline of the Melson house are unique examples of a truly expressive ornamentation unlike anything else in Griffin's American work.

While the serious scholar may find some vague references in Griffin's mature architecture to earlier designs by Frank Lloyd Wright, the overwhelming impression it produces is one of defiant originality. Surely few would disagree that, in these buildings which Griffin designed between 1910 and 1915, he created an architectural style of considerable originality, a modern style that equalled and perhaps exceeded the achievements of the few Europeans actively searching for personal versions of a modern architecture. And without question, Griffin was also ahead of his colleague Frank Lloyd Wright in this regard. Wright did not manage to catch up with Griffin's vision of a modern architecture until he designed Midway Gardens early in 1914. Even then, Wright took the wrong turn in the road toward modernism by embracing an ornamented expressionism which later, at the end of the 1920s, he found it necessary to abandon in order to return to the mainstream of modern architecture. By contrast, Griffin's severe geometric style, minimally ornamented but expressively organised, seems in retrospect to have been more attuned to the inevitable direction that modernism took in the 1920s. Whatever the case, the new style that Griffin invented in 1910 demonstrates his innate qualifications as an imaginative and creative architect who deserves to be recognised along with Louis Sullivan and Frank Lloyd Wright as one of the three founders of modern architecture in America.

Above: Gilbert Cooley house, Monroe, Louisiana, designed by Walter Burley Griffin about August 1908, built in slightly revised form in 1925–1926. Detail of drawing by Marion Mahony Griffin.
Courtesy the Mary and Leigh Block Museum of Art, Northwestern University, Illinois, 1985.1.32.

Right: Norval Hawkins house, Detroit, Michigan, designed by Marion Mahony Griffin about October 1913, not built. Drawing by Marion Mahony Griffin with monogram 'MMG'. Formerly in the Taylor Woolley collection. Photo from microfilm frame 199, Special Collections, Library, University of Utah. The location of the original drawing is now unknown.

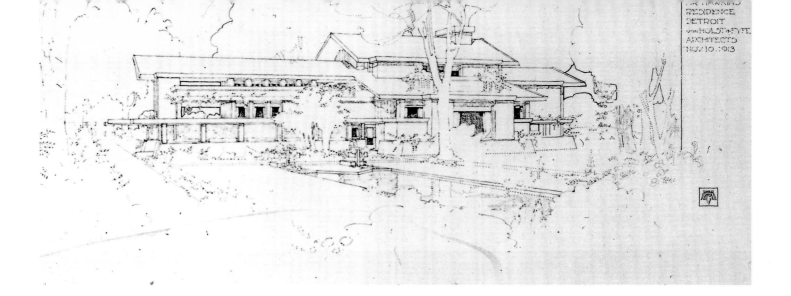

Notes

1. As Professor Kruty and I will argue in the book we are preparing about the American work of Walter Burley Griffin, his early designs were not nearly so dependent upon Wright as is generally supposed and, in fact, they displayed many individualistic characteristics not found in Wright's work, some of which Wright actually incorporated into his own architecture.

2. Today it is known as the Prairie School, a name derived from the visual characteristics of Wright's houses of the first decade of the twentieth century, whose long, low proportions Wright had characterised as reflecting the level character of the midwestern prairie. The problem with continuing to use this term is that the mature styles of Sullivan, Griffin and other architects who sought to create individual styles not based on the historic styles, cannot be crammed into the visual concept of a horizontal ground-hugging building from which the name 'Prairie School' is derived. Even Wright's non-residential buildings, especially such flat-roofed geometric abstractions as his Unity Temple, are visually unrelated to the levelness of the midwestern prairie. It is hoped that some day this visually-inspired term will give way to a more historically precise designation, such as the 'Sullivan School'.

3. H Allen Brooks, 'The Prairie School: the American spirit in midwest residential architecture, 1893–1916', PhD dissertation, Northwestern University, 1957, p 58.

4. Janice Pregliasco, 'The life and work of Marion Mahony Griffin', in *The Prairie School: design vision for the midwest* (issued as *Museum Studies*, vol 21, no 2), The Art Institute of Chicago, Chicago, 1995, p 175.

5. Ibid.

6. Ibid, p 179 and note 31, p 192.

7. For feminist critiques, see Donna Ruff Munchick, 'The work of Marion Mahony Griffin: 1894–1913', MA thesis, The Florida State University, School of Visual Arts, December 1974; Susan Fondiler Berkon and Jane Holtz Kay, 'Marion Mahony Griffin, architect', *Feminist Art Journal*, vol 4, Spring 1975, pp 10–14; Susan Berkon, 'Marion Mahony Griffin', in Susanna Torre, ed, *Women in American architecture: a historic and contemporary perspective*, Watson-Guptill, New York, 1977, pp 75–79; Anna Rubbo, 'Marion Mahony Griffin: a portrait', in J Duncan and M Gates, eds, *Walter Burley Griffin: a re-view*, Monash University Gallery, Victoria, 1988, pp 15–26.

8. H Allen Brooks, *The Prairie School: Frank Lloyd Wright and his midwest contemporaries*, University of Toronto Press, Toronto, 1972.

9. Ibid, p 262.

10. *The Prairie School*, 1957, p 40.

11. The source for this date is given in 'Findings of fact and law', 19 March 1917, Ford archives, Dearborn, Michigan. A detailed discussion of the Ford commission will appear in the book Professor Kruty and I are preparing on the American work of Walter Burley Griffin.

12. David Van Zanten, 'The early work of Marion Mahony Griffin', *The Prairie School Review*, vol 3, Second Quarter, 1966, p 21.

13. Clearly the date of 1912 was added sometime after the drawing was finished when the year in which it was made had been forgotten. If it had been appropriate to date the drawing when finished, the person who drafted it — surely Marion Mahony Griffin in this case — would have given the day, month and year. The date occurs on a rendering of the Ford house now at Northwestern University, inventory number 1985.1.119.

14. 'The Prairie School', 1957, p 41.

15. Ibid, p 51.

16. *The Prairie School*, 1972, p 247.

17. Brooks does not mention the library in his dissertation because he limited its scope to residential buildings, as the subtitle, 'The American spirit in midwest residential architecture', makes clear.

18. 'Findings of fact and law', op cit.

19. *The Prairie School*, 1972, p 159.

20. Pregliasco, 'The life and work of Marion Mahony Griffin', p 171, op cit.

21. Of the scholars who have written about the Adolph Mueller house, only Donald Leslie Johnson seems to have noticed the relationship between that house and Griffin's work. In his *The architecture of Walter Burley Griffin*, Macmillan, Melbourne, 1977, p 12, he writes that the Mueller house 'was a complex design so very similar to the reserved, more refined J. B. Cooley House by Griffin in the same year [actually the Cooley House was designed in 1908]. Griffin must have had some, if not a great deal of influence on the design of at least this house … Elements of the Niles Club, Mason City houses, the Mess house and other stylistic evidence suggest a close collaboration with Griffin'. Johnson is incorrect, however, in citing the Mason City houses and the Mess house as sources for the Mueller house as all were designed after it.

22. It is certain that Marion made the design as her monogram appears on the rendering of the Hawkins house. Microfilm images of the original drawings, formerly owned by Wright's draftsman, Taylor Woolley, are in the Taylor Woolley collection at the Library of the University of Utah.

23. A photograph of a rendering of the Ralph Griffin house dated '1906' is in the collection in Sydney of Marie Nicholls, daughter of Griffin's Australian partner, Eric Nicholls.

24. Marion Mahony Griffin, 'The magic of America', manuscript at the New York Historical Society, 4 volumes, vol 4, 1949, p 236.

25. Ibid, vol 4, p 339.

26. Lippincott to Van Zanten, 24 September 1965, as partly quoted in 'The early work of Marion Mahony Griffin', p 22.

27. Usually dated 1901, the house was actually designed in 1903.

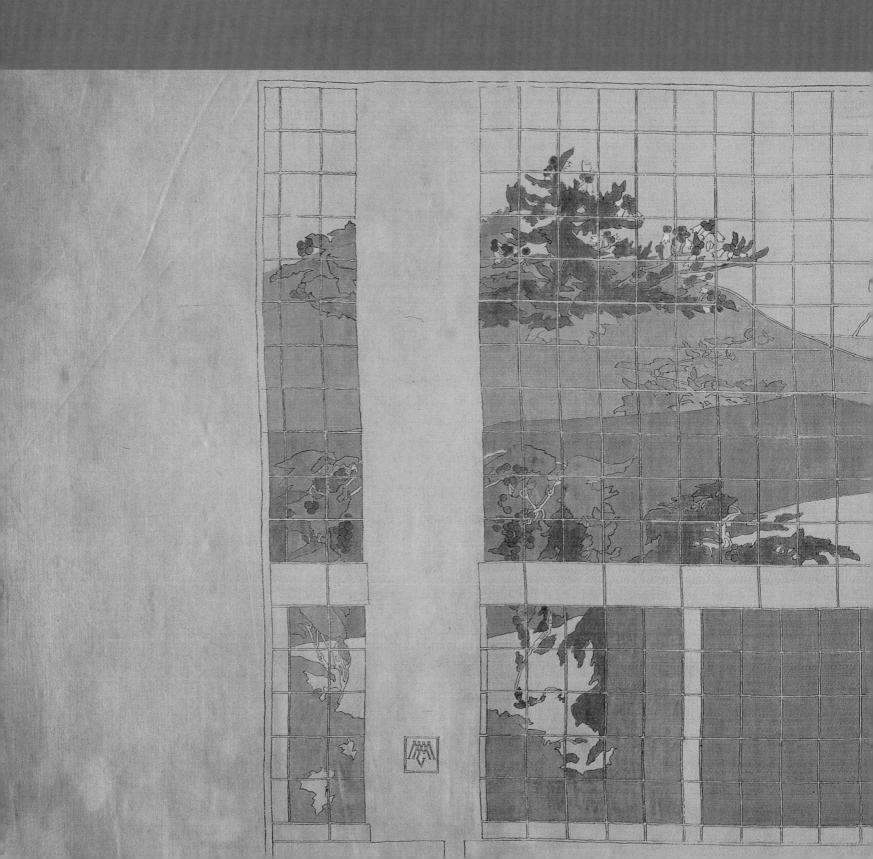

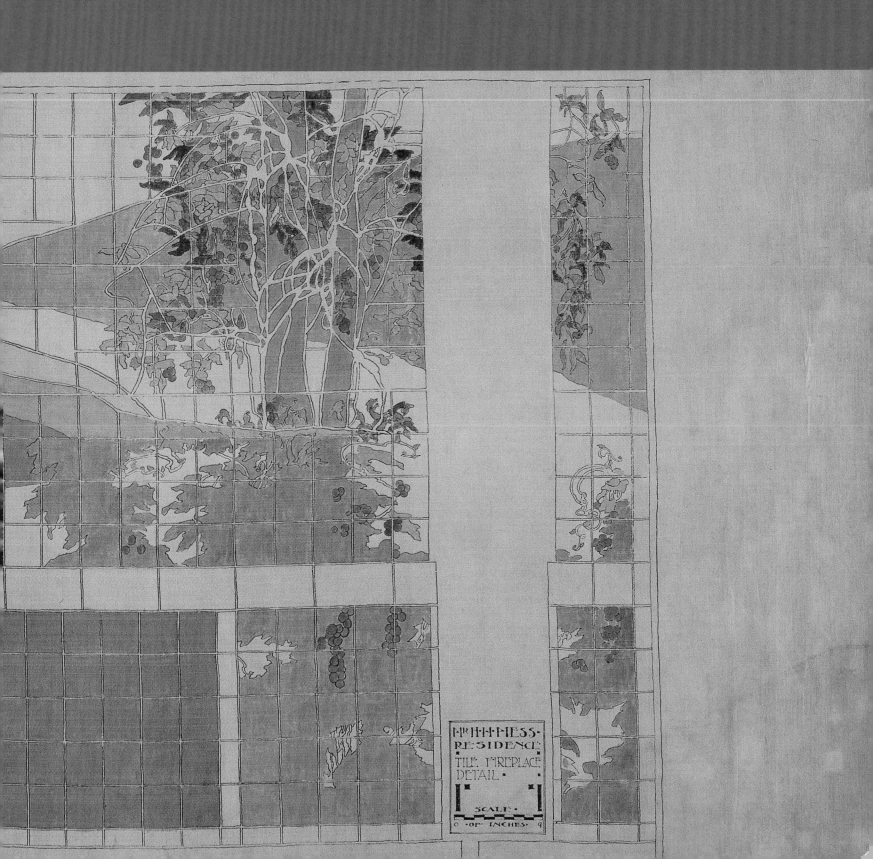

Mr H H HESS
RESIDENCE
TILE FIREPLACE
DETAIL

SCALE
0 ·OF· INCHES· 9

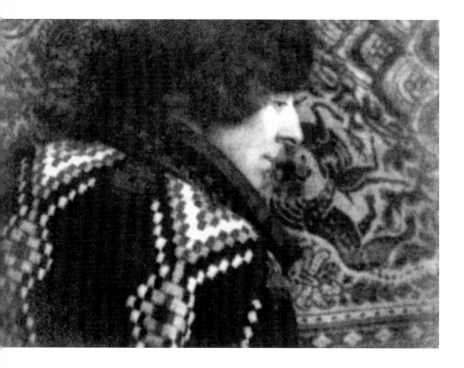

Marion Mahony Griffin and her husband Walter Burley Griffin have yet to be fully recognised for their contribution to the theory and practice of architecture in the first half of the twentieth century. Outspoken and often passionate in her convictions, Marion was simultaneously larger than life and quite modest. When it came to taking credit for her own achievements she seemed almost disinterested. She claimed to be shy in 'self-expression' but throughout her life she espoused intense intellectual friendships. She played second string to Walter and deferred to his ability as a designer. In later life, however, Marion erased his name from a significant number of drawings, and the meaning of this action has been speculated upon but never properly deciphered.

It is through Marion's own writing that we get glimpses of this modesty but also insights into her forceful character and remarkable achievements. This essay explores some of these contrasting facets of her character, looking at the ideas and experiences that influenced her thinking, and at their expression in one of the most creative architectural partnerships between a married couple this century has seen.[1]

The partnership between Marion Mahony and Walter Burley Griffin began with their marriage in 1911, and endured until his death in 1937. As the second woman to graduate in architecture from MIT in Boston in 1894, Marion helped pioneer women's participation in architecture in the United States. In her role as a designer she contributed to the development of the Prairie School which revolutionised American architecture, and through her superb drawings helped disseminate those ideas worldwide. Her pursuit of artistic, democratic and spiritual ideals through art, architecture and community planning in Australia and the United States is significant, and she was outspoken on a broad range of topics, including architecture, planning, nature, education, the environment, politics (and politicians), and women as professionals. In her middle and later years she spoke at length on anthroposophy, which knitted all her other passions together and linked her personal, professional and political views. It was through the lens of anthroposophy and its promise for developing the creative and spiritual aspects of humankind that Marion made sense of the world.[2]

Throughout their long association the Griffins engaged in work across three continents, ranging in scale from the very large to the very small: city and community design, public, commercial and private buildings, furniture, murals, tableware, and even menu design. Marion played a central role in that architectural and artistic production in an active professional life that spanned over 50 years: the early years as a young architect in Chicago (1894–1914), the middle years in Australia and India (1914–1938), and the later years back in Chicago (1938 to about 1944).

Marion Mahony Griffin's unpublished magnum opus, 'The magic of America', provides a key to understanding the Griffins' intellectual and creative contribution to architecture. There was nothing modest about the 'Magic' project, which Marion undertook

Above: Marion Mahony Griffin about 1930.
Reproduced from David Van Zanten, *Drawings of Walter Burley Griffin architect*, the Prairie School Press, Palos Park, Illinois, 1970, p 2.

Right: J G Melson house, Rock Crest–Rock Glen, Mason City, Iowa, 1912.
Photograph courtesy Mati Maldre, Chicago, 1990.

Previous pages: Fireplace design, H M Mess house, Winnetka, Illinois, 1912. Lithograph and watercolour on silk sateen with 'MMG' monogram, 61.8 × 116.8 cm.
Courtesy Avery Architectural and Fine Arts Library, Columbia University, New York (1986.002.00001).

BEYOND ARCHITECTURE

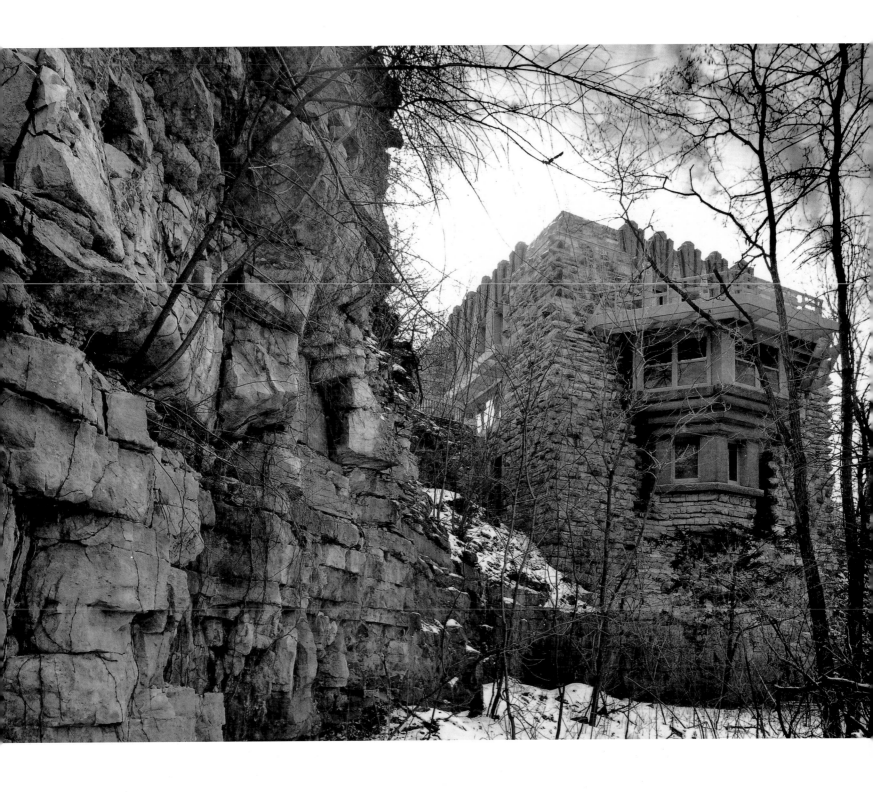

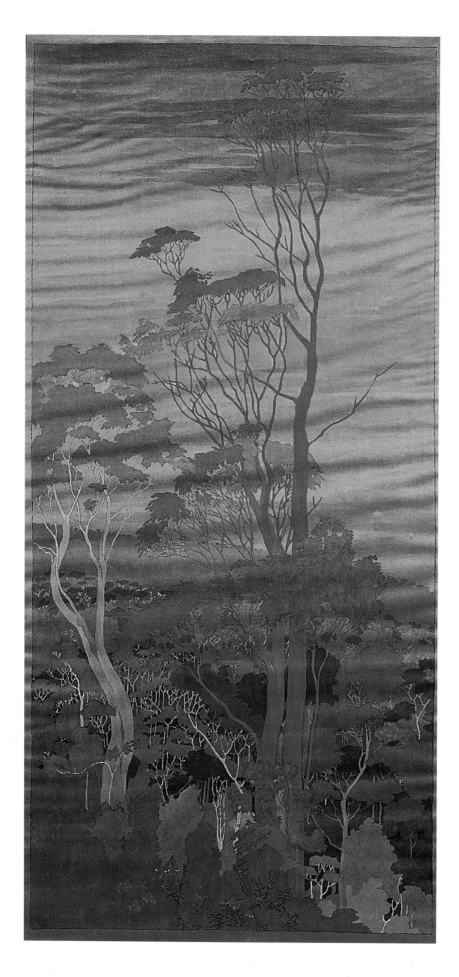

Left: 'Eucalyptus urnigera', ink and watercolour on silk sateen, 112 × 55 cm. The original drawing for this tree study was made by Marion on a trip to Tasmania in 1919. She wrote of her impressions of it: 'The eucalyptus urnigera growing along the coast of Tasmania, a slender tree, vivid red, shooting like a flame straight up into the sky' ('The magic of America', vol 3, p 345). Photographs of many of Marion's pen and ink or watercolour on silk tree studies appear in 'The magic of America' and a number of original renderings survive in American and Australian private collections.
Courtesy the Mary and Leigh Block Museum of Art, Northwestern University, Illinois (1985.1.117 — 'Tropical Vegetation').

Right: 'Three flat building', lot 86 The Rampart, Castlecrag, about 1930, unbuilt. Ink and watercolour on cloth, 61.2 × 45.7 cm, artist unknown. As in a number of drawings, reference to Walter Burley Griffin has been blocked out.
Courtesy Avery Architectural and Fine Arts Library, Columbia University, New York (1000.015.0041).

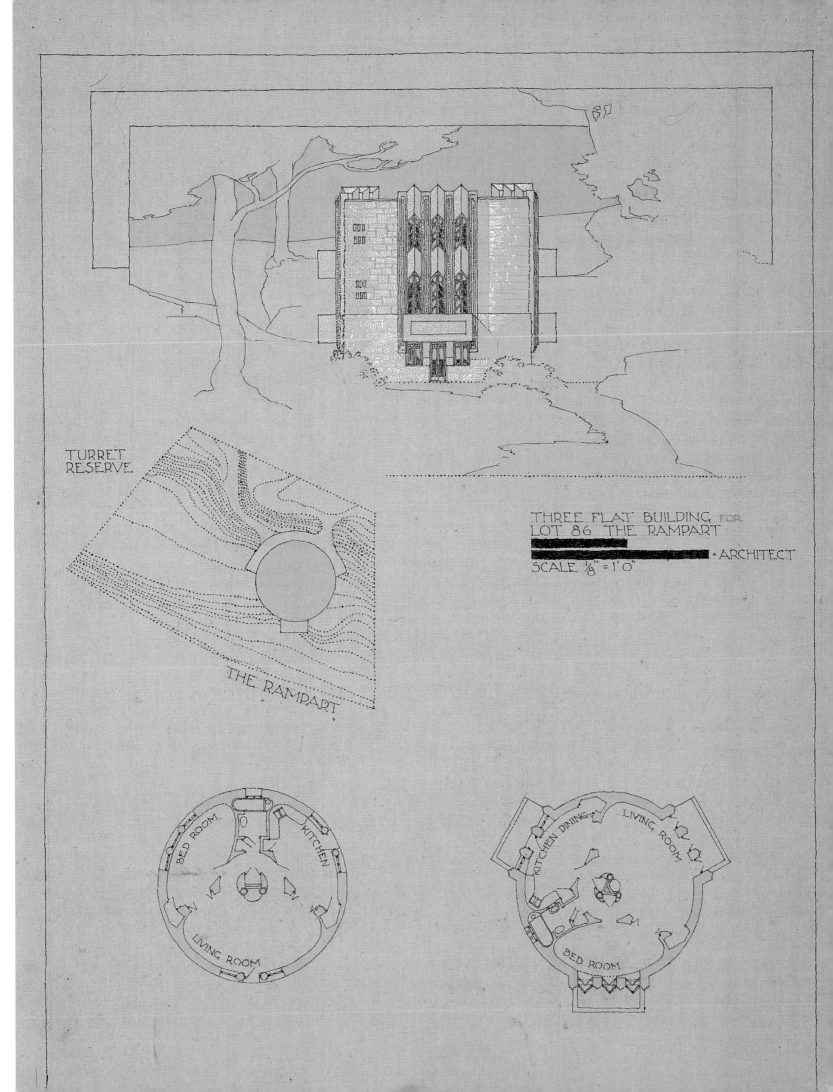

TURRET
RESERVE

THE RAMPART

THREE FLAT BUILDING FOR
LOT 86 THE RAMPART

ARCHITECT

SCALE ⅛" = 1' 0"

BED ROOM

KITCHEN

LIVING ROOM

KITCHEN DINING

LIVING ROOM

BED ROOM

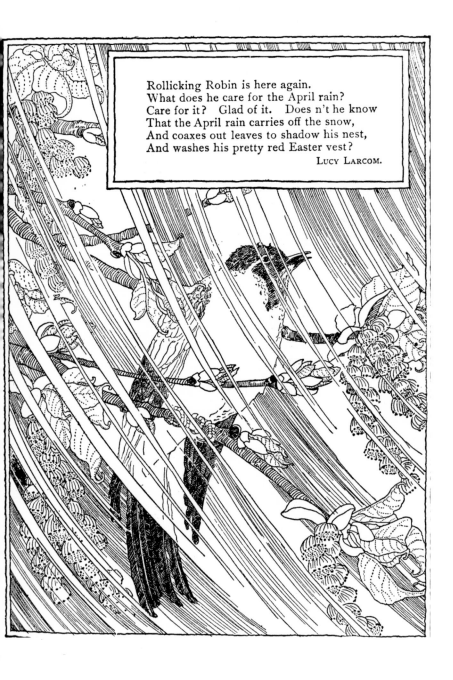

Rollicking Robin is here again.
What does he care for the April rain?
Care for it? Glad of it.   Does n't he know
That the April rain carries off the snow,
And coaxes out leaves to shadow his nest,
And washes his pretty red Easter vest?

LUCY LARCOM.

Above: Illustration by Marion about 1910 from *The children's year book* by Maud Summers, published by Stoll & Edwards, New York, 1923. Marion's lively Japanese-inspired style is very different from other more traditional drawings in the book by Marion's cousin Lucy Fitch Perkins. Courtesy Library of Congress, Washington (PZ5 S95 Ch).

Right: Thomas P Hardy house, Racine, Wisconsin, 1904. Plate xv (c) of *Ausgeführte Bauten und Entwürfe von Frank Lloyd Wright*, the folio of drawings published by Ernst Wasmuth, Berlin, 1910. Lithograph, 63.5 x 40.5 cm. Marion was responsible for this and many other renderings in this very influential publication.

Courtesy Frank Lloyd Wright Foundation, Scotsdale, Arizona (0506.038).

primarily to secure Walter Burley Griffin's place in architectural history, but there is a certain modesty, in conventional historical terms, about the form it took. 'Magic' is some 1000 pages long and is an assemblage of drawings, photographs, essays, speeches, letters, newspaper clippings and commentary by Marion. Walter had died suddenly in India in 1937, and in the following year Marion returned to Chicago. She began writing at age 67 in 1938, and finished some ten years later.

As an epitaph to their lives together this work is both a public record and a personal history. It is revealing of them as a couple but also of her as an individual. 'Magic' shows that Marion Griffin lived a feminist principle well ahead of her time in the way she was able to integrate the various aspects of her life into a whole. Work, or the public, merged with the private, which in turn merged with the political dimensions of their lives. The fact that the Griffins had no children made possible their single-minded devotion to their work; it did not mean however, that they were not interested in children. 'Magic' is full of details about the children in their lives: the Castlecrag children, and later Marion's nephews and nieces with whom she lived. A considerable amount of her creative energy went into illustrating children's books, and to the major mural project in the Rogers Park elementary school in 1931. This mural, 'Fairies feeding the herons', has an avowedly pedagogical and anthroposophical purpose.

In 'Magic' she organises their lives as four 'battles', and each has elements of the public, the private and the political. She begins with the 'Empirial [*sic*] Battle' (or as she sub-titled it, 'An American architect's year in India'). This is followed by the 'Federal Battle' (their struggles over the design for Canberra), the 'Municipal Battle' (the story of their utopian suburban development in Castlecrag), and the 'Individual Battle' (the battle ground of their personal lives). Their ruling passions — architecture, community planning, landscape architecture, the protection of the environment, anthroposophy, and their abiding commitment to democracy — run through the four battles.

While 'The magic of America' is a key source of information about this important early twentieth-century architectural practice in the United States, Australia and India, its value as a historical record has not been fully explored. Its postmodern fragmentary quality, and the interpretative task the text demands may partly explain this. However, it is the quasi proselytising religiosity of 'Magic' that has probably done most to make it a contentious document in the eyes of many Griffin scholars, who by and large have resisted the idea that Walter Burley Griffin was also deeply involved in anthroposophy, and that these beliefs were perhaps nearly as central to his life and work as they were to hers.[3] Marion was introduced to anthroposophy in the 1920s when she read Rudolf Steiner's *Outline of occult science*, and in 1930 she joined the Sydney Anthroposophical Society. Griffin joined in 1931. The Griffins were, as the historian Jill Roe has said, the theosophists' favourite planners, 'not simply because they were theosophists but because they tried to resolve the problems of individualism communally'.[4]

There are two slightly differing versions of 'The magic of America' in existence: one is held at the Burnham Library in the Art Institute of Chicago (AIC), the other is in the New-York Historical Society Library (NYHSL). One of the surprises in the NYHSL copy is a swatch of the silk Marion Mahony Griffin used for some of her most famous drawings. The small sample of smooth beige glossy fabric must have been tucked away amongst Marion's possessions, a reminder of when she put pen to silk with such precision and delicacy in the early days of this century.

Together, 'Magic' and the drawings tell a good part of Marion's and Walter Burley Griffin's story; the other necessary part is the first-hand experience of the buildings and cities they created.[5] Rock Crest–Rock Glen in Mason City, Iowa (*see p 96*), and Castlecrag, Sydney, are accessible in terms of 'reading' the design ideas and philosophy. They are both dramatic and beautiful settings. Rock Crest has a river coursing through it; Castlecrag is a promontory jutting out into Sydney's Middle Harbour. These projects are great achievements in community planning, expressing vividly the democratic aspects of community, and its inter-dependence with the built and natural environment. Of particular importance is the responsiveness to the site and the social intention which is achieved through design. In the case of Rock Crest–Rock Glen, buildings flank a communal meadow which all residents can enjoy. In Castlecrag the roads follow the contours and a system of public pathways runs between the roads from ridge to waterline, making the water's edge easily accessible. Thus the special beauty of each site is enhanced and made accessible to the community.

Castlecrag was a utopian vision for a suburb developed between 1920 and 1935 by the Griffins through the Greater Sydney Development Association. James Weirick writes of it: 'The greatest achievement of the Griffins' Australian career was undoubtedly Castlecrag'. He describes it as 'an attempt to remake Australian society'.[6]

Walter and Marion grew up with an appreciation of nature and community. It is useful here to look at Marion's childhood to see where some of her later thinking must have taken root. Marion Mahony was born in Chicago but spent the first few years of her life in Hubbard Woods, to the north of Evanston. She described it as 'the loveliest spot you can imagine, beyond suburbia — four houses and no others within a mile in any direction … at the head of a lovely ravine'.[7] She recalled how she wept when the trees on the allotment next door were cut down, and that if there had been any true democracy then the 'whole wonderful ravine would have been left'. Her father died when she was twelve, and she and her four brothers and sisters spent the rest of their childhood in a woman-headed household. Her mother, Clara Mahony, was a respected educationalist and for many years was principal of the radical Komensky school, located in a poor, immigrant neighbourhood of Chicago. Through her mother's circle Marion was surrounded by a network of influential women, some of whom were educational

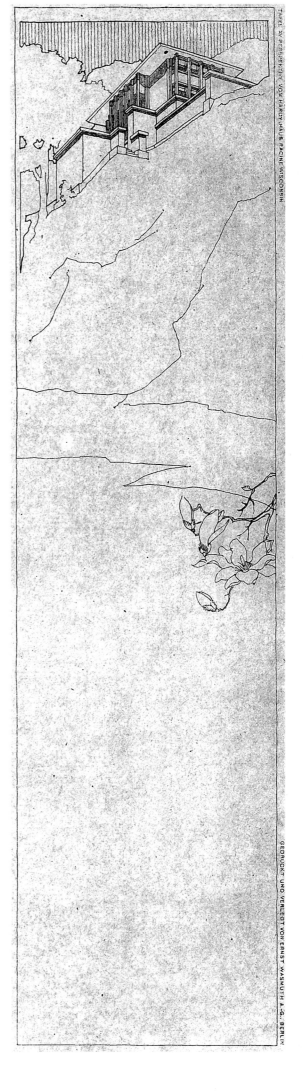

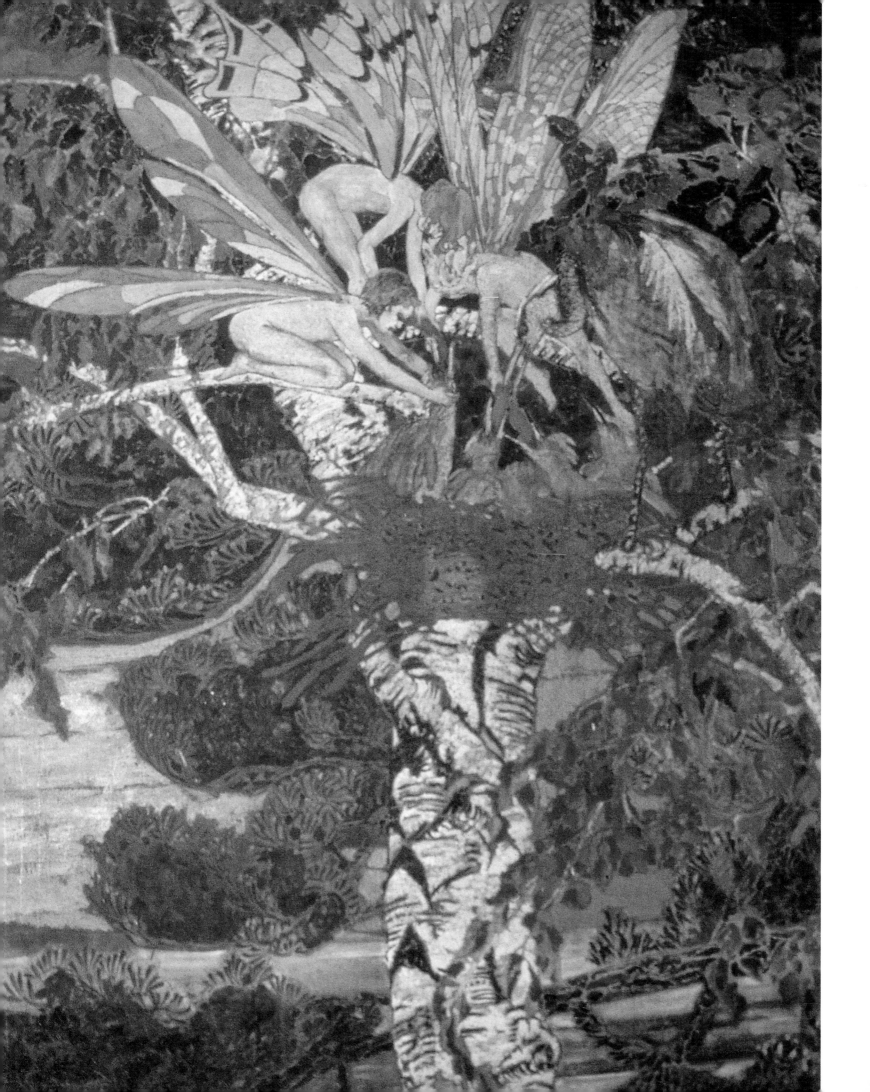

reformers or involved with Jane Addams' Hull House.[8] Marion's aunt Myra moved in with the family, and Marion recalls that it was her aunt who taught her that 'one of the greatest schools for thinking is friendship'.

Marion Mahony studied at MIT in Boston where she received, by today's standards, a very liberal architectural education. In addition to architectural courses she studied languages, political history, political economy, anthropology, and literature. She refers to her discussions with a fellow student on Kant's *Critique of pure reason*, and it is possible that Kant's views were influential in her growing interest in the transcendental as an agent for progress. She showed her independence of mind in her choice of thesis topic of a house and studio for a painter. Most students chose grander projects favoured by the Beaux Arts instructors, but Marion's project was very innovative and anticipated a home–work building typology.[9] While at MIT Marion developed a strong interest in theatre and performed in several college plays. Later in Castlecrag she would produce more than twelve plays in the open-air Haven Scenic Theatre designed by the Griffins, a theatre which is still used today.

Marion Mahony returned to Chicago in 1894. Her first job was with her cousin, MIT graduate Dwight Perkins, a reform-minded architect who saw the potential of architecture to address social and environmental issues. In 1895 she joined Frank Lloyd Wright's Oak Park studio and began eleven years of intermittent employment with Wright. Between 1900 and 1909 Wright, the main protagonist of the Prairie School, completed some 120 commissions in the midwest. Historian G C Manson considered Mahony to have been the key figure in the practice up till 1909. His view was that 'If the studio had been organised along more conventional lines she would have held the rank of "head designer" … She was not only a skilled designer but a gifted draughtswoman'.[10] Wright held 'informal competitions' at 'our little University', as he liked to refer to the studio. The competitions were for parts of projects, such as murals, fireplaces, windows, furniture, even complete interiors. Marion often 'won' these competitions, but she is best known for her renderings of Wright's designs. Her style was inspired by Japanese printmaking, an interest she and Wright shared. *Studies and executed buildings by Frank Lloyd Wright*, also known as the 'Wasmuth folio', was published in 1910, and became one of the most influential architectural publications of the twentieth century.[11] Of the one hundred plates in the 'Wasmuth folio' Mahony prepared more than half the underlays. The extraordinary drawings in this publication of the Hardy house in Racine are amongst the best examples of Marion's delicate linework. She also prepared the drawings of Unity Temple (*see p 62*) and the Cheney house, two well-known Oak Park buildings. The Como orchard perspective carries her characteristic 'MLM' (Marion Lucy Mahony) monogram, as does *The Ladies Home Journal* perspective, 'A Fireproof House for $5000' (*see p 21*).

When she was not working at Wright's studio Marion painted and taught, studied horticulture and carried out some private architectural work. Her first project on her

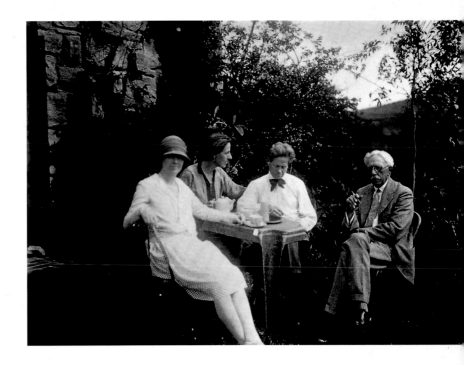

Above: Walter and Marion in their garden at Castlecrag with architect Louise Lightfoot and Walter's father George, about 1927.
Courtesy National Library of Australia, Canberra (PIC P490/1–7).

Left: Detail of mural 'Fairies feeding the herons', painted by Marion for a Chicago elementary school in 1931. The 1.5 × 6 metre mural depicts fairies in a subtropical setting inspired by the Castlecrag landscape. For Marion, the ability to see fairies held great significance: 'For the same faculty that enables one to see the fairies is the faculty which enables one to do original work in all human realms, and to transform our community… into a civilization thereby attaining great and worthwhile ends' ('The magic of America', vol 4, p 232).
Photograph courtesy Mati Maldre, Chicago, 1995.

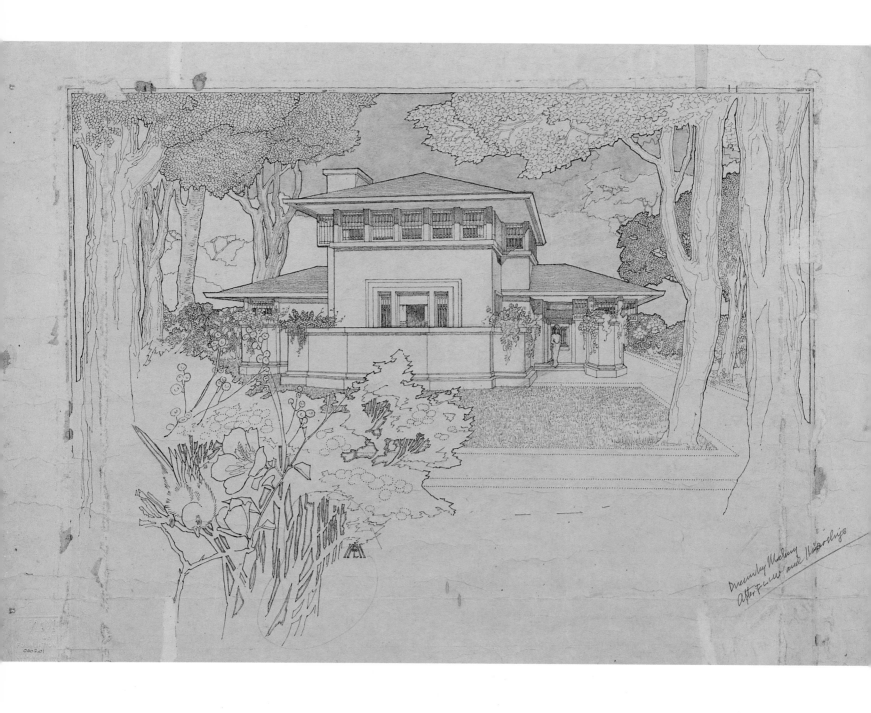

Above: Marion's rendering of Frank Lloyd Wright's K C De Rhodes house, South Bend, Indiana, 1906. Ink and watercolour on paper, 48 x 65 cm. Note the inscription by Wright: 'drawn by Mahony after FLW and Hiroshige'.

Courtesy Frank Lloyd Wright Foundation, Scottsdale, Arizona (0602.001).

own was the Unitarian Church of All Souls in Evanston, Illinois, in 1903. Her original and quite radical design, which linked three geometric forms, was rejected and the final project was more gothic, and more conservative. The interior, however, retained much of the original design and included a mural by Marion, an art glass ceiling over the chancel and delicate light fittings (see p 23).

Marion Mahony made a strong impression on people in Australia and in the United States. She was a forceful character; a former apprentice, Louise Lightfoot, recalled: 'I can still hear the sound of her ring scratching as she scrubbed out the mistakes in my drawing'.[12] Castlecrag residents remember her vividly and described her climbing the steep slopes of Castlecrag 'like a mountain goat', extolling the virtues of the area to prospective buyers.[13] They remember her exotic clothes and the plays she produced at the open-air theatre. Artist Bernard Hesling recalls her looking across the water to the suburb of Northbridge and exclaiming, 'It's hoorabul, hoorabul. Wahlter an' I wanna keep the Crag voigin bush'.[14] In the United States Barry Byrne, a fellow employee in Wright's office, found her rather larger than life, even in her twenties:

> She had a fragile frame and walked as though she was falling forward. She was a good actress, talkative and when Wright was around there was a real sparkle … Her mordant humour always attracted me as a fellow Celt, and I can well remember welcoming her advent because it promised an amusing day. Her dialogues with Frank Lloyd Wright, who as we all know is no indifferent opponent in repartee, made such days particularly notable. In all a rather fiery, spectacularly brilliant person.[15]

Wright himself rarely offered praise but called Marion a 'talented apprentice',[16] and Brendan Gill mentions Marion in his biography on Wright: 'Mahony was one of the few people whom Wright appears not to have dared patronise, at least to her face. Behind her back he was braver; when praising her art somebody compared it to Japanese printmaking, Wright said at once that, while Mahony copied Japanese prints, he was inspired by them'.[17]

During Griffin's tenure in Wright's studio he and Griffin had argued vehemently, and Marion never forgave him for his treatment of Griffin.[18] So when Wright asked Marion if she would like to take over his practice shortly before his departure for Europe in 1909, she refused. Hermann Von Holst, however, did accept Wright's offer. In 'Magic' Marion wrote:

> after Wright had gone Mr von Holz [sic] … asked me to join him so I did on a definite arrangement that I should have control of the designing. That suited him. When the absent architect didn't bother to answer anything that was sent over to him, the relations were broken and I entered into a partnership with von Holz and Fyfe. For that period I had great fun designing.[19]

She made good use of the time when she was not in the shadow of a 'great man', although Wright's office had provided her with a challenging environment in which she grew professionally and creatively. Working with Hermann

Von Holst as a relatively independent practitioner was important in establishing her architectural credentials. Her most significant projects at that time were the David Amberg house in Grand Rapids (1909), and the Adolph Mueller house in the Millikin Place, (see p 37) Decatur community (1910). The strong vertical surfaces and the sophisticated planning and detailing of the Mueller house are evidence of a mature and sure designer. In both the Amberg and Mueller houses the art glass ceilings are used to advantage, and resemble the Church of All Souls ceiling of 1903. There is a vivacity in the internal spaces in the Amberg house which is in contrast to the more measured spatiality of Wright's Meyer May house, located only a block away. Marion had written: 'For that period I had great fun designing', and there is certainly a sense of fun in these houses. The dramatic living room in the Adolph Mueller house, the whimsical bird coop, or the attention to the detail of the stable have a lightness of touch that is worth noting. The E P Irving house (1910), Millikin Place, Decatur, has some odd, even humorous details: for example, a section of the attic stair was cut away and replaced by glass to allow light into the hall through an art glass ceiling. The external decoration on the Amberg house renders it rather painterly, fanciful and even feminine, and the internal spaces are made more dramatic by the elevation of the building above the sidewalk level. Janice Pregliasco describes the entry to the Amberg house well: 'Inside the low dark vestibule is a stairway that, upon ascending, turns to face a wall of delicate yellow and clear glass windows. For someone living in this house, this sequence — of first being exposed to light, then sheltered from it, and finally ascending into it — made the everyday act of coming home a transcendental experience'.[20]

Walter and Marion had worked on a number of projects together, in Wright's office and then on the Millikin Place project where Walter designed the landscape. They married in June 1911 in Michigan City, and Marion became a partner in Walter's Steinway Hall office. The office expanded, and the commissions flowed in. Marion developed the characteristic single board presentation of plan, section and perspective set in a beneficent and often orientalised landscape. Her drawings for the Stinson Memorial Library, their own house and the H M Mess house illustrate this to perfection. These drawings, together with the Mason City Rock Crest–Rock Glen perspective and the Canberra drawings allow the viewer to appreciate the virtuosity of her work.

In 1912 the Griffins' entry for the design of Canberra was selected by the competition jury, and in 1914 they left the United States for Australia. They set up offices in Sydney and Melbourne; the latter was to deal with the Canberra project and the Sydney office was for their private work. Marion supervised the Sydney office and she was assisted by American colleagues Roy Lippincott, Genevieve Lippincott (Walter's sister) and George Elgh. Until 1917 many commissions were handled in the Sydney office including the Leeton and Griffith town plans in New South Wales, the Tuggeranong town plan in the Australian Capital Territory,

Collins House, Newman College, Cafe Australia in Melbourne and the Sydney University campus plan. Griffin spent considerable time in the Melbourne office working on Canberra but still had time for the projects in the Sydney office. Marion was the driving force behind many projects (the Capitol Theatre, Cafe Australia and Newman College), and it has been generally acknowledged that she was responsible for the brilliant, geometric Capitol Theatre ceiling. She provides an insight into Griffin's role:

> We did get hold of him [Walter Burley Griffin] for moments, usually late at night. One day he came in with a sketch on a usual small sized envelope which he made on the train ... He had been given the job of doing the Newman College at Melbourne University. The whole thing was there on that envelope plus what he had in his head. It was settled and so it was built but that was war to the finish for everything was totally different from anything anybody had in mind.[21]

Throughout 'Magic' Marion gives Griffin most of the creative credit, and takes very little herself. However, she was intimately connected with the practice and very much responsible for its operation. It was Marion who taught the young apprentices in Australia and in India, a role she took very seriously and which in no small way was inspired by the model of her mother. It was Marion who worked long hours without complaining, and who often did battle with the authorities. This letter to Griffin's sister in May 1916 gives some idea of her daily life:

> The only thing I take any interest in is doing the work and I keep at it long after I have a curl in my back bone, and am sick with fatigue. I don't know what will happen unless some of you folks come over and play with me. It's a queer kind of life Walter and I are living full of a kind of satisfaction but altogether too intense but with all its strenuousness there is a peace of soul which after all is all that is necessary. The currents we are pulling against have not yet proved too strong for us and we'll paddle on as long as we can. I have a notion we're helping clear a way through the jungle but Lord how the beasts do bite and snap. At present I am doing mostly listing of native plants for planting now for both private work and the Federal Capital. I ought to have a go at it now but guess I'll go stretch on Walter's desk and go to sleep instead.[22]

It would be remiss to leave the 'larger than life' theme without referring to Marion Mahony Griffin as a public person, and this was a role she took on with gusto throughout her life by writing articles and giving speeches and public lectures. A year after she arrived in Australia she spoke to the National Council of Women at the Royal Society's rooms on the topic of 'Women as architects'. Her strong message made quite an impression and it was reported in the Sydney *Daily Telegraph* on 12 October 1915:

> Mrs Walter B. Griffin said that she could talk indefinitely about architecture, but about women in architecture there was nothing really to say except what one would say of women in any field that was not a matter of pure routine. The notion that 'women can't do this and can't do that' was all of a piece that it required special genius on the part of certain men to do this or that. It was a theory that truckled to the vanity of some and the laziness of others. Those experienced in modern methods of teaching children would have seen how all children could do anything their elders were willing or have the opportunity to do so. All that was necessary was to rouse interest and effort.

> The first essential was to be sure we had outgrown the belief in slavery, which was but another way of saying that we had outgrown the belief in privilege in any form, or the right of any party of a community to dictate to any other part of the community. All our troubles arose from that same fundamental false standard. So long as men considered they were superior to women and so privileged to work, or women considered themselves superior to men and so privileged not to work it would perpetuate the same standard in other fields brought about ...

> It was necessary for women to take up work in the same spirit as men did. If we wanted anything in the world we must pay the price for it, and to succeed in the more interesting lines meant the greater effort. Women could not expect to take up a profession like architecture because it was specially fitted to ladies. As a man did so a woman must — work day times, night times. It must form the basis of her dreams. She must give it her Saturdays and her Sundays and go without holidays. There might come a time when with a better social system some of the burden for not earning a living might be removed, but any real accomplishment would always mean a life's devotion. Women could not expect to accomplish it with less than the men had to give. At present men had to give up practically all social life, and women must expect to do the same. That did not mean she had no relation with her fellow creatures, but those relations would be in connection with and in relation to her work.

> To solve an architectural problem satisfactorily you must consider it as an element in a community to be considered in connection with its neighbours said the speaker, 'not only the community plan is part of your problem, but the landscaping and planting of the grounds. You are still unfinished till you have designed the furniture, and the pottery and draperies, which must be totally different from the old handicraft so beautiful in handicraft times, but so unfit in the midst of work done by greatly superior tools, which we have barely begun to make proper use of'.[23]

I have focused here on Marion Mahony Griffin's role in the making of architecture over a period of some 45 years, touching on her creative contribution to Frank Lloyd Wright's studio, her leading role in the office of Von Holst and Fyfe, and her collaboration with Walter Burley Griffin. As I have suggested earlier, Marion Griffin was ahead of her time in the way she integrated the various aspects of her life, and while childless herself managed to involve the world of children in her own. The advice she offered women in this speech of 1915 was also ahead of its time. If women wished to succeed there was no reason why they should not, but they had to be prepared to dedicate themselves to the task. She believed that 'the civilisation of a people is expressed in many of its arts but recorded most permanently in its structures', and she dedicated most of her life to that

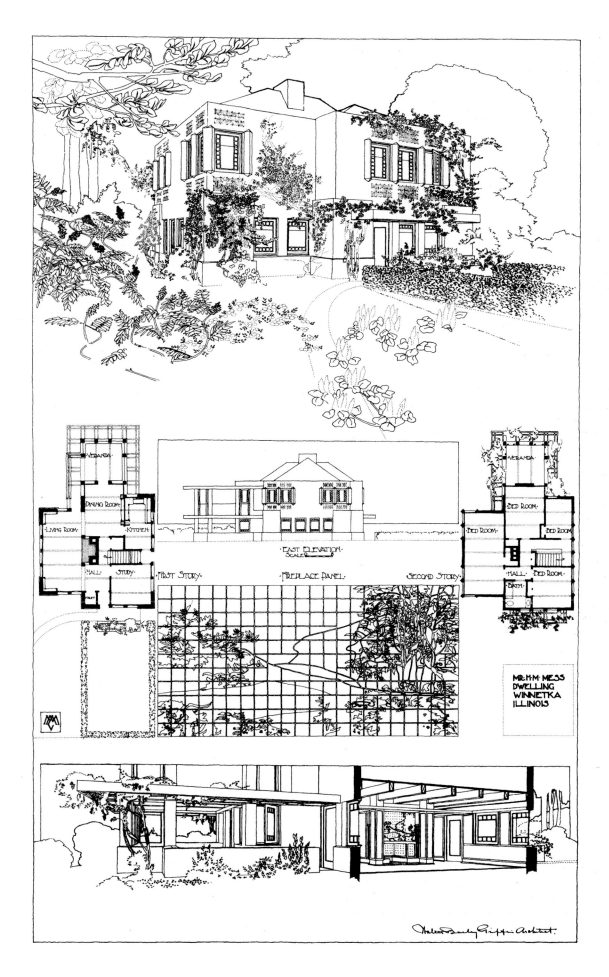

EAST ELEVATION
SCALE

FIRST STORY   FIREPLACE PANEL   SECOND STORY

·VERANDA·

·DINING ROOM·

·LIVING ROOM·   ·KITCHEN·

·HALL·   ·STUDY·

·VERANDA·

·BED ROOM·

·BED ROOM·   ·BED ROOM·

·HALL·   ·BED ROOM·

·BATH·

MR·H·M·MESS
DWELLING
WINNETKA
ILLINOIS

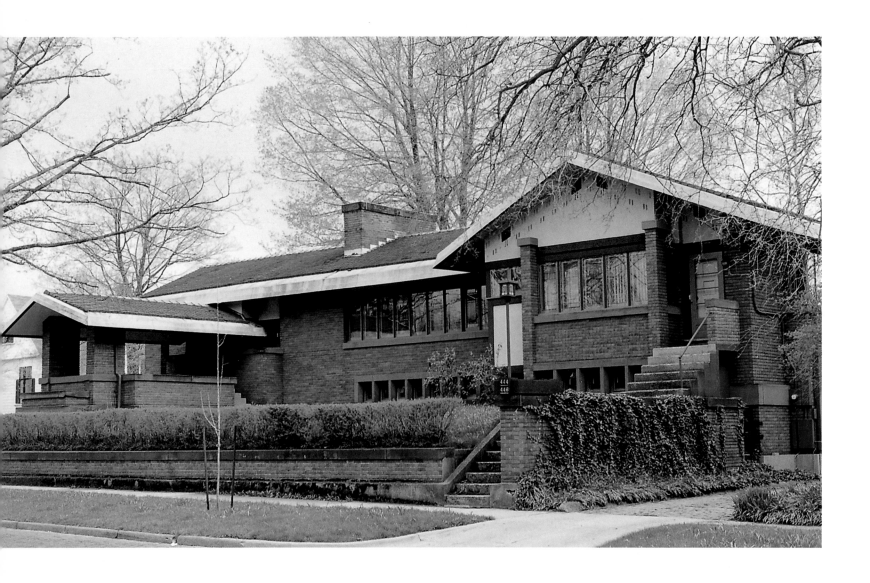

purpose. Returning to Chicago after Griffin's death in 1937 and after almost a quarter of a century in Australia she wrote in 'Magic': 'Now I left Castlecrag, truly a bit of paradise on earth to take on the next adventure, the return to the land where I was born, to put my shoulder to the wheel of moulding the destiny of my country to break down its barriers in economic thinking, transform it, the only democratic community in the world into a wholesome community'.

Marion spent the rest of her life writing and on occasions designing. Her keen intelligence and her many contributions to the making of architecture and its representation assure Marion Mahony Griffin a place in architectural history and in women's cultural history. In an age characterised by competition, and the desire to create stars or 'heroes', the collaboration between Marion and Walter Burley Griffin (along with other famous architectural partnerships such as the Mackintoshes or the Eames) provides another paradigm through which creative activity can be viewed. Marion Mahony Griffin emerges as larger than life but not as an architectural hero.

Above: D M Amberg house, Grand Rapids, Michigan, 1909. Designed by Marion while working with Hermann Von Holst, this substantial house reflects something of Wright's Prairie style as well as her own unique sense of design.
Photograph courtesy Anna Rubbo, Sydney, 1993.

Previous page: H M Mess house, Winnetka, Illinois, 1912. Ink on linen, 96 × 59 cm, with 'MMG' monogram. This beautiful style of presentation, devised by Walter and Marion about 1910, has left a unique legacy of ink on linen and watercolour on silk architectural renderings.
Courtesy the Mary and Leigh Block Museum of Art, Northwestern University, Illinois (1985.1.109).

Notes

1. For a fuller discussion of their partnership see A Rubbo, 'Marion and Walter Burley Griffin: a creative partnership', *Architectural Theory Review*, vol 1, no 1, 1996, journal of the Department of Architecture University of Sydney, pp 78–95. See also W Chadwick and I de Courtrivron, eds, *Significant others: creativity and intimate partnership*, Thames & Hudson, London, 1993.

2. New religions such as theosophy attracted a number of architects in the late nineteenth century including Sullivan, Bragdon, Wright and the Griffins in the United States, and Lethaby, Gaudi, Lutyens, Berlage and Behrens in Europe. The Griffins were influenced by theosophical ideas, and like many of their contemporaries were also drawn to the nature philosophies of Whitman and Emerson. Through the Theosophical Society eastern thinking became popular, and theosophy appealed to people seeking truth and freedom of thought. Walter Burley Griffin contributed articles to the society's monthly magazine, *Advance! Australia*, on such topics as 'The outdoor arts in Australia' and 'Building for nature'. In 1913 Rudolf Steiner broke away from theosophy and founded the Anthroposophical Society. Steiner conceived of anthroposophy as a path of knowledge to guide the spiritual in the human being to the spiritual in the universe. One of Steiner's concerns was that materialism and the state were increasingly dominating the spiritual aspects of life, and this was a view that the Griffins shared. Steiner's educational philosophies, for example, were directed at the spiritual and artistic development of children in their early years, ideas that Marion took up enthusiastically.

3. See P Proudfoot, *The secret plan of Canberra*, University of NSW Press, Sydney, 1994, where he suggests that the design for Canberra is first and foremost an ancient cosmic schema.

4. J Roe, 'The magical world of Marion Mahony Griffin: culture and community in Castlecrag in the interwar years', in Shirley Fitzgerald and Garry Wotherspoon, eds, *Minorities: cultural diversity in Sydney*, NSW State Library Press, Sydney, 1995, p 96. For further discussion on Marion Mahony Griffin and anthroposophy see A Rubbo, 'The numinous world of Marion Mahony Griffin: architect, artist, writer' in *Spirit and place: art in Australia 1861–1996*, Museum of Contemporary Art, Sydney, 1996, pp 123–31.

5. For further excellent photographs of the American work see Mati Maldre and Paul Kruty, *Walter Burley Griffin in America*, University of Illinois Press, Illinois, 1996.

6. See J Weirick, '*The magic of America*: vision and text' in J Duncan and M Gates, eds, *Walter Burley Griffin: a re-view*, Monash University Gallery, Victoria, 1988, pp 5–15.

7. Marion Mahony Griffin, 'The magic of America', vol 4, p 130.

8. Hull House was established in 1889 by Jane Addams and Ellen Gates Starr. Modelled on London's Toynbee Hall settlement house, its charter was to serve the sick, the poor and the oppressed, and to investigate and improve housing and working conditions in the industrial districts of Chicago. Hull House became a centre for civic and social life for working men and women, immigrant groups and children, and attracted reformers and professionals to its causes. Educationalist John Dewey maintained a long connection with Hull House as did Marion's cousin, the architect Dwight Perkins. Frank Lloyd Wright gave his famous address, 'The art and craft of the machine', at Hull House. Jane Addams was awarded the Nobel Peace Prize in 1931.

9. James Weirick suggests that Frank Lloyd Wright may have been influenced by Marion's student project when embarking on the extensions to his Oak Park studio. See J Weirick, 'Marion at M.I.T.', *Transition*, RMIT, Melbourne, Winter 1988, pp 49–54

10. G C Manson, *Frank Lloyd Wright to 1910: the first golden age*, Van Nostrand, New York, 1985, p 217.

11. *Frank Lloyd Wright: studies and executed buildings*, reprint of the 1910 edition with foreword by Vincent Scully, Rizzoli, New York, 1986. Originally published as *Ausgeführte Bauten und Entwürfe von Frank Lloyd Wright* and *Frank Lloyd Wright: Ausgeführte Bauten*, by Ernst Wasmuth, Berlin, 1910 and 1911 respectively.

12. Louise Lightfoot, 'Memories of the Burley Griffins', no date, unpublished, Willoughby Library, New South Wales.

13. A Rubbo, 'Marion Mahony Griffin: a portrait', in J Duncan and M Gates, eds, p 18.

14. P Harrison, *Walter Burley Griffin: landscape architect*, National Library of Australia, Canberra, 1995, p 82.

15. H Allen Brooks, *The Prairie School: Frank Lloyd Wright and his midwest contemporaries*, University of Toronto Press, Toronto, 1972, pp 79–80.

16. Letter from Frank Lloyd Wright to Robin Boyd, 14 June 1946, J P Getty Museum, Los Angeles.

17. B Gill, *Many masks: a life of Frank Lloyd Wright*, Putnam, New York, 1987, p 187.

18. See A Rubbo, 'Marion Mahony Griffin: a portrait', in J Duncan and M Gates, eds, pp 15–24, for a more extended discussion.

19. Marion Mahony Griffin, 'The magic of America', vol 3, p 172.

20. J Pregliasco, 'The life and work of Marion Mahony Griffin', in *The Prairie School: design vision for the midwest* (issued as *Museum Studies*, vol 21, no 2), the Art Institute of Chicago, 1995, pp 164–81. While useful this article makes claims for sole authorship for a number of buildings by Marion Mahony Griffin for which no evidence is given, for example, the Griffins' own house in Winnetka, the Cafe Australia, Newman College and the Capitol Theatre.

21. Marion Mahony Griffin, 'The magic of America', vol 2, p 240.

22. Ibid, vol 2, p 27.

23. *Daily Telegraph*, Sydney, 12 October, 1915.

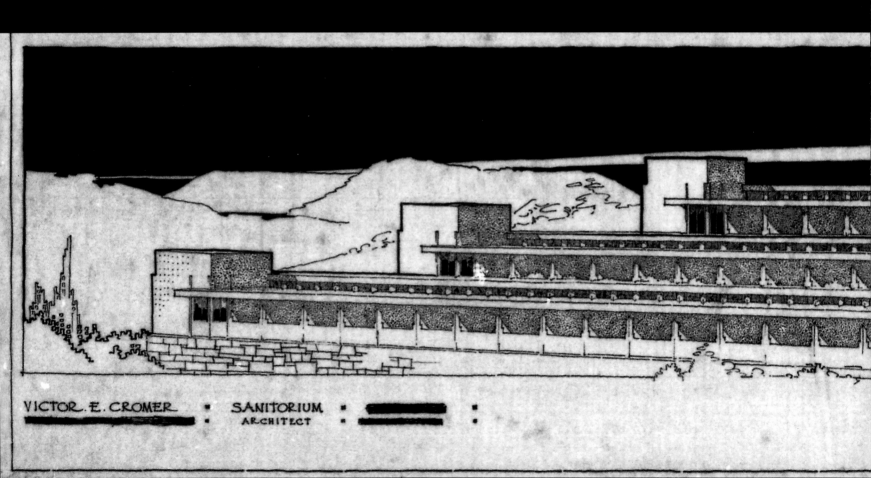

VICTOR. E. CROMER ▪ SANITORIUM ▪ ▬▬▬▬ ▪
ARCHITECT ▪ ▬▬▬▬ ▪

WORK OF THE GRIFFINS   JAMES WEIRICK

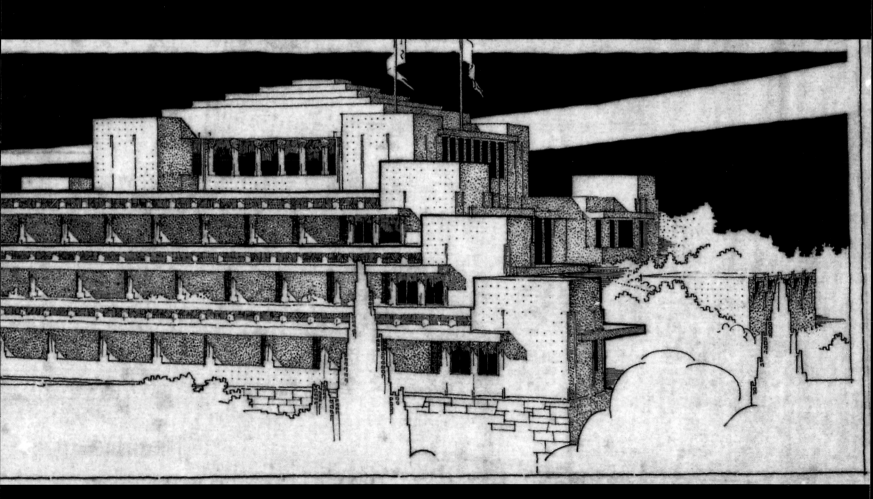

... their architecture is the fruit by which ye shall know them. It is the hero of every epoch. Into it can be read the destiny, doctrines and predispositions of a time, a being, a place, a material ... A building is a language which tells us all. It cannot cheat.

This first reference to Walter Burley Griffin in contemporary fiction can be found in a little-read novel of the late 1960s, Lawrence Durrell's *Tunc*: 'violet the Saronic Gulf, topaz Hymettus, lilac bronze the marbles' — the scene is the steps of the Parthenon — in the half light of evening an audience is assembled to hear an expatriate architect, Caradoc, deliver a lecture on his art:

'"All day," he said on a hoarse and delphic note, "I have been locked in meditation, wondering what I was going to tell you tonight about this ... Wondering how much I would *dare* to reveal of what I know." He had unwittingly fallen upon a splendid opening gambit. The hint of mysteries, of the occult, was most appropriate to the place as well as the gathering. There was a stir of interest ...' And indeed, before the sudden end of this scene, the rambling but occasionally lucid Caradoc adds to the mystery of the moment by revealing a most unexpected source for his ideas: 'in the smallest thing we build is buried the lore of centuries. All this and much more occurred to me in my youth as a prentice architect playing about among the foundations of Canberra with Griffin, one of Sullivan's lads'.[1]

The conjuring up of Canberra, Walter Burley Griffin and Louis Sullivan at this fictional moment is extraordinary, even for Lawrence Durrell, but the allusions are surprisingly accurate. Griffin and Sullivan passionately believed that architecture is a language which tells us all. Griffin's Canberra plan was an ambitious extension of this idea; and there were 'prentice architects' who long remembered the experience of working with Griffin on the beginnings of the city:

> We his staff — ten of us, perhaps — tried to help him make his dreams come true. Visionaries all, we were said to be men chasing the shadows of a dream! Canberra — the mythical city — could never take on form and substance, we were told. Pessimists and obstructionists did their best — or their worst — but the work went on. Inspired by our leader, we calculated and drew — gave the best that was within us, and put on paper those abstruse notes he handed us. Infected with his energy and indomitable patience, we grew like him ... And so by degrees, with calculations and drawings, we put our leader's dreams and poems into that completed whole which we call Canberra.[2]

Canberra, the mythical city — there is something about Griffin's work, particularly the work which has come to us from his long collaboration with Marion Mahony —which seems to carry with it a hint of mysteries, a hint of the occult. Was Durrell right in sensing this? The subject has excited considerable speculation but the evidence is difficult to weigh. Essentially there is the evidence of the work and there is the evidence of the lives — and on the face of it, they do not correlate. The Griffins' strange architecture and powerful city plans date from a time when they had no known links with esoteric or occult groups and no known interest in esoteric thought. The situation changes dramatically in Sydney in the 1920s. From 1926 onwards, both Walter and Marion were closely associated with esoteric groups — theosophists, anthroposophists and others — but there is no discernible change in the design work of their practice, at least until they went to India in the mid 1930s.

There are two explanations for this conundrum. The first advances the notion that there is an occult conspiracy behind the Griffins' early work: it is not possible to document their esoteric sources because they kept everything secret. According to this argument, there is a 'secret plan of Canberra' based on the 'cosmic canon of the ancients' which the Griffins guarded 'just as the medieval master masons guarded their secrets'. In Australia, this explanation shows alarming signs of becoming the conventional wisdom.[3]

The second explanation, based on a close study of the Griffins' lives, argues that although their work is characterised by strong geometries and expressionist forms, there is nothing specifically esoteric or 'theosophical' about this, indeed quite the reverse. The Griffins were opposed to an architecture 'left to a priestcraft of its own'[4] and sought to employ straightforward symbolism. It was their life experiences in Australia which led them into new realms — as American idealists under constant challenge, they found themselves on a spiritual journey which, by 1930, had brought them to the anthroposophy and 'occult science' of Rudolf Steiner (1861–1925).

When Walter and Marion became interested in theosophy and anthroposophy they made no secret of it — they publicly proclaimed their enthusiasms and allegiances in public lectures, radio broadcasts, published articles, community discussion groups, plays and festivals. The Griffin office undertook a number of design projects for 'theosophical' clients from 1926 onwards. Prior to that date, there are no known theosophists among the many remarkable people who commissioned work from their practice. In terms of formal links, the Griffins supported many causes championed by the Sydney lodge of the Theosophical Society in the 1920s, such as the Crusade for a Beautiful Australia, *Advance! Australia* magazine and the *Advance! Australia* Round Table — but they did not actually join the Theosophical Society itself. In 1928, Walter Burley Griffin was a foundation member of the New Renascence Society, a 'New Age' group established in Sydney by the theosophist and spiritual healer Victor Cromer. The New Renascence Society does not seem to have survived the death of Victor Cromer in 1930, however by that date the Griffins had established contact with the small group of Rudolf Steiner's followers in Sydney. This had a profound effect on both Walter and Marion. From 1930 onwards, Steiner's esoteric philosophy became central to their lives. In Sydney, both Griffins formally joined the St John Group of the Anthroposophical Society, Marion in September 1930 and Walter in September 1931.[5]

As a progression in time, the Griffins' spiritual journey moves from Emersonian beginnings in Chicago, to high social and political idealism at the time of their entry in the Canberra competition; a testing of that idealism in their first seven years in Australia; defeat over Canberra and suppressed despair in the early 1920s; a new beginning in Sydney in 1925 associated with the Castlecrag venture, a new circle of friends and the Sydney theosophists; a search for inner direction which the Theosophical Society does not fulfil; and then the discovery of Steiner and anthroposophy.

As a progression in belief, this represents a movement from liberal protestantism to a distinctive form of occultism. In Chicago, both Walter and Marion were associated with the stream of religious thought which flowed from the providential and revelatory beginnings of the Puritan experience in New England, through the religious fervour of the Great Awakening in the years before the American Revolution, to the liberal ideals of transcendentalism in the 1830s — the teachings of Ralph Waldo Emerson, William Ellery Channing, Theodore Parker and others — and following the Civil War, the Free Religious movement and the embrace of comparative religion at the World's Parliament of Religions hosted in Chicago in 1893.[6]

The details of the Griffins' respective religious backgrounds in Chicago have never been studied in depth, but they are highly relevant to their design work.

From the 1890s until she left Chicago for Australia in 1914, Marion Mahony was a member of the Church of All Souls, Evanston — a Unitarian congregation of decidedly independent stamp whose pastor throughout this period was the Reverend James Vila Blake — poet, philosopher and 'poetic preacher of the soul'. James Vila Blake (1842–1928) was one of the leaders of the liberal wing of the Unitarian Church in the midwest. As a young man, he had been called to succeed Theodore Parker (1810–1860) in his congregation in Boston and so represented in life and character a point of continuity with the philosophical beginnings of American transcendentalism.[7]

One of liberal protestantism's great inheritances from New England transcendentalism was the conviction that the source of religious authority was to be found within the individual. This was the lesson of Emerson's 'Self Reliance' and the heroic cause of Theodore Parker, who did not resign his pulpit like Emerson but worked within the Unitarian fold. To independent thinkers in the Unitarian movement, Theodore Parker was as significant as Luther — just as Luther had transferred the authority of the Christian creed from the Church to the Bible, it was argued, so Parker had transferred it from the Bible to the soul.[8] In Chicago in the 1890s, James Vila Blake preached this doctrine in accordance with his commitment to 'Natural Religion':

> anything professing to be religious truth must appeal to the soul to be justified. And as the religious nature grows clearer and higher, age by age, like all the human powers, no dictum of the past can override its clear decision in the present … Natural Religion does away with the pretence of divine authority. The religious nature is not created by any institution, nor depends on a form, nor is bound to a doctrine. In its divine activity it neither awaits nor permits an authoritative book. It is itself the source of all form and creeds.[9]

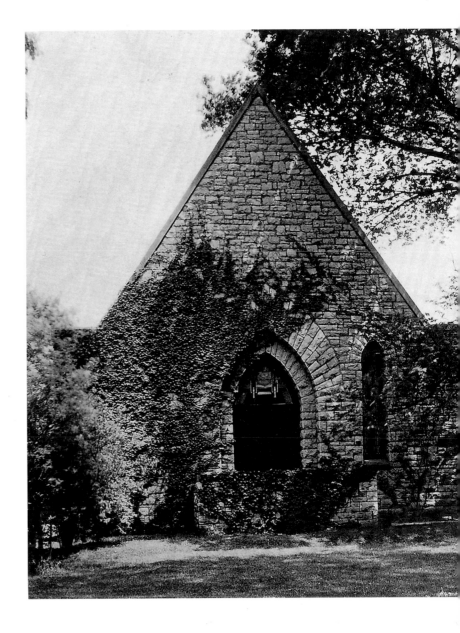

Above: West-front view Church of All Souls, Evanston, Illinois, 1902 — 1904, designed by Marion Mahony. From *The Western Architect*, vol XVIII, no 9, September 1912. Courtesy James Weirick

Previous pages: Victor E Cromer Sanitorium [*sic*] for Spiritual Healing, Covecrag, Sydney, 1927, designed by Walter Burley Griffin. Ink on linen, 13 × 72 cm. Courtesy Mary and Leigh Block Museum of Art, Northwestern University, Illinois (1985.1.74).

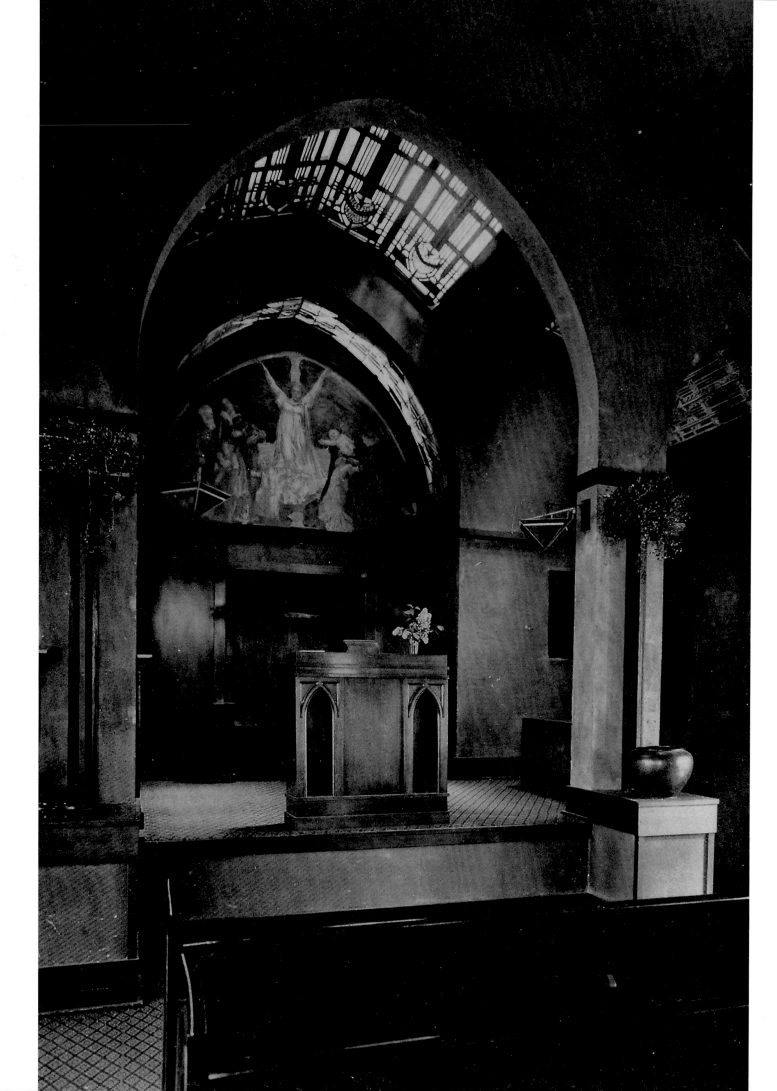

To James Vila Blake, there was a common basis to the great faiths of the world which institutional authority would always deny. 'After a time', he wrote, 'a new prophet is needed and arises, to bring forth religion once more into *the simplicity of the spirit and the authority of the soul*'.[10]

The Church of All Souls was organised in 1891 by a group of Unitarian women in Evanston, then a suburban village on the northern outskirts of Chicago. The first service was led by the Reverend Jenkin Lloyd Jones (1843–1918), the uncle of Frank Lloyd Wright. In 1892 James Vila Blake agreed to be the regular minister for this small but active congregation which included Marion's mother, Clara Hamilton Mahony and her aunt, Myra Perkins. The group met for more than a decade in homes and rented rooms until they raised the funds to build their church. Through worship and 'friendly fellowship' the life of the church was filled with poetry, theatre, song — it was a group devoted to discussion, reading circles, musical performances, play readings and progressive political causes.

In 1902 Marion Mahony was commissioned to design the first permanent place of worship for the Church of All Souls. This small stone chapel was her first independent work as an architect and the only building she ever published under her own name. The site was a narrow suburban lot on Evanston's Chicago Avenue. Hemmed in by High Victorian frame houses, the scheme that was built was a simple, traditional form, exquisitely scaled. An earlier concept, more adventurous but awkwardly resolved, was rejected by the building committee. In its neighbourhood setting, Marion's Church of All Souls combined a still, strong presence with a sense of inner energy, an effect created by its elemental gothic forms, the attenuated triangle of its gable front, the balanced asymmetry of its central entranceway set against a single lancet window and its rough-hewn masonry walls. The entrance, deep-set under the dramatic voussoirs of an indented, pointed arch, was approached indirectly from the street to reveal the chapel as a sculptural composition within the confines of its lot. The auditorium, designed for a congregation of 110, was a simple space, rectangular in plan under the open trusses of a timber panelled roof. The chancel was divided from the auditorium by a structural screen wall which repeated the arch motif of the entranceway. The floor of the chancel was raised as a stage above the congregation with the pulpit in burnished oak centrally placed, top lit by patterned skylights and backed by a figurative mural. This was located in the lunette of the east wall, above a tall-backed speaker's bench. There was no altar. The mural, somewhat Pre-Raphaelite in expression, was also the work of Marion Mahony and had as its central figure an angel, wings outstretched, encompassing 'all souls' in spiritual embrace. The composition was ringed with a glory of radiant light from a band of illuminated glass and crowned by a higher abstraction of angel forces in the art-glass patterns of the central skylight.

The interior surfaces in tinted stucco were trimmed with oak skirtings, rails and planter brackets to articulate the form and inner nature of the simple structural system of

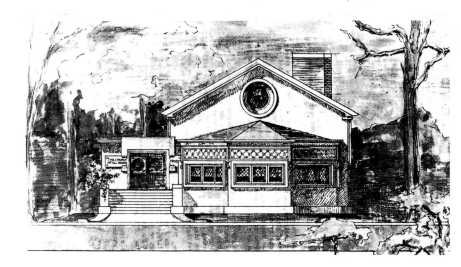

piers, buttresses and load–bearing walls. The auditorium was illuminated by prismatic lights, suspended in pairs from the roof beams — inverted pyramidal forms in glass which glowed in gold–green hues and cast expanded patterns of light upward, above the assembled congregation.

The simplicity, strength and inner depth of the design was in total harmony with the Covenant of Faith which the congregation adopted in 1894:

> These things are commonly believed among us, but are to be reasoned by each one for himself, conscientiously, with the freedom of the spirit:
>
> That religion is natural, helpful, needful, the witness within us of the Infinite and Eternal;
> That the many things of the Universe have their being in One Life, the One-in-All, the 'Power not ourselves that makes for righteousness,' the Eternal God, Our Father;
> That the Universe is beautiful and beneficent Order;
> That we ought to give reverence to all Prophets of religion, who 'have wrought righteousness,' whose teachings are holy and inspiring Scriptures;
> That we ought to work for the good of man, to make the world better;
> That character is the supreme matter — not the beliefs we hold, but what we are *in heart and life*;
> That in the soul of man awakes the sense of things eternal, and of belonging unto them, whereby we have the earnest of immortal life;
> That we ought to hold fast to the freedom of the spirit for ourselves and for all men.[11]

The key to Marion Mahony's life and work is to be found in this statement of faith, to which she committed herself as a young woman in the 1890s.

Walter Burley Griffin shared a similar experience of liberal protestantism in his Chicago upbringing. The Griffin family — of Puritan descent — were members of First Congregational Church, Oak Park until 1893. In that year, the family moved to the semi-rural suburb of Elmhurst on

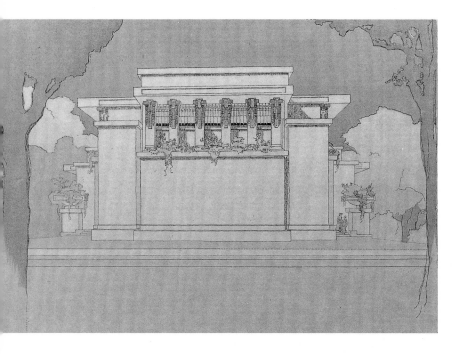

the western fringe of the metropolis. There they joined a small Congregationalist Church, which was named Christ Church in 1897 and re-organised on non-denominational lines in a radical but generous-hearted spirit 'for the purpose of uniting as far as possible, all the representatives of truly Christian faiths in vital membership and active work'. In the American tradition of the covenanted community, a new constitution was established which retained the essential 'congregationalist' principle that governance of the church was 'vested in the body of believers who compose it'.

The church, which stood across the road from the Griffin family home, was built in 1890, a Shingle-style structure — gothic in spirit — with a high pitched roof, half-timbered gables and a shingle-clad spire. The original architect is unrecorded but around 1900 Walter Burley Griffin designed a scheme for its austere auditorium which included a stencilled frieze, Sullivanesque in inspiration. The pattern consisted of a series of flowing, intertwined lines, stem-like and luxuriant, punctuated periodically by re-entrant vees, suggesting the embedded presence of pure form in nature. Painted in gold on a dull green background, Griffin cut the stencils and carried out the work himself. The effect was to bind the room together in accordance with the congregation's first article of faith: 'This Church is established in faith in God for the spiritual welfare of this community'.[12]

In doctrine, Christ Church, Elmhurst was not as liberal as the Church of All Souls. Unlike the Evanston Unitarians' embrace of comparative religion and the conspicuous absence of Christian references in their Covenant of Faith, Christ Church, as its name proclaimed, stood steadfast in its mission 'to propagate the essential teachings of Jesus of Nazareth'. Unlike James Vila Blake's declaration of independence from biblical authority, the constitution of Christ Church called for belief that 'the Bible is the God-given record of principle and example for spiritual growth, and the true interpretation of life and nature'. However, in terms of an active social mission, Christ Church seems to have been more progressive than James Vila Blake's congregation. The Church of All Souls may have been renowned for its advanced political views but it was not involved in social outreach or a 'settlement' program. The constitution of the Elmhurst congregation, on the other hand, called for Christ Church to 'take an active part in works of true moral reform, benevolence, and charity; and especially seek to benefit the poor, the afflicted, and the stranger'. An outreach program, in which Griffin's mother played a prominent part, culminated in the construction of a widely acclaimed Community House in 1913.[13]

Walter Burley Griffin did not receive the commission to design this building but he was a member of Frank Lloyd Wright's office during the long campaign to design the most radical 'community house' in Chicago, the Abraham Lincoln Center, a project conceived by Wright's uncle, Jenkin Lloyd Jones, as an independent expression of the 'ethical sense of the community'.[14] The preliminary designs for Unity Temple and Unity House in Oak Park were also in preparation in the

Above: Unity Temple, Oak Park, Illinois, 1905–1908, designed by Frank Lloyd Wright. Perspective drawing by Marion Mahony. Lithograph, 46 × 68 cm.
From *Ausgeführte Bauten und Entwürfe von Frank Lloyd Wright*, Ernst Wasmuth, Berlin, 1910. Private collection, Sydney.

Previous pages left: Church of All Souls, Evanston, Illinois. Interior view to chancel showing leaded stained-glass skylights and the mural painted by Marion.
From *The Western Architect*, vol XVIII, no 9, September 1912. Courtesy James Weirick.

Previous pages right: First version of the Church of All Souls, Evanston, Illinois, 1902, designed by Marion Mahony. Elevational study, west front.
From *The Prairie School Review*, vol III, no 2, 2nd quarter, 1966, p 7. Courtesy of the New-York Historical Society

period before Griffin left Wright's studio to establish his own practice at the beginning of 1906. These projects, together with the Larkin building in Buffalo, are similar in spirit to the corner-piered, cubical buildings Griffin designed throughout his career. Of course, Marion Mahony was also a member of Wright's Oak Park studio at that time. Her involvement in the Unity Temple project is documented in the perspectives she prepared of this profoundly significant building which were considered to be among her finest work from the moment they were drawn.[15]

The current of liberal protestantism which was so much part of the lives of Walter Burley Griffin and Marion Mahony in their Chicago years was combined in more than equal measure with that other dimension of America's destiny, the 'civic religion' of democracy and freedom.[16] Here a long strand of influence can be traced from Walt Whitman back to Thomas Jefferson — but the immediate source of inspiration for the Griffins was Louis Sullivan and his over-arching conception of democracy as the highest form of emancipation in all spheres of life. This view was publicly proclaimed for the first time in Sullivan's celebrated address 'To the Young Man in Architecture', delivered in June 1900 to the Architectural League of America in the Auditorium building in Chicago — with Walter Burley Griffin in the audience. The influence of Louis Sullivan would be seen in Griffin's work and writings from that time. As Griffin stated in 1913:

> Democracy, as I define it, is independence of thought. Democracy in politics is independence of action, but action must be dominated by thought, and unless our thought is independent we are still in a feudalistic environment ... Feudalism, as Louis H. Sullivan has expressed it ... is carrying into a time of democracy ... the real essential mental attitude of the Middle Ages, looking to authority for our beliefs and thought.[17]

In 1914, Marion Mahony advanced similar views fused with the values and beliefs of James Vila Blake. 'Democracy is a fundamental world-principle which is simply a belief in authority from within, instead of from without. It depends on the superiority of the spiritual element: that one element which lifts human beings out of the animal kingdom'.[18] Both these statements were made in Australia and of course, the circumstance which had brought Walter and Marion so far from their midwest milieu was their success in the Australian Federal Capital competition — and after some delay, the opportunity for Walter to direct the design and construction of the city. Their next seven years in Australia would submit their idealistic view of democracy to the severest of tests.

To begin to understand the Griffins' spiritual journey, we must see the preparation of their entry in the Australian Federal Capital competition as the central experience of their lives. Produced in a great flow of creativity in nine weeks at the end of 1911, the Canberra plan is the Griffins' masterwork. The scheme is remarkable for the ideas which informed it, the resolution of those ideas and their artistic expression. Work on the Canberra plan began within months of the Griffins' marriage and it is the first great

achievement of their personal and professional partnership, a perfect expression of their complementary talents and personalities. This was described in memorable terms many years later by Eric Nicholls (1902–1965), their Australian partner: 'Walter has been characterised as the "thought" and Marion as the "will". As soon as Walter produced one of his many remarkable ideas then Marion set about imple-menting it, and Griffin with his tenacious nature would not depart from it'.[19]

Although we cannot trace the actual evolution of the design — none of the preliminary studies are known to have survived — it is clear that the principal planning ideas behind the Canberra scheme can be attributed to Walter Burley Griffin and the superb set of presentation drawings to Marion Mahony. The extensive architectural proposals for the city appear to be a collaborative achievement. Indeed the brilliance of the scheme derives from the sense that ideas and their representation came together in a controlled outpouring of creative energy. This is nowhere more apparent than in the great rendering of the city plan and the endlessly inventive building designs schematically indicated in Marion's sectional elevations and perspective from Mount Ainslie. The light of inspiration shines through these drawings — glowing, confident, unique. From their Chicago office, the Griffins envisioned 'a city not like any other city in the world',[20] not just a new city for a new nation — a democratic city for a democratic nation. Griffin made this very clear when he arrived in Australia for the first time in 1913:

> Australia, of most democratic tendencies and bold radical government, may well be expected to look upon her great future, and with it her Federal capital, with characteristic big vision ... Australia has ... so well learned some of the lessons taught through modern civilisation, as seen in broad perspective from her isolated vantage point, that we may be justified in believing that she will fully express the possibilities for individual freedom, comfort, and convenience for public spirit, wealth and splendor of the great democratic city ideal for which her capital offers the best opportunity so far.[21]

At the time they planned Canberra, both Walter and Marion were political idealists, American progressives imbued with a Jeffersonian commitment to freedom and democracy. Their Canberra was conceived very much in the American tradition of liberal and progressive thought.

To indicate how this American spirit can find physical form in the city, we need only consider New York's Central Park, designed in the mid-nineteenth century by Frederick Law Olmsted (1822–1903), the doyen of America's first generation of landscape architects. Initially, Central Park seems to be little more that the re-creation of an English romantic landscape in the middle of Manhattan. Yet no matter where one enters from the crush and tumult of the city, the various winding paths lead through an evocation of 'nature' to The Mall: a plaisance, a long formal promenade under a canopy of elms. There on The Mall, the citizens of the city are together again — but everyone is different for the experience of nature they have had. In this great public space, a democratic society re-creates itself, reaffirms its values, experiences the reality of the abstract principles it proclaims.

This is what Griffin hoped to achieve with his plan for Canberra, to embody in the everyday life of the city, the reality of the democratic experience. Here he was clearly inspired not only by the Jeffersonian tradition but also by a specific injunction in Louis Sullivan's *Kindergarten chats*, addressed to the young man in architecture: 'Current ideas concerning democracy are so vague and so shapeless, that the man who shall clarify and define, who shall interpret, create and proclaim in the image of Democracy's fair self, will be the destined man of the hour: the man of all time'.[22]

Walter Burley Griffin — in his own words, a 'radical democrat' — was a member of the Jefferson Club, the politically progressive City Club of Chicago, and the Chicago Single Tax Club.[23] He was an enthusiastic Single Taxer, a committed follower of America's most radical political economist, Henry George (1839–1897), who had a wide following throughout the world, including Australia where he had conducted a highly successful lecture tour in 1890.

With a knowledge filtered through the Single Tax literature of the day, Griffin imagined Australia to be:

> a vast potentially productive undeveloped insular continent … with a people cherishing the highest standards of human rights, with no dire poverty or political corruption … a democracy already in the vanguard of political progress setting a standard for the entire world in its struggle against private monopoly and exploitation.[24]

Griffin's belief that Australia was some sort of new, vital social laboratory generally reflected progressive opinion in America at that time. One source for his ideas was almost certainly an article which appeared in the progressive journal, *The Independent*, about the time the Griffins started work on their entry in the competition:

> in dealing with questions involving the general welfare, in holding the scales even between the rights of men and money and in forecasting the requirements of future generations, Australia has shown a distinct superiority over America. Its social and industrial legislation, has by its humanity and its success, made Australia a hope and inspiration to all English speaking countries.

This article, entitled 'What Australia can teach America', was written by Elwood Mead, an American irrigation engineer who was Chairman of the State Water Supply Commission of Victoria. His appointment, in itself, was indicative of professional opportunities for Americans in the new democracy across the Pacific and his conclusion was compelling:

> The great lesson of Australia to America is … that the people have learned that they can act together wisely and efficiently in carrying out great works for the common good and that, in the development and use of their resources, it is the welfare of the many, rather than the enrichment of the few, which is the governing principle.[25]

Evidence of this commitment to social equity could be seen in the Commonwealth Government's land policy for the Federal capital — the 1901 decision, supported unanimously, to purchase all land in the Federal Territory and hold it in public ownership in perpetuity.[26] Walter Burley Griffin drew particular inspiration from this decision. Public ownership, leasehold tenure and land rent would make possible comprehensive community planning and, in accordance with the principles of Henry George, ensure that 'land earnings, increased from rural to urban proportions purely through the advent of the capital population, will accrue not to private individuals but to the community as a whole'.[27] As Griffin explained in a letter to the Minister for Home Affairs, King O'Malley, after he won the competition:

> I … entered this Australian event to be my first and last competition, solely because I have for many years greatly admired the bold radical steps in politics and economics which your country has dared to take, and which must for a long time set ideals for Europe and America ahead of their possibility of accomplishment … yours is the greatest opportunity the world has afforded for the expression of the great civic ideal. Your advantages are not only in the characteristic Australian idealism and interest in Government activity, but in the fundamental land policy of the Capital … freed from land speculative selfish interest, the natural instincts of the community will guarantee higher aesthetic and social standards.[28]

These were Griffin's ideals and values. For a nation he believed to be 'in the vanguard of political progress', he designed a capital city which was intended to express in its physical form, the true nature of the democratic experience. Everyday activities and the functions of government were so arrayed in the landscape that by simply moving about the city, engaging in everyday life, the powers and responsibilities of government institutions together with the rights and responsibilities of each individual would become manifest. The city would be charged with self-evident truth, its public landscape would have meaning for every citizen.

Griffin's competition entry was essentially a diagram, a set of principles presented in a way 'to force the emphasis of the underlying ideas'. Given the basic structure, a society which Griffin imagined shared his values and particular vision of the democratic experience, would be quite able to develop the city in detail. As conceived in Chicago, the Griffin entry in the Australian Federal Capital competition was a classical utopia: an icon in which, Griffin clearly believed, Australia would see its own tendencies perfected.

Walter Burley Griffin had remarkable abilities as a landscape architect. From the material available to him in Chicago he was able to grasp the significance of Canberra's regional setting, to completely visualise the site; to seize the strategic points; develop great vistas; adjust to subtle changes in relief; work with water, land, sky; and introduce as a constant theme, the life-force of nature. However, the controlling idea of Griffin's Canberra was its social and political symbolism.

This was expressed most forcefully in the design for the central area of the city.[29] Across the broad valley of the Molonglo, Griffin inscribed a great triangle aligned on the

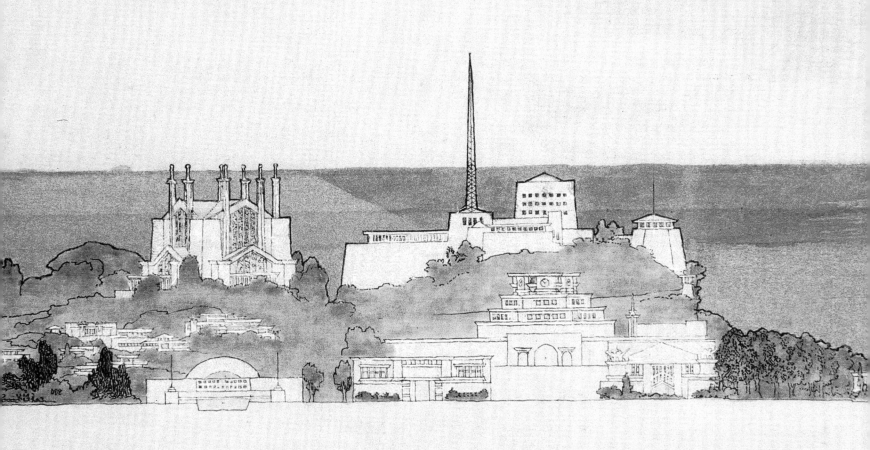

Above: Sectional elevation through the city, submitted in the Federal Capital competition, 1911. Designed by Walter and Marion Griffin. Detail showing the cathedral, main railway station and military college. Ink, watercolour, gouache and gold oil paint on linen.
Courtesy National Archives of Australia (CRS A710, item 45).

mountains which rose above the site. The triangle was defined by tree-lined avenues and spanned the central basin of an impounded lake. For the base of the triangle, Griffin envisaged a continuous zone of activity — a commercial terrace which would be the premier address of the nation, backed by the premier shopping street and a residential district of courtyard apartments. The commercial terrace would overlook the central park of the city, which would reach down to the northern shore of the lake. Various public institutions and cultural facilities would be sited within this park — the national stadium, the opera house, auditoria for music and drama, museums of art, science and technology — in the same way the Art Institute and Field Museum were sited in the public open spaces of Chicago's lakeshore. With its walks and drives along the water's edge, its cultural institutions, its national sporting venue, its vital links with the everyday life of the city's business district — the central park of Griffin's Canberra was conceived as the people's park, the principal place of spontaneous congregation in the capital. The park and the street, freedom and enterprise, would form the base of the triangle. In Griffin's scheme, the base of the triangle would be the People.

Looking across the lake to the Government Centre, the completion of the triangle — the convergence of the

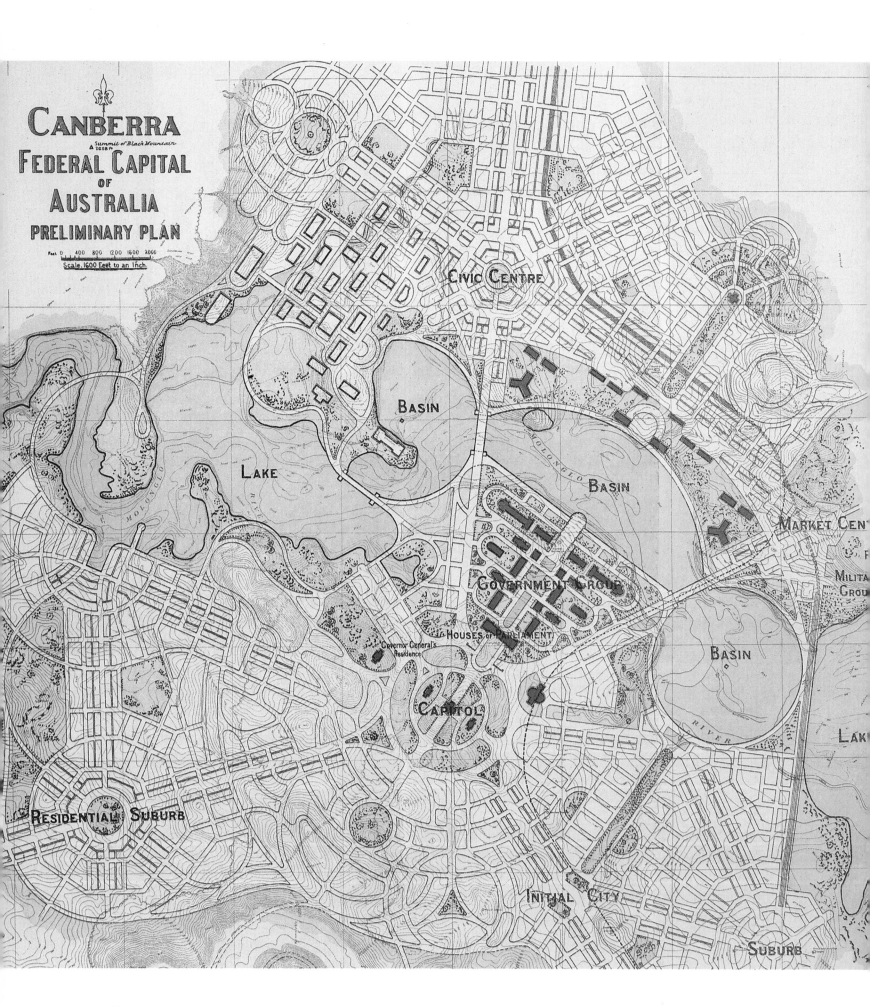

CANBERRA
FEDERAL CAPITAL
OF
AUSTRALIA
PRELIMINARY PLAN

Summit of Black Mountain
△ 2658 ft

Feet 0 400 800 1200 1600 2000
Scale. 1600 Feet to an Inch

CIVIC CENTRE

BASIN

LAKE

MOLONGLO BASIN

MARKET CENTRE

GOVERNMENT GROUP

HOUSES OF PARLIAMENT

Governor General's Residence

MILITARY GROUP

CAPITOL

BASIN

RIVER

LAKE

RESIDENTIAL SUBURB

INITIAL CITY

SUBURB

avenues — would express in compelling physical form, the will of the People.

On the far lakeshore, between the people and their government Griffin sited the Federal Judiciary. Behind this front rank of judicial buildings, the various government departments were symmetrically grouped as a contained bureaucratic entity around a formal court — a Court of Honour. Raised above the Bureaucracy on a natural podium was the Legislature, the Houses of Parliament sited on axis with both chambers clearly expressed, a visible presence in the city.

In the Griffin plan, the Houses of Parliament, though prominent, would not crown the ensemble of government buildings, as a higher hill stood on axis beyond. Kurrajong — or Capital Hill as it is known today — was the climax of the entire scheme. There the convergence of the avenues was resolved in a rotary sweeping around the crest of the hill, marking out the site of three significant buildings. Two of these, though small in scale, gained presence by their function and setting. The first was the official residence of the Governor-General; the second, the official residence of the Prime Minister. Both were sited at the apex of the triangle to emphasise the central place and importance of the Executive. With the two official residences given equal prominence, Griffin also managed to express the curious disposition of executive authority under the Australian Constitution. The view over the Houses of Parliament to the central park and business district of the Capital, affirmed that the Executive required the support of a parliamentary majority and ultimately, the support of a majority of the people.

The central triangle of Griffin's Canberra thus arranged the functions of the government in relation to the life of the city to express the very nature and workings of representative democracy. At one level, this exercise in civic design was a timeless, universal statement on the meaning of the democratic experience. But it was fixed in the Australian context by two devices: the alignment of the great triangle on the Australian landscape, the bushland preserves of Mount Ainslie and Black Mountain — and the focusing of the avenues on a building uniquely expressive of Australia. This was the building Griffin designated the 'Capitol', the third structure planned for Capital Hill. Sited in the most prominent position at the apex of the triangle between the two official residences, Griffin envisioned this building to be a place of popular assembly, a repository of the national archives and an institution commemorating national achievements. Shown in Marion Mahony's drawings as a stepped pyramid with a vast vaulted interior, the Capitol was conceived as a temple dedicated to the national spirit, an expression of the collective genius of the Australian people, a creation of the imagination and will of the entire community. The Capitol would stand at the focal point of the city plan and become the focus of national consciousness, a physical embodiment of all that was unique and distinctive in the Australian experience.

In responding to the larger landscape of the Canberra valley, Griffin saw the city as a theatre with the government on stage:

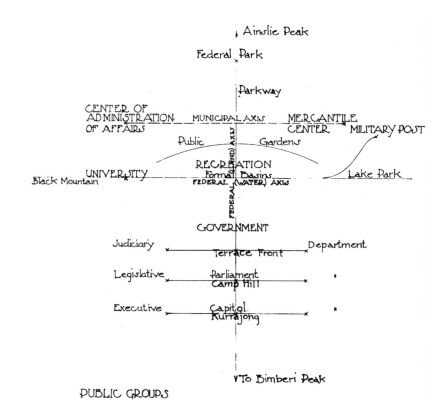

Above: Principles diagram prepared by Griffin to explain the Public Groups, Canberra, appearing in 'The magic of America', vol 2.
Reproduced from David Van Zanten, *Drawings of Walter Burley Griffin architect*, Prairie School Press, Palos Park, Illinois, 1970, pp 10–11. Copyright New York Historical Society.

Left: This published version of Walter Burley Griffin's revised plan first appeared in a federal capital report in October 1913 and is usually referred to by its title 'Preliminary Plan'.
From *Commonwealth of Australia Federal Parliament House architectural competition*, Department of Home Affairs, Melbourne, 1913. Courtesy James Weirick.

Taken altogether, the site may be considered as an irregular amphitheatre — with Ainslie at the north-east in the rear, flanked on either side by Black Mountain and Pleasant Hill, all forming the top galleries; with the slopes to the water, the auditorium; with the waterway and flood basin, the arena; with the southern slopes, the terraced stage and setting of monumental Government structures, sharply defined, rising tier on tier to the culminating hill of the Capitol; and with Mugga Mugga, Red Hill and the blue distant mountain ranges, sun reflecting, forming the back scene of the theatrical whole.[30]

However, the city was conceived as a living entity, not a set piece. Movement through the landscape would engage everyone in the actual workings of democracy. With public and private institutions set in specific relationship to each other, the bounded domains of their powers and responsibilities, their inter-relationships and dependencies would be always apparent. What Walter Burley Griffin was offering was a Rousseauist dream, 'the dream of a transparent society, visible and legible in each of its parts, the dream of there no longer existing any zones of darkness'.[31] But in the great scheme of things, there would be one mystery. In a landscape offering everywhere the possibility of transcendent experience, there would be one place of immanence. The inner space of the Capitol would suggest the possibility of unity, of oneness — it would offer above all, a place of psychic repose and resolution.

The sense of meaningful space — sometimes subliminal, sometimes self-evident — would not be restricted to the monumental centre of the capital. Throughout the city, Griffin's subtle adjustment of geometry to terrain, land use to circulation, parkland to built form would create endless opportunities for abstract ideas to be fused with concrete experience. The National University, for example, was to have the most theoretical disciplines sited at the centre of the campus, and the most applied — the professional schools — sited on an outer ring, where the university met the city.

One of the most intense sequences of spatial and symbolic experiences was set out along 'Prospect Parkway', the urban element which extended along the Land Axis on the northern side of the lake. In the Griffins' Canberra, this was both drawn and planned as a cross-section of city life. Prospect Parkway would extend from the National Stadium on the lakeshore to the forested slopes of Mount Ainslie. Griffin described the parkway as a 'formal plaisance' and Marion Mahony's perspective from the summit of Mount Ainslie clearly shows a sweep of space, lined on both sides by informal drifts of trees, which merge into formal avenue plantings. This urban element was conceived as a grand promenade in the tradition of The Mall in Central Park, except that it would be a meeting place in the heart of the city rather than a meeting place in a park.

Served by an underground station on the city railway line, and the streetcar network Griffin imagined would set the horizontal scale of his city, the parkway would be filled with crowds of people spilling onto its concourse to go about their daily business; to attend sporting events in the National Stadium; to visit the opera, theatre, or museums; to go shopping. Residents from the nearby courtyard apartments would use this slice of green in the midst of high density housing as their urban park — a human scaled, modulated space under a canopy of trees, opening to exhilarating prospects along the sweep of its central greensward.

Griffin's plaisance was intended to be a natural funnel of activity, a meeting place for people from the neighbourhood, the city, the nation, a truly vital place in the life of the capital. To be caught up in its energy, to walk along the central axis of the city, would be to experience an extraordinary transition from the public to the private. To stand, first, on the northern shore of the lake, would be to experience the full impact of Griffin's symbolic schema — the brilliant, sun-lit ensemble of public institutions — in all its power. This great prospect would also be visible from the stands of the National Stadium, where the contained spectacle of the sporting contest and the roar of the crowd, projected across the lake, would set the dynamics, the immediacy, the flux of contemporary life against the *gravitas* of national government. To turn 180 degrees, to turn from this set-piece and be drawn along the axial line of the plaisance, would be to experience a series of transitions from the civic, formal and spectacular to the private, informal and relaxed. From the Capital's great cultural institutions — the theatre, the opera, the galleries — a promenade along the parkway would cross at right angles the main commercial and retail streets of the city, cross the city railway line above the station, then proceed through the apartment belt to reach the forest preserve on the slopes of Mount Ainslie. To encourage people to use the full length of The Mall, Griffin sited a casino at its upper end, a facility for popular entertainment and relaxation, somewhat like McKim, Mead and White's casino in Newport, Rhode Island or the Midway Gardens which Frank Lloyd Wright subsequently designed for a similar site on the Midway Plaisance in Chicago.

Beyond the casino, the formal walks of a commemorative park would lead to bushland paths on the mountain slopes. As one climbed the mountain, the intimate scale and subtle qualities of the natural forest would contrast with the dramatic sense of the city provided at every outlook. Stretched out in the valley below would be a compelling geometric form, aligned on the mountain itself, containing the centre of national government. To climb the mountain and look out upon this scene of order, balance and control would be to experience the tension between nature and the city, between the spiritual and the intellectual, between the unique, perceptive qualities of each individual and the controls and mechanisms of society.

In this way, nature would be embedded in the lived reality of the city, for inspiration and individual empowerment in the true Emersonian sense:

> The world is emblematic ... the whole of nature is a metaphor of the human mind ... life in harmony with nature, the love of truth and virtue, will purge the eyes to understand her text. By degrees we may come to know the primitive sense of the permanent objects of nature, so that

the world shall be to us an open book … 'every object rightly seen, unlocks a new faculty of the soul.' That which was unconscious truth becomes, when interpreted and defined … a part of the domain of knowledge — a new weapon in the magazine of power.[32]

In Chicago, the Griffins' great success in the Australian Federal Capital competition was seen as a triumph for the city's small but spirited band of progressive architects, and was consciously presented as such by the journal most dedicated to their cause, the *Western Architect*. The September 1912 issue of this magazine published a complete set of the competition drawings, with accompanying text, laid out within a photographic survey of some of the Griffins' Chicago architecture. The work which Walter and Marion chose at that time to illustrate their principles is most revealing. First came Marion Mahony's Church of All Souls, then came the Canberra drawings, followed by Griffin's most urban building — the Store and Flat building for the Cornell Estate on the southside of Chicago — and finally a photograph of Marion's coloured rendering on satin of their most radical design, the Solid Rock house, Winnetka. There was also an article, 'Walter Burley Griffin, Progressive', by William Gray Purcell, a fellow architect of the 'Sullivan School'.[33] This selection of projects and executed work, clearly polemical, must be understood in the broader context of Chicago's architectural development.

The Griffins' experience in architecture at the turn of the century coincided with a significant realignment of political and economic forces in the United States, the result of new concentrations of capital and the emergence of corporate ideology.[34] The domestic architecture with which Walter and Marion were principally involved, in Frank Lloyd Wright's office and in independent practice, held out the possibility of refuge from the social conflict and contradictions of the time for a certain segment of middle-class society. Given sufficient expert attention, the home could become a total work of art and craft, in spite of an industrial system which was alienating increasing areas of human activity from creative, individual involvement.[35]

The art and craft of the home, however, was torn between sentimental artistic associations and a radical challenge which began to embrace abstraction, the machine and the processes of production. The progressive architects in Chicago — Frank Lloyd Wright, the Griffins and others — like secessionist architects in various parts of the world, were poised on the edge of negating, not complementing the bourgeois sense of refuge from the realities of the industrial age. The situation which made Chicago unique was the intersection at this point of mass corporate culture, implied by that other Chicago architectural genre, the skyscraper. The vast business organisations which occupied the standardised space of the tall office building valued managerial conformity above individuality. For a brief period at the turn of the century unusual homes were built for a small clientele of successful individualists, but the emerging managerial class wanted something everybody else had. Thus, as corporate culture grew in power and influence,

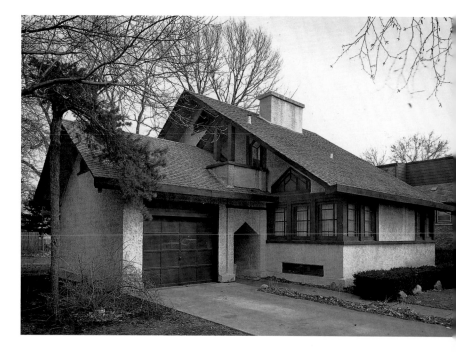

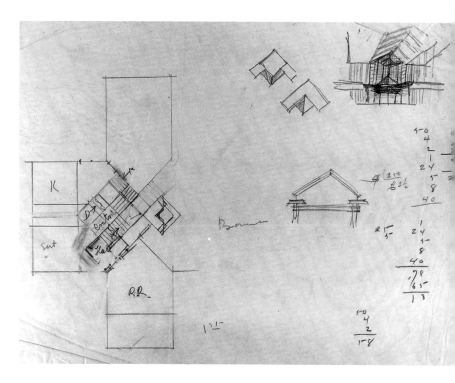

Top: Harry V Peters house, Chicago, Illinois, designed by Walter Burley Griffin in 1906.
Photo courtesy Mati Maldre.

Above: A rare surviving example of a design development drawing by Walter Burley Griffin. Unidentified project, undated (about 1906), pencil on tracing paper, 24 × 36 cm.
Courtesy Nicholls collection, Sydney.

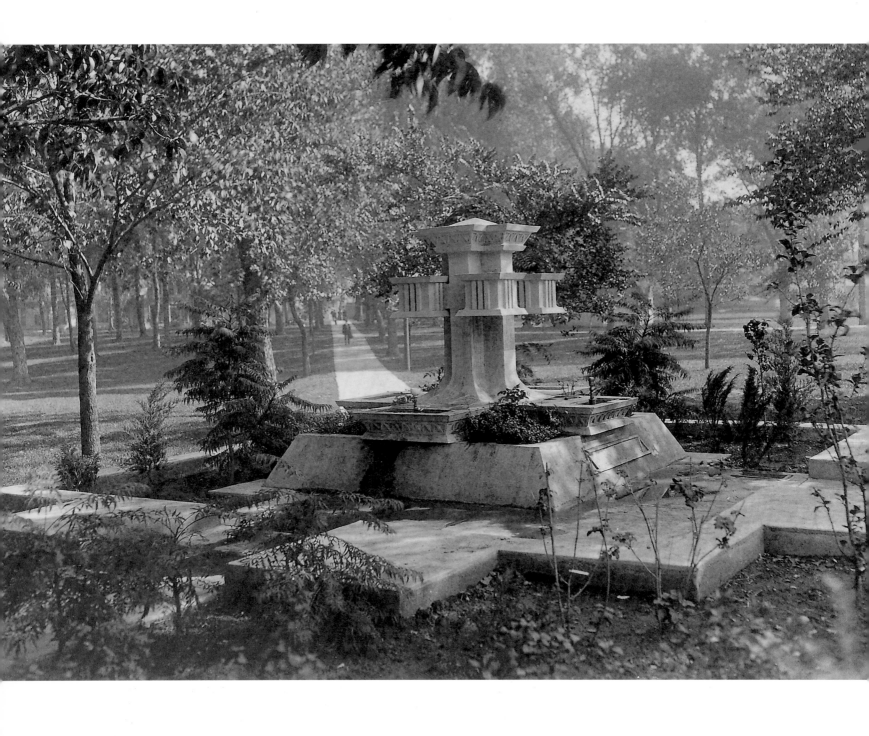

Above: Clark Memorial Fountain, Grinnell, Iowa, designed
by Walter Burley Griffin in 1910.
Courtesy Nicholls collection, Sydney.

the domestic architecture of Chicago began to reject progressive tendencies and subside into standardised sentimentality, the architecture of revival styles.[36] These were the critical forces at work in American architectural life when the Griffins resolved to enter the international competition for the Australian Federal Capital in 1911 and project their ideas into a new realm.

At the time of their marriage in June 1911, the Griffins were beginning to experiment with a severely abstract aesthetic, the direction implied by the superposed planes and masses of Wright's Larkin Building and Unity Temple. This is what European modernism took from Wright — De Stijl, early Gropius, early Mies — but the Griffins did not continue in this direction. The Solid Rock house is their only essay in severely planar forms, thereafter their architecture incorporated rough-hewn masonry, crystalline structural members and decorative elements, spandrels with incised patterns, flaring cornices, exaggerated voussoirs. They turned from stripped, abstract forms of uncompromising severity to an architecture of complexity, richness and emotional power. By September 1911, when they began work on the Canberra competition, this new approach to design had been anticipated in some small-scale works — the faceted lanterns of the Clark Memorial Fountain in Grinnell, Iowa; the concrete belvedere of a display pavilion for the Universal Portland Cement Company — but in the Canberra drawings, these decorative elements were extrapolated to the scale of an entire city. The Griffins' new aesthetic in its full power came out of the experience of producing the Canberra drawings. In a few weeks of intense activity Walter and Marion developed a complete design vocabulary, undoubtedly flowing from the freedom of imagining a new city in Australia but really responding to the pressures on progressive design in America. Abstraction threatened to negate bourgeois society, to bring it too close to the reality of industrial production. To complement the growing conformity of the new corporatism in America, a fundamentally anti-modern aesthetic was emerging, hence the twentieth-century gothic of the businessmen's club, the country club, prep school, private university, corporate boardroom.[37] This is what the Griffins were responding to in their Canberra drawings, finding ways to vivify this aesthetic while retaining its aura of Arthurian commitment to the commonweal.

At the time of the Canberra competition, the work of public architecture which most clearly expressed this aura was Marion Mahony's Church of All Souls, hence its prominence and precedence in the issue of the *Western Architect* which published the Canberra project. However, in the month this issue appeared — September 1912 — the Griffins completed the working drawings for the first work to be built in their mature style, the J G Melson house in Mason City, Iowa. This was followed by other expressive works — the Griffins' own house projected for Trier Center, Winnetka, the Holahan house proposal for Mason City, the Stinson Memorial Library, the projected house for Henry Ford. The Griffins' distinctive approach to architecture, heralded in the Canberra drawings, would achieve its most complete expression in the design of Melbourne's Newman College — and its most suggestive resolution at the scale of the Australian city in the residential architecture of Castlecrag.

The true basis of this mature style is to be found in the dynamics of the partnership between Walter and Marion. They began to work together, on a consultant basis as architect and landscape architect, a year or more before their marriage. It is not possible to identify the precise moment they began to collaborate on architectural design, but it is clearly some time in 1910. Walter helped Marion on her 'Wrightian' projects for Von Holst and Marion helped Walter on his austere experimental houses in reinforced concrete. In formal design terms, Griffin's skill was in plan generation and the manipulation of geometric solids — cubes and prisms — endlessly inventing ways to inter-relate mass and void. Marion lacked this ability, as evidenced by the unresolved massing of her first design for the Church of All Souls, but she was supremely adept at working with motifs — and she could draw anything.

Walter lacked Marion's drawing ability, and Marion lacked Walter's almost limitless capacity for ideation. Together they could see and test, enrich and resolve each other's ideas. In a set of Griffin's own architectural sketches, undated but probably surviving from the early years of his independent practice, there is a pencil drawing, repeatedly over-worked, in which he is struggling to express the idea of rotating a fireplace mass 45 degrees in the centre of a room with a tent ceiling — a design move which would create a prismatic mass in a prismatic void. Griffin could imagine this and he could build this — it is similar to the entranceway of the Harry Peters house of 1906 — but he could not draw it.[38] Once Marion was beside him, there was no such problem. Marion's independent work had some affinity with Walter's. Her completed design for the Church of All Souls incorporated triangular and prismatic elements. So, for example, did Walter's design for the Peters house. But Marion's church lacked articulation in its massing and spatial complexity; while Walter's house lacked repose and refinement of detail. Combine the two and we begin to see the possibilities of a richly articulated crystalline architecture — the architecture of the Canberra plan.

The competition drawings of 1911 contain literally hundreds of architectural proposals. As an ensemble, the immediate source for this profusion of ideas was the architecture of the World's Fairs. The pavilions and exhibition halls at Chicago 1893, St Louis 1904 and countless other expositions of that era, incorporated architectural elements from all over the world — classical, romanesque, gothic, Mayan, eastern and more. All these are detectable in the Griffins' vision for Canberra, they just happened to be synthesised in a new way. Fascinating as it is to speculate on specific sources, the mystery key to the Griffin aesthetic resides in architectural principles. The first is geometry, the basis of all the Griffins' work with modular grids and pure form. The second is expression, the quality that comes from the fusion of program, form and site so that

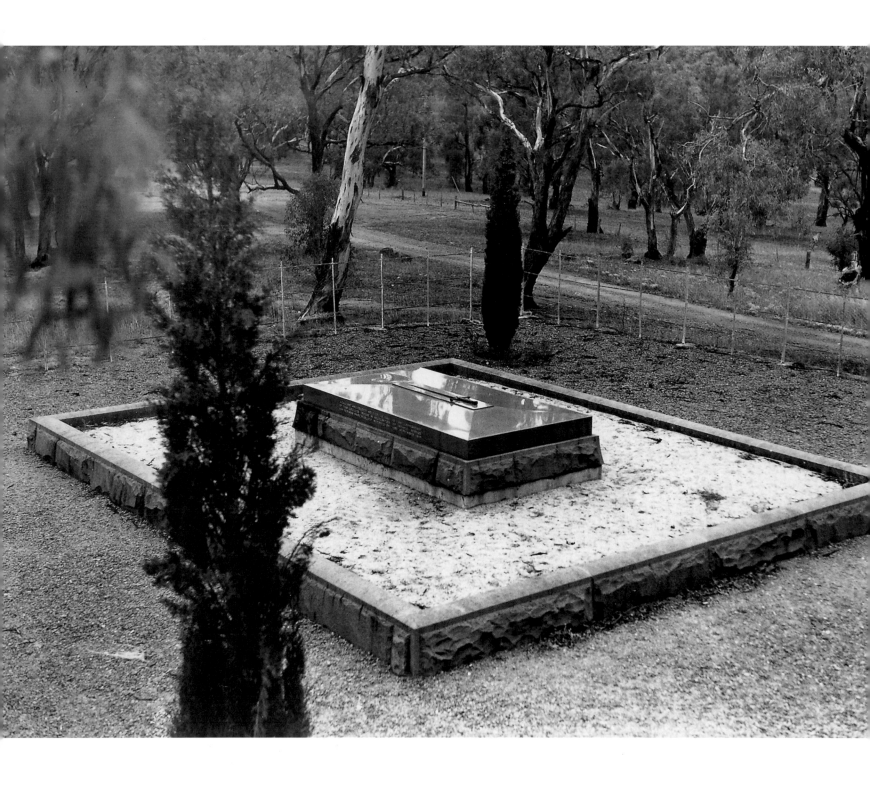

a building communicates its inner meaning. The third is structure and materials — here the Griffins saw the potential of the age, particularly in the use of reinforced concrete. Linking these principles is movement through space and time — the direct experience of ephemeral qualities which has the potential to heighten our awareness and understanding. All this can be found in the work of Sullivan, Wright and other members of the 'Sullivan School', but the Griffins' unparalleled achievement was to undertake a design exploration of this intensity at the scale of the modern city.

Alas, they did not have the opportunity to realise any architectural work of substance in Canberra. The only permanent work in the city attributed to Walter Burley Griffin is a tomb, a memorial to Major–General Sir William Throsby Bridges (1861–1915), the Australian general killed at Gallipoli in 1915. The Bridges tomb is sited in a cypress grove on the eastern slopes of Mount Pleasant overlooking the Royal Military College, Duntroon, which Bridges had founded and directed as commandant in the years before World War I. The tomb is a simple rectangular slab of grey–green trachyte, polished and cut in the form of a low truncated pyramid, set on a single course of rough-hewn ashlar which rests within a plane of raked gravel. The gravel is contained by a kerb formed from another single course of ashlar, laid four-square. A soldier's sword lies on the top plane of polished granite. The care of the grave in its gravel bed requires a continuing commitment of discipline and duty by the cadets of Duntroon, the qualities Bridges instilled in the college.

Griffin had little affinity with the military or militarism but in his official capacity as Federal Capital Director of Design and Construction, had worked with Bridges on plans for Duntroon in 1914. To honour the loss of a great soldier in the service of his country, Griffin managed to combine in this memorial the character of the man and the character of the country. The disciplined precision of the polished stone, enscribed in letters of gilt 'a gallant and erudite soldier' and cut as if by the sword, distils a sense of duty and honour. The stepped profile of the stone masses abstracts the low, rolling form of the hills on the far side of the Molonglo River. And the polished surface of the low-pitched pyramid reflects in geometric planes the endless progression of cloud formations across the Canberra sky.

The Bridges tomb was completed in 1920 just prior to the visit of the Prince of Wales to the Canberra site which included a pilgrimage to the grave of the only Australian from 60,000 war-dead whose body had been returned to Australia from the battlefields of World War I. On that day, the Prince also laid the foundation stone for the Capitol on the summit of Capital Hill, a simple granite slab designed by Walter Burley Griffin inscribed with gilded letters:

His Royal Highness
Edward
Prince of Wales
Laid this Stone
21 June 1920

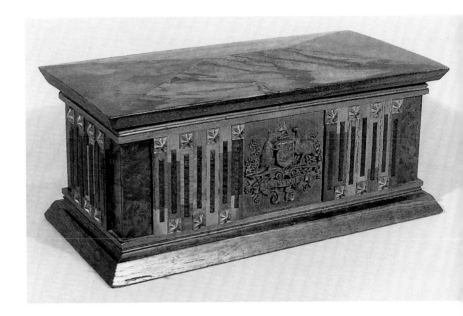

Above: Casket designed by Walter Burley Griffin to hold the mallet used by the Prince of Wales at the ceremony for the laying of the foundation stone for the Capitol, Capital Hill, Canberra on 21 June 1920. Myrtle beech, blackbean and other Australian timbers, gold, velvet, 16 × 32 × 14.5 cm. Made by the H Goldman Manufacturing Company, Melbourne.
Courtesy Parliament House Art Collection, Canberra.

Left: Tomb of Major-General Sir William Throsby Bridges, KCB, CMG, Mount Pleasant, Canberra. Designed by Walter Burley Griffin in 1920 as a memorial to the Australian general killed at Gallipoli in 1915.
Photo courtesy Australian War Memorial, Canberra.

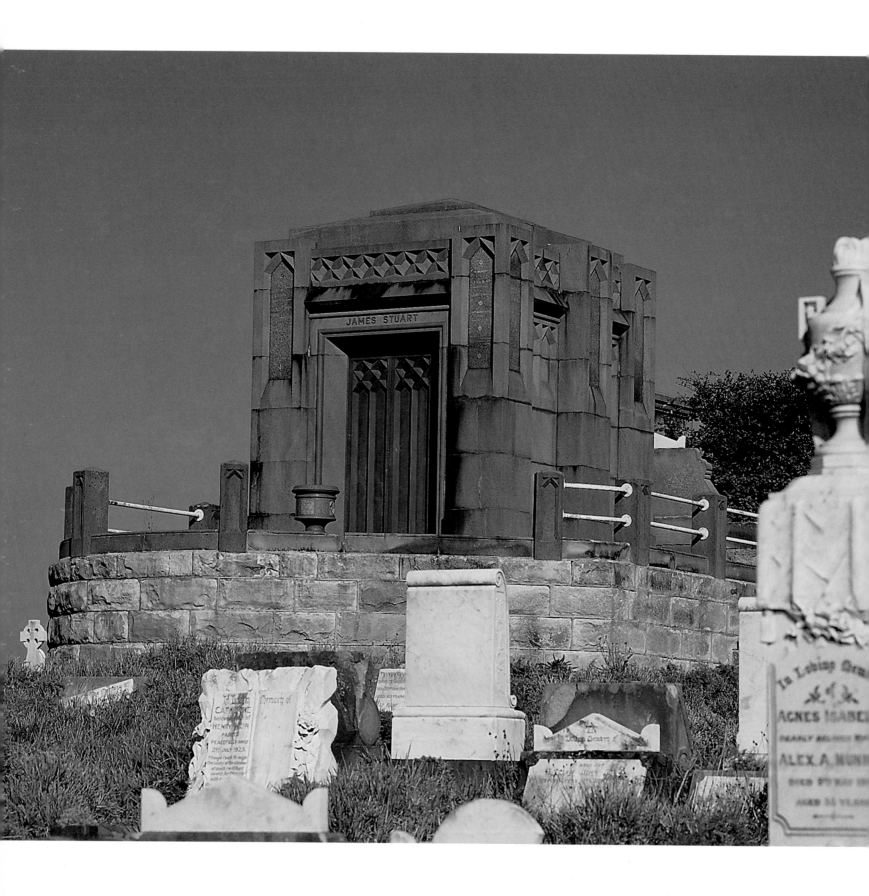

An incised dot in the middle of the letter 'o' in 'Prince of Wales' marked the precise point of the survey datum from which the city plan had been laid out — but at that time, apart from some unsurfaced road formations and preliminary plantings, there was virtually nothing on the site. The only tangible expression of the Griffins' 'democratic architecture' lay momentarily in the Prince's hands. The inlaid casket designed to hold the mallet used by the Prince of Wales in the stone-laying ceremony is an exquisite fragment of the Canberra drawings realised in Australian timbers and solid gold — a representation in miniature of the monumental architecture the Griffins had envisioned for Canberra.[39]

Another architectural fragment from the Canberra drawings was built as a tomb, not in Canberra but in Sydney: the Stuart tomb in Waverley Cemetery which dates from 1914 to 1916 is a surviving work of the Griffins' brief partnership with Sydney architect J Burcham Clamp (1868–1931). The tomb is a granite vault, built for the family of James Stuart (1862–1914), founding partner of Stuart Bros, pre-eminent master builders of Edwardian Sydney and contractors for the Australian Picture Palace designed by Griffin and Clamp, then in construction.[40] The Stuart tomb is undoubtedly the best built work of the Griffins' Australian practice. Superbly sited in the broad amphitheatre-like valley of Waverley's nineteenth-century cemetery, poised above the sea, the tomb stands on a prow-like *temenos* at the meeting of two long retaining walls — a terminal element on a long horizontal terrace. Gothic in spirit, the tomb is built in grey granite, buttressed against the elements to the north and south, with a suppressed pyramidal roof built from solid slabs of stone. Twin doors in heavy bronze sit sealed on hidden pivots facing the vastness of the ocean to the east. They are cast in a prismatic pattern which interlocks at head height to form a double set of diamond-shaped vents, open to the interior darkness of the tomb. On the west wall, a round-ended cross is formed at the meeting of four granite blocks, its four equal arms narrow slits cut through to the interior chamber, inlaid with a bronze plate drilled for ventilation. Glimpsed through the openings in the east doors, the drill holes create beads of light in a paternoster pattern as a cross within a cross. Memorial tablets, gold lettered in polished granite, are set as vertical shields within the buttresses, which are topped with a diaper pattern of prismatic elements incised in the granite cornice of the vault.

The heaviness of the overall massing seems to carry with it a mood and memory of profound grief but in the clear air of the coast, the play of light and shadow across the prismatic surface of the vault, the glint of gold and polished quartz in the memorial tablets, give the deadness of the rough-sawn granite the miracle of life. Each morning the first rays of the sun penetrate the darkness of the tomb through the grill-like openings in the east facing doors; each evening the last rays of the setting sun burst through the pin holes of the paternoster cross as a last pulsation of light and life. At sunrise on the summer solstice, the shaft of first light pierces the inner chamber to fall directly on the cross and in

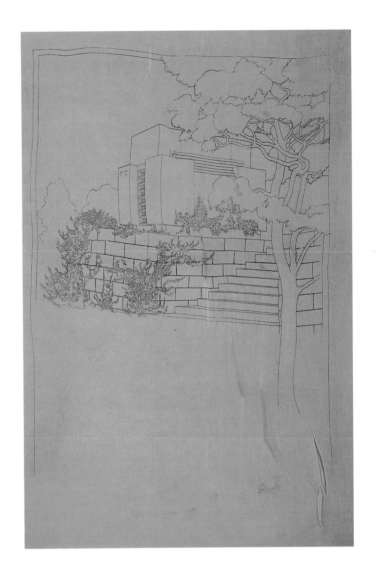

Above: First version of the James Stuart tomb, Waverley Cemetery, Sydney. Designed by Walter Burley Griffin and built in a revised form 1914–1916. Ink on silk sateen, 96.8 x 66.4 cm.
Courtesy Avery Architectural and Fine Arts Library, Columbia University, New York (1000.105.00034).

Left: James Stuart Tomb, Waverely Cemetery, Sydney, 1914–1916. Designed by Walter Burley Griffin in partnership with J Burcham Clamp.
Photo by Geoff Friend, Powerhouse Museum, 1998

the resting place of the dead, illuminate the symbol of resurrection. Every day, every year the cycle will repeat — until the Day of Last Judgement. The tomb is a silent temple to the immortality of the soul.

James Stuart was not a Freemason and neither was Walter Burley Griffin but this memorial to a master builder has a 'masonic' presence — clearly, openly — not veiled in mystery or secret lore. It stands as a clear expression of its symbolic purpose and a clear expression of the master mason's craft, the 'operative craft' which is the basis of all great architecture: 'in the smallest thing we build is buried the lore of centuries'.[41] This knowledge is not limited to the initiated, its principles are simple and self-evident — geometry, expression, materials, location in space and time. To Griffin, design as the synthesis of these principles involved 'rational deductions for the actual facts and conditions of our times', the specialised skill of architects in the modern world but a skill shared by all in 'primitive' and pre-modern societies. He believed that architecture is 'an abstract appeal to fundamental human capacity to judge of time and space, of rhyme and proportion, as in music'. He wanted to re-awaken this capacity 'held back by too much dogma' in modern civilisation, in the case of architecture by academicism: the dogma of historic styles. He believed the ability to judge 'those beauties that are poetical' is an 'intuitive quality in the human mind' which could be re-awakened by an architecture based on independent thought, a democratic architecture based on authority from within, not authority from without. This is the same thinking as James Vila Blake and the American transcendentalists in religion. Addressing the New South Wales Institute of Architects in 1913, Griffin defined architecture in transcendentalist terms as 'an art which must appeal directly to the soul'.[42]

In the archive of Griffin drawings at the Avery Architectural and Fine Arts Library, Columbia University, there is an earlier design for the Stuart tomb which is more abstract in its composition, consisting of severe rectilinear solids — a central mass contained by four corner piers in the manner of the Larkin building. The rejection of this noble but uncompromising design in favour of a more decorated, traditional scheme illustrates the trend away from early modernism's machine age moment to the standardised sentimentality of revival styles. The memorial to the successful builder suggests nothing of the commercial world in which his fortune had been made or the industrial reality of the foundation pit. It evokes, instead, romantic associations of medieval guilds, Crusader quests and Arthurian honour. This may be appropriate for a cemetery located in a suburb named for the novels of Sir Walter Scott, but it is in no way avant-garde. The Griffins were not part of the revolutionary trajectory of twentieth-century modernism — they were interested in the poetic and spiritual dimensions of architecture as an art.

The rejection of the earlier scheme may also have resulted from tensions in the partnership with J Burcham Clamp, which was dissolved during construction of the tomb. Clamp, a quirky but conservative architect of the Australian arts and crafts movement, was closely associated with George Augustine Taylor (1872–1928), editor of Sydney's highly opinionated *Building* magazine, who initially championed the Griffins then turned against them. Taylor also championed Sullivan and Wright but turned against them too after a visit to the United States in 1914. When he saw the Larkin building in reality, Taylor found it repelling, 'a huge mausoleum-like building ... too uninviting to enter'. Standing before its 'forbidding aspect', he was led to speculate: 'Convention is often the law of the majority, and the man who would be original enough to dare such a thing as that might dare to break conventions in other things and be dangerous to somebody'.[43]

This was a criticism of Wright, but it was aimed at Griffin, who by that time had arrived in Australia and was experiencing extreme difficulties in his campaign to implement the Canberra plan. Following the outbreak of World War I, the cultural values represented by the Griffins' work appeared somewhat disturbing to conservative interests in Australia. George Taylor led the campaign by drawing attention to 'German' tendencies in the Griffins' architecture and planning, a theme taken up by no less a public figure than the Governor-General, Sir Ronald Munro Ferguson, who in a speech at the opening of a town planning conference in 1918 observed that 'a banal, clumsy German architecture, typical of German "Kultur" had recently been disseminated over a suffering earth, and was reaching Australia via America'.[44] Walter Burley Griffin was in the audience on this occasion and there was just enough truth in Munro Ferguson's statement for it to have struck home. The Griffins' architecture does have a formal affinity with the early expressionist work of Peter Behrens, Max Berg, Bruno Taut in Wilhelmine Germany, together with the work of the secessionist architects in Vienna, Otto Wagner, J M Olbrich, Josef Hoffmann. Griffin had contacted Otto Wagner (1841–1918) just prior to the outbreak of World War I with the invitation to join the design jury for the Parliament House Competition. And Marion Mahony's most significant work in terms of world culture — her presentation perspectives of Frank Lloyd Wright's architecture — had been published in Berlin by Ernst Wasmuth in 1910. The comment by Munro Ferguson merely confirmed the feelings of isolation and alienation the Griffins were experiencing in Australia. As Marion noted at the time:

> A foreigner is a person to be feared, to be hated, to be despised ... A foreigner is one whose honesty, intelligence, industry are things to be deadened as establishing bases of comparison threatening established methods of muddling and monopoly. The whole community unites to hound, to cheat, to defame the foreigner wheresoever he may come from. These methods are common to business, professions and unions.[45]

The cause of this bitterness was the campaign Marion termed the 'Federal Battle': Walter Burley Griffin's long and frustrating struggle to have Canberra built according to his plan. Griffin's difficulties were caused by the fact that the departmental officials who advised the Australian Government to hold an international competition for the design of Canberra, never intended that the winner would be involved in building the city. They were not looking for an ideal city plan, they were looking for ideas for a city plan. In the aftermath of the competition they proceeded to produce their own plan, a very bad amalgam of elements appropriated from a number of the winning schemes. Only a change of government and intervention by the minister resulted in Walter Burley Griffin being brought to Australia in August 1913, almost six months after the foundation stone for the city had been laid and construction started, not according to the Griffin plan but the plan of the departmental officials. The new minister attempted to reverse this situation by appointing Griffin Federal Capital Director of Design and Construction but unfortunately, despite the grandiloquence of his title, Griffin was dependent on the departmental officials for all the information he needed to carry out the work — the Permanent Secretary of the Department of Home Affairs, the Director General of Works, the Commonwealth Surveyor-General, the Commonwealth Architect, senior engineers and others. From this group he experienced implacable opposition and obstruction.

Thwarted at every turn, the one avenue of appeal open to Griffin was to go over the heads of the officials to the responsible government ministers, which in desperation, is what he did. However, this totally politicised the issues. During World War I, the instability of Australian political life led to a rapid succession of governments and ministries. In his seven–year term as Federal Capital Director of Design and Construction, Griffin had to deal with no less than ten different ministers. Support for Canberra fluctuated wildly and Griffin found his work subjected to a bewildering series of policy reversals. After seven difficult years — including a Royal Commission of Inquiry into Federal Capital Administration — his position was abolished. Griffin was offered a place on a five-member advisory committee, which included several of the officials he had battled so long. Given the man of principle that he was, he declined the offer and severed all official connection with the city.

Three years after being forced from the Canberra project, Walter Burley Griffin put forward the following judgment on Australian public life, in a devastating address to the Henry George League in Melbourne entitled 'The Menace of Governments': 'Politicians ... are the agents of the actual privileged classes whom governments serve. Knowing politicians and officials and their habits, character and means of place holding should be sufficient to forever preclude anything but grave suspicion as to any real human welfare from such a source or under such control'.[46]

There is a profound sense of disillusionment in this statement. The Griffins' idealised vision of Australia had been totally destroyed. The 'civil religion' of democracy and freedom which was so much part of their American background was completely alien to Australian public life. Walter expressed no anger at what had happened to him, his nature was imperturbable, but there is evidence that in the early 1920s he suffered from inner despair. In a 1923 talk to architecture students at the University of Melbourne published as 'The modern architect's field — its limits and discouragements', he reflected on the fate of the creative individual in the modern world 'condemned to one of three states — a parasite, a pander or a recluse'. Although it was possible for some artists to carry on 'to a small degree' as a recluse, he argued: 'the architect cannot so carry on at all, and the fact that he is driven to be either a parasite or a pander is enough to account for the obvious absence of creative architecture today'.[47]

Significantly, the cynicism and suppressed despair which lies behind this vision dates from a time in Griffin's life when he and Marion were beginning to develop a successful commercial practice in Melbourne with the Capitol Theatre on the boards, the largest and most spectacular project of their Australian practice. Yet for all its brilliance, the Capitol was a place of escape from the pressures of modern life, an architecture of illusion not an architecture of emancipation and individual empowerment. Denied the opportunity to build a truly democratic architecture in Canberra, the Griffins poured all their creative energies into the Capitol cinema. The crystalline interior is breathtaking and has a formal affinity with the high moment of German expressionism — the fantasy projects of Bruno Taut, the Grosse Schauspielhaus in Berlin by Hans Poelzig, the cinematography and set design of *The cabinet of Dr Caligari*. The Griffins in Melbourne in the early 1920s may not have seen images of this work but they almost certainly read evocative descriptions of it by the German-American critic Herman George Scheffauer (1878–1927) who was a regular contributor to *The Freeman*, a New York literary journal of a 'Georgist' persuasion, to which they subscribed.[48] In articles with arresting titles such as 'The vivifying of space' and 'The architecture of aspiration', Scheffauer painted dramatic word-pictures of the aesthetic content and social ideals of German expressionism as it developed in the aftermath of World War I. He reviewed the 1919 book by Bruno Taut (1880–1938), *Die Stadtkrone* (The City Crown), which includes among its illustrations the Griffins' Canberra plan:

> In his book 'The City Crown', Taut expounds his plans for the creation, the culture of organic cities of the future, the functional parts grouped round a central structure of monumental proportions raised on an eminence — a temple of the people, a cathedral of the communal soul. All the needs of the modern day, nay, of the future municipality are considered and a harmonious entity is projected, developing naturally like a crystal or a flower, instead of morbidly like industrial cancer ... It is architecture applied to the landscape and the planet, it is the spiritualization of the environment.[49]

From this description, the Griffins could recognise in Taut's utopian dreams, the content of the Canberra plan with its central vision of the Capitol as the physical embodiment of all that was unique and distinctive in the Australian experience. Despite all that had happened in

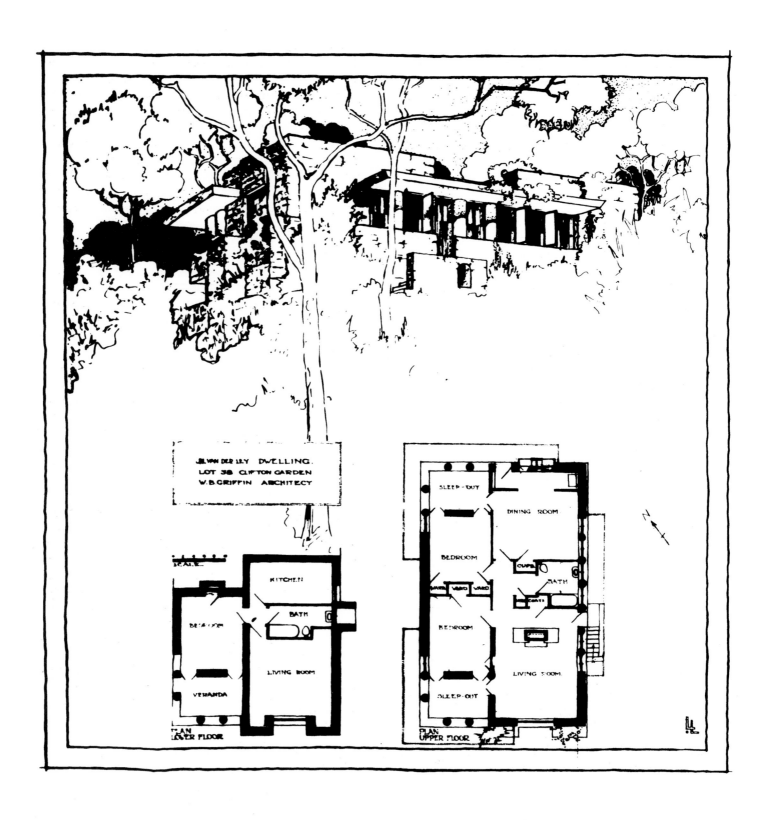

Above: J N van der Ley house, Clifton Gardens, Sydney, 1927–1929. Designed by Walter Burley Griffin but now substantially altered. Ink on linen drawing by Louise Lightfoot. This perspective is one of the many missing Griffin drawings now known only through microfilm copy. Courtesy Ian Griggs, Sydney.

Europe, the 'Architecture of aspiration' in Germany was on an ascendant path, whereas the Griffin vision of a public architecture in Australia, imbued with democratic values, had been defeated. The foundation stone ceremony on Capital Hill had been no more than an empty political gesture. The Capitol in Canberra would never materialise. Instead, the Griffins had a commercial project in Melbourne — a city cinema to seat two thousand, and it is not without significance that it was named in memory of the centrepiece of their Canberra plan.

Judging by his public utterances, the years 1923 and 1924 were a period of spiritual crisis for Walter. Marion had suffered great isolation and bitterness during the Canberra struggle, but by the 1920s she had developed a supportive network of friends, particularly among the Melbourne suffragists, Vida Goldstein, Ina Higgins, Adela Pankhurst Walsh. She also threw herself into the formidable task of detail design for the Capitol interior, the ultimate expression of her capacity to elaborate motifs. After the triumphant opening of the cinema — with the Melbourne premiere of Cecil B de Mille's *The Ten Commandments* — the Griffins took a holiday, they made their first return visit to the United States. There is a graphic description of Marion at that time in the social pages of the Melbourne press:

> Amid the beautiful surroundings of the Botanic Gardens, the Quarterly Club met on Saturday to bid farewell to Mrs W.B. Griffin prior to her departure for America. The guest of honour was attractively gowned in a mastic colour knitted silk frock with a cape effect and a Tutankhamen turban and carried presentation bouquets of brilliant hued poppies. Tea was served in the pagoda, and Mrs Griffin, with her dynamic personality, gave a graphic outline of her future plans.[50]

Walter and Marion left Melbourne to travel in the United States for three months then returned to Sydney and settled at Castlecrag. There they focused their energies on promoting the physical growth and community development of the bushland suburb on Sydney Harbour Griffin had designed in 1920, which had languished in the years they had not been able to give it their full attention.

Castlecrag offered a way out of Griffin's inner impasse of the early 1920s. As a commercial venture, it was controlled by Griffin himself; community development involved gathering together a stimulating group of like-minded people; and the very site of Castlecrag, the forested heights of Middle Harbour, provided a constant source of inspiration.

Between 1925 and 1935, the Griffins' energy and idealism did indeed attract a fascinating group of people to Castlecrag, from little theatre, the arts, bushwalking and conservation, radical politics, alternative medicine and alternative religion. However, at the same time, the commercial aspect of the venture became extremely difficult, partly due to the Griffins' unusual aesthetic ideas, partly due to the fact that their friends had little money — but mainly due to the onset of the Great Depression. In this situation the Griffins sought solace in the one community enthusiasm which extended their ideals and values — alternative religion.

In 1926, the Griffins came into contact with members of the Theosophical Society in Sydney. Prior to that date, there is no evidence that theosophy played any part in their lives at all. The Theosophical Society, founded in New York in 1875 by Madame Helena Petrovna Blavatsky (1831–1891) and others, established its international headquarters in India in the early 1880s and chartered its first lodge in Australia in 1891. Progress over the next 30 years was not without incident but the society entered a new phase in 1926 with the arrival of George Sydney Arundale from the international headquarters in Adyar, Madras to take up the position of General Secretary of the Australian Section. Arundale (1878–1945) had ambitious plans to 'theosophise Australia', to increase the influence of theosophy in the cultural life of the country. He established a magazine of liberal opinion, *Advance! Australia*, with a Round Table of literati and cultural identities as its advisory group; a theosophical broadcasting service with its own radio station, 2GB; and a civic betterment movement, the Crusade for a Beautiful Australia, launched by no less a personality than Anna Pavlova.

The Griffins' direct contact with the Theosophical Society can be dated with precision to the middle of 1926. In February that year one of the new generation of intellectuals in the theosophical movement, the Dutch philosopher Dr J J van der Leeuw (1893–1934) — who had been resident in Sydney since 1921 — returned from a three-month overseas visit. He brought with him the special issues of the Dutch architectural magazine *Wendingen* devoted to the work of Frank Lloyd Wright, which had been published in Amsterdam in 1925. A member of the Kuring-gai Lodge of the Theosophical Society, Ula Maddocks (1896–1976) was so inspired by this presentation of Wright's work that she made a special window display of the *Wendingen* magazines in the shop front which her group rented by the railway station in suburban Roseville in May 1926. There they were seen by a nearby resident, Edward Beeby, who was Walter Burley Griffin's attorney and an enthusiastic supporter of the Griffins' broad-ranging interests. Beeby pointed out the contribution Walter and Marion had made to Wright's early work and promptly arranged an introduction.[51] In June 1926, a party of theosophists made an expedition to Castlecrag[52] and in August, J J van der Leeuw met Griffin for the first time, as a letter records:

> This morning I went to see the houses built by an architect called Griffin, the architect of Canberra who at present is building and planning what will practically be a new suburb on Middle Harbour, Castlecrag. He is an American, and is the first architect whose work I have seen in Australia and really liked ... Personally I have decided that whatever more I build here ... whether Guest house, Masonic Temple or Church is going to be built by Griffin, he is the only architect in Australia whose work is really modern and beautiful.[53]

This was a significant endorsement of Griffin's abilities. J J van der Leeuw's family held the controlling interest in the Van Nelle Company, tea, coffee and tobacco merchants in Rotterdam, which was managed by his brother, the 'industrial magnate' C H van der Leeuw, one of the most influential patrons of modern architecture in the world in the 1920s and 1930s.[54] As it turned out, J J van der Leeuw did not build anything to Griffin's design, although he persuaded several other members of the Theosophical Society to do so. This led to a series of domestic commissions, the A E Creswick House at Castlecrag, the J N van der Ley House at Clifton Gardens and a projected house for Madame Eva Marie Wolfcarius at Castlecrag. Theosophical connections also played a part in the decision of Dr E W Rivett (1894–1962) to settle at Castlecrag in 1928 and establish his private hospital 'Cabarisha' there.[55] In all this work, Griffin's design solutions are interesting but not significantly different from his earlier proposals for non-theosophical clients. Griffin was a kindred spirit, not a theosophical architect.

The most 'theosophical' project from this period in terms of its program was the Cromer Sanitorium [sic]. Victor Eugene Cromer (1883–1930) was a theosophist who practised as a spiritual healer in Sydney from 1926 until his premature death in 1930. Cromer had a clairvoyant capacity to sense the invisible aura which surrounds each individual and a capacity to channel healing energies to the auras of patients with disease. He termed this energy a 'vrillic force', a form of magnetism which produced etheric vibrations and dramatic physical effects, at times audible — generating a sound like 'a loud electrical discharge ... easily heard over a large room'; at times muscular, stimulating spontaneous body movements; and at times visible across a wide range of the colour spectrum:

> Even people who are not 'psychic' in any way can soon see the force ... Heliotrope, mauve, gold, lilac, pink, sky blue and magenta are some of the colors which are frequently seen. The diseased conditions on the other hand, appear in the aura of the patient as dark blotches or patches of red or brown ... When the healing force is directed towards a diseased condition the beautiful healing colors are seen in conflict with the darker colors of disease, and after a while, the more beautiful color can be seen gradually dissipating the diseased conditions, and physical healing results ...[56]

The demonstrations and healing practices were recorded on motion picture film to calibrate the treatment for each patient, with X-rays used as 'diagnostic adjuncts'.[57]

For Cromer to carry out his healing practices, Walter Burley Griffin designed one of his most serene and restrained essays in monumental composition.[58] Sited at Covecrag with long views over bushland reserves to the upper reaches of Middle Harbour, the Sanitorium [sic] for Spiritual Healing was to have been a stepped pyramidal structure built from Knitlock, Griffin's patented concrete block system, rising as fluted colonnades in tiers above retaining walls in sandstone. The horizontality of the overall composition was emphasised by cantilevered roofs in reinforced concrete contained by a series of powerful corner piers.

The principal public rooms were located in the central pyramidal element. At the entry level, an inwardly-focused demonstration hall, circular in plan, was ringed by twenty cubicles which radiated from the central stage to receive the dramatic channelling of Cromer's healing power. An auditorium with expansive views was located in the tower element above. Patients' suites were ranged on the north side to catch the sun, each clerestory-lit room opening on to a generous 'sleep out' verandah bounded by planter beds which turned the tiered terraces into hanging gardens. Kitchens and utility rooms were located on the south side together with the dining room, which would have extended the length of a sunlit courtyard. Everything about the scheme was supremely rational, except its rationale. The Griffin proposal had a seriousness and sense of dignity which invested Cromer's project with a distinct air of credibility. As an exercise in monumentality at a human scale, the Cromer Sanitorium [sic] was an updated version of the Griffins' architectural proposals for Canberra — as strange a commission as they ever received, yet openly innovative, not hermetic and secret.

The highpoint of Walter Burley Griffin's involvement with the Sydney theosophists was his address to their annual convention in 1928, 'Architecture, landscape architecture and town planning'. Press accounts at the time described it as a 'scathing indictment' of the design and construction of Canberra in the 1920s.[59] Subsequently published in *Advance! Australia*, the tone and content of this talk make clear Griffin's despair over what had happened to his Canberra plan, together with his appreciation in finding a group of Australians with whom he could communicate on the subject. Griffin published another article in *Advance! Australia* in 1928, 'Building for nature' and in 1932 contributed 'Architecture and the economic impasse' to *The Theosophist* published in Adyar.[60] None of these articles draw upon theosophical doctrine, theosophical texts or theosophical thinkers — they are Griffin's own statements worked out from first principles.

Theosophy as it had developed in the Theosophical Society had some affinity with the Griffins' philosophical beliefs — its universalism, pantheism, engagement with higher consciousness — but in its central tenets, it differed significantly from the Griffins' long-held principles. The doctrine of the Theosophical Society was hierarchical and secret, not democratic and open. Derived from Madame Blavatsky's codification and projection of occult lore under instruction from mysterious 'Masters', theosophical thinking combined western esoteric traditions with nineteenth-century spiritualism and various eastern religions, particularly Hinduism and Buddhism. In the 1920s, the international theosophical movement was dominated by two figures, Annie Besant (1847–1933) and Charles Webster Leadbeater (1854–1934), who had become committed to an adventist expectation of a new World Teacher, a vision of a coming Christ. In 1909, Leadbeater had identified a young Indian boy, J Krishnamurti (1895–1986), as the 'vehicle' for this role and over the next twenty years considerable energy was invested in the project. Secret groups were created within secret groups to prepare adepts for the Coming — the Order of the Star of the East, the Universal Co-Masonic Order. This was particularly the case in Sydney where

Leadbeater settled in 1914. A clairvoyant and occultist of peculiar genius, Leadbeater was an Anglican curate when he joined the Theosophical Society in 1883 and never lost his enthusiasm for the priesthood and High Church ritual. In 1917 he was instrumental in establishing the Liberal Catholic Church as a parallel organisation to the Theosophical Society with himself consecrated to the episcopate as Regionary Bishop of Australasia through an appropriately authenticated form of Apostolic succession.[61]

If there is one explanation for Walter and Marion Griffin not joining the Theosophical Society, it is almost certainly embodied in the person and personality of Bishop Leadbeater. A greater contrast to a liberal Unitarian such as James Vila Blake could not be imagined. In his spiritual mission, Leadbeater's arch conservatism was paramount, he sought the return of religious authority to the Church, the re-establishment of authority from without, not from within.

The Griffins turned instead to Rudolf Steiner and anthroposophy. As a way station, Walter served on the foundation committee of Victor Cromer's New Renascence Society, which espoused a form of Christian mysticism.[62] However in 1929, the Griffins met Edith Williams, General Secretary of the Anthroposophical Society in Australia, and were formally introduced to Steiner's ideas and teachings.[63]

Anthroposophy, which Steiner described as 'a path of Knowledge, to guide the Spiritual in the human being to the Spiritual in the universe',[64] originated as an independent current of thought within the German Section of the Theosophical Society in the first years of the twentieth century. Led by Rudolf Steiner, then General Secretary of the German Section, the 'anthroposophists' formally broke with the Adyar Theosophists in 1913. The Anthroposophical Society then established its centre at Dornach, near Basel in Switzerland, where the 'Goetheanum' was built to Steiner's design, one of the most remarkable achievements of German expressionism.

Essentially a form of Christian theosophy, Christ is recognised within anthroposophy as the one great spiritual teacher whose death and resurrection revealed the world beyond the realm of the senses and set free the divine essence within each individual. Anthroposophy offers a path to gain knowledge of higher realms and free the divine element from within, not through mystic experience — a sudden epiphany or revelation — but through Steiner's version of occultism which offered techniques and procedures to gain 'knowledge of higher worlds' through imagination, inspiration and intuition.[65] To the Griffins, this provided a way to revitalise their creativity and energy, to re-charge the 'authority from within' which was the essence of their life philosophy — and raise it to new realms.

In 1930, Walter Burley Griffin spoke before the New South Wales Institute of Architects for the first time since 1913. After years of travail and professional isolation, his message was a profound extension of the idea he had put before his peers seventeen years before, that architecture is 'an art which must appeal directly to the soul':

> In my boyhood Herbert Spencer's synthetic philosophy had essayed the summation of human wisdom, and so by aid of

the index, I sought his view of architecture and was much surprised to learn that he interpreted it as a form of religious expression. It took me many years to appreciate the force of this observation, but all experience confirms the opinion ... We have to look to every individual architect to develop insight, imagination, intuition, the permanent qualities of the spirit ... The more directly and honestly each ... individual invokes and applies his inner spiritual qualities to the direction of his peculiar, economic, intellectual and emotional capacities the sooner will he reinstate creative architecture.[66]

This is an encapsulation of Griffin's intellectual journey from rational enquiry to the realisation that architecture is a form of religious expression — and then to the philosophy of Rudolf Steiner. In his principal writings after 1930, Griffin always acknowledged his debt to Steiner.[67] However, in his architecture the influence is not immediately apparent. This is because his architecture always had a strong symbolic content through the influence of the American transcendentalists and Louis Sullivan. Only two works from the final years of his Australian practice exhibit any overt trace of Steiner's influence — the Pyrmont incinerator of 1932–1935 and the Eric H Pratten house of 1935–1936. And in both these works, the 'occult' content is subservient to the grand themes of Griffin's architecture — expressive monumentality at human scale and emotional power — themes which had been established in the Canberra drawings twenty years before the Griffins discovered anthroposophy.

The Pyrmont incinerator, the largest of the unique industrial structures which Griffin designed in the Depression years, was originally intended for an alternative site in metropolitan Sydney at Moore Park. Community opposition forced its relocation to the industrial suburb of Pyrmont and completion was long delayed. The original concept dates from 1932 and was almost certainly developed by Walter and Marion on board the SS *Monowai* while crossing the Pacific from the United States. Marion had left Sydney in November 1930 for an extended sojourn in Chicago, two months after she had joined the Anthroposophical Society. Walter followed her to the United States in July 1932 on a tour otherwise devoted to investigating large-scale incineration plants in various American cities prior to submitting the all-important tender for the Moore Park destructor. This was due one month after the scheduled date of their return. Walter had joined the Anthroposophical Society in Sydney during Marion's long absence. The incinerator project was the first opportunity to work together for two years — and the first opportunity to work together as anthroposophists. Time was of the essence — and inspiration was to hand in a major anthroposophical treatise on cosmology which had just been published in English translation: *The etheric formative forces in Cosmos, Earth and Man* by Guenther Wachsmuth (1893–1963), one of Rudolf Steiner's principal successors. There is some evidence that the Griffins had this book with them on their return journey. In any event, the geometric symbolism representing the 'etheric formative forces' identified by Wachsmuth formed the basis of the complex ornamental system the Griffins developed for the exterior surfaces of the incinerator to express the building's inner purpose: the creation and dissolution of matter.[68]

The notion that a building should communicate its inner meaning was not 'anthroposophical': it was Griffin's greatest inheritance from Louis Sullivan. Similarly, the incinerator was not 'anthroposophical' in its architectonic presence — it fulfilled another of Griffin's long-held notions, dating at least from the time of the Canberra competition, that a monumental architecture in reinforced concrete should integrate 'immensity in spans and masses with contrasting delicacy in plastic ornamentation'.[69] In terms of architectural expression, Steiner's ideas were no more than an overlay on Griffin's fundamental principles.

The house built for Eric H Pratten (1903–1965) on a generous suburban estate at Pymble on Sydney's North Shore shows a similar relationship between Griffin's design ideas and Steiner's spiritual insight. The Pratten house was the largest domestic commission Griffin received in Australia and was one of a series of works which he and his partner Eric Nicholls carried out in the 1930s for the Pratten family, prominent Sydney printers with no known interest in esotericism or the occult. Nevertheless, Steiner motifs can be detected in this major work. The house is formed from powerfully articulated sandstone masses with battered walls, triangular prows and deep reveals set beneath a series of over-sailing roofs in a re-interpretation of the Wrightian Prairie house. The ground floor window reveals, cut in to the sandstone batters, have lintels dressed in a low triangular profile. The effect is somewhat Tudor gothic — but it is also reminiscent of the trapezoidal windows which characterise much of Steiner's work at Dornach. These set up fivefold figures which Steiner equated with an extension of the fourfold dimensions of human life — the four elements, the four temperaments — into the fifth dimension of the Spirit Self, the inner divine.[70]

Prismatic and trapezoidal elements were expressed more vigorously in an earlier scheme for the Pratten house — a flat-roofed proposal with parapet-piercing voussoirs like the Melson and Holahan houses designed for Mason City so many years before.[71] This was rejected by the client in favour of the more Wrightian scheme that went into construction in 1935. Indeed, there are distinct references in this Pymble house to some of the projects in rough hewn masonry overseen by Griffin in Wright's Oak Park studio — the Hillside Home School, the projected house for Thaxter Shaw — which must be considered among the sources for the Griffins' mature style. However the heavy fascias and block-like massing are distinctively Griffin's. The Pratten house, although designed at the highpoint of Griffin's Steiner phase and incorporating some Steiner motifs, is in fact a reprise of the central design problem of the Griffins' Chicago years: how to create a radical house for a conservative client.

The real value of anthroposophy was to give the Griffins new insight into the inner processes of imagination, inspiration and intuition, to revitalise their creativity, re-affirm the value of their life's work after years of struggle in Australia. All this would find its moment of high expression in India — in a new synthesis of spiritual and symbolic content nowhere more graphically displayed than in the scheme for the United Provinces Industrial and Agricultural Exhibition, designed by Walter, drawn by Marion[72] and in the process transmuted into a creative achievement greater than the sum of its parts, just like the Canberra plan.

In 1968, the writer Lawrence Durrell incorporated a telling allusion to Walter Burley Griffin in his novel *Tunc*, the first work he wrote after the spectacular success of *The Alexandria quartet*. A satire of the modern world, *Tunc* is set within the vast system of commodification which controls the marketing, packaging, distribution of art, and individual creativity in general. Caradoc the architect, once a young man in Griffin's Federal Capital office, now works for the 'Merlin Corporation', a global conglomerate which controls all creative production. He escapes only by staging his death, fleeing to a remote island and abandoning architecture. As Griffin stated in 1923, the creative individual has the choice to be 'condemned to one of three states — a parasite, a pander or a recluse'.[73]

In the sequel to *Tunc*, *Nunquam*, where Canberra is again alluded to in Caradoc's musings, the mood is even bleaker. To escape from the firm as Caradoc says, was a matter of then or never, 'aut Tunc aut Nunquam'. The first novel was infused with the hopeful, rebellious spirit of escape — but the escape fails. In *Nunquam*, Caradoc is found out and brought back into the firm; he is tempted with a project he cannot resist, 'aut tunc aut nunquam', it was then or never, but never wins — and the novel ends with the sense that creative individuals have no choice but to surrender their freedom.[74]

This is the condition Griffin identified. An architect cannot function as a recluse — the dilemma is whether to be a parasite or a pander. The shared life of Walter and Marion Griffin was an heroic attempt to overcome this dilemma, to seek inner freedom — authority from within, not from without — and live authentic lives of principle. Their dream of a democratic architecture — of a democratic city — was essentially mystical. They believed that through clear symbolic intent they could influence the way people experience the physical world. The individual would be empowered through a sudden epiphany, a revelation, in Emerson's terms 'every object rightly seen, unlocks a new faculty of the soul'.[75] Their approach to design was therefore open and transparent, not esoteric or hermetic. However, their idealism was shattered by the Canberra experience and further challenged by the commercialism of the 1920s. They found solace in alternative religion, choosing to follow Rudolf Steiner into a form of occultism which yielded insight into their own creativity. This did not change their architecture, however, it did infuse new energy into their design practice. And when the opportunity presented itself in India, Walter and Marion experienced again the creative outpouring of ideas which had produced their masterwork, the Canberra plan.

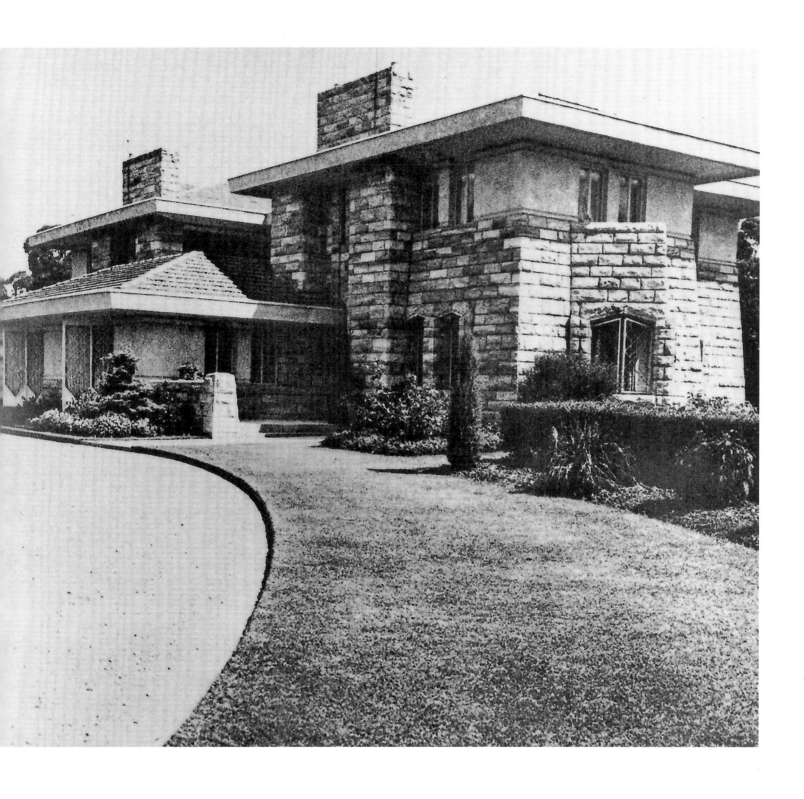

Notes

Sections of this essay have been published in *Transition* and the Monash University Gallery catalogue, *Walter Burley Griffin: a re-view*; they appear here in revised form with the kind permission of the editors.

1. Lawrence Durrell, *Tunc*, Faber & Faber, London, 1968, pp 65, 67–69, 77. I am indebted to a great and true friend of Griffins, the late Ula Baracchi, for bringing this reference to my attention.

2. Cecil V Quinlan, 'Walter Burley Griffin: how a great dream came true', *Australian National Review*, vol 1, no 4, 1937, pp 24–25.

3. Peter Proudfoot, *The secret plan of Canberra*, University of New South Wales Press, Sydney, 1994; Peter Proudfoot, 'The symbolism of the crystal in the planning and geometry of the design for Canberra', *Planning Perspectives*, vol 11, no 4, 1996, pp 225–57; John Arnold and Deirdre Morris (gen eds), *Monash biographical dictionary of 20th century Australia*, Reed, Port Melbourne, 1994, pp 221, 312.

4. W B Griffin, 'Town planning and its architectural essentials', *Building*, 11 October 1913, p 52.

5. *Advance! Australia*, vol 1, no 4, pp 185, 191; *Art in Australia*, no 17, September 1926, pp 66–67; *Federal Independent*, August 1928, Supplement p iv; Membership files, Marion Mahony Griffin 57/1930, 29 September 1930, Walter Burley Griffin 66/1931, 1 September 1931, Allgemeine Anthroposophische Gesellschaft Sekretariat, Dornach, Switzerland; the Griffins are not recorded in the membership files of the Theosophical Society in Sydney, NSW; Wheaton, Illinois; or Adyar, Madras (now Channai).

6. Winthrop S Hudson, *Religion in America: an historical account of the development of American religious life*, 2nd ed, Scribner's, New York, 1973.

7. George R Gebauer, 'James Vila Blake', *Christian Register*, vol 104, no 2, 28 May 1925, p 534; 'James Vila Blake', *National cyclopaedia of American biography*, White, New York, 1929, pp 283–84.

8. Stow Pearson, *Free religion: an American faith*, Yale University Press, New Haven, 1947, p 20.

9. James Vila Blake, *Natural religion*, Kerr, Chicago, 1892, pp 168–69.

10. Blake, *Natural religion*, p 191, emphasis in the original.

11. Historical records file 21: Church Covenant, Unitarian Church of Evanston, Evanston, Illinois. I am indebted to Doris Overboe for this reference.

12. *Manual of Christ Church, Elmhurst, Ill*, Oliphant, Chicago, 1897, p 18. A full-scale pencil drawing of a section of the frieze and a sketch of its interior location survives in the E M Nicholls collection, currently held by the Nicholls family; see also Gertrude Griffin Sater, 'Walter Burley Griffin', ms notes dated 7 & 8 November 1953, Elmhurst Historical Museum.

13. William E Danforth, 'The story of a church that believes in a town', *American City* (*Town and Country* ed), vol 12, no 1, 1915, pp 22–26.

14. Joseph M Siry, *Unity Temple: Frank Lloyd Wright and architecture for liberal religion*, Cambridge University Press, Cambridge, 1996, pp 34–35; Dwight Heald Perkins (1867–1941) was also involved in this project and brought it to completion.

15. Charles E White jr, letter to Walter Willcox, 4 March 1906, Nancy K Morris Smith (ed), 'Letters, 1903–1906 by Charles E. White jr from the studio of Frank Lloyd Wright, Oak Park', *Journal of Architectural Education*, vol 25, Fall 1971, p 110.

16. For a typical statement on this theme by a Chicago progressive of Griffin's day, see Charles Zueblin, *The religion of a democrat*, Huebsch, New York, 1908.

17. W B Griffin, 'Architecture and democracy', *Building*, 11 October 1913, pp 63–64.

18. M M Griffin, 'Democratic architecture — I: its development, its principles and its ideals', *Building*, 12 June 1914, p 101.

19. Eric M Nicholls, letter to Peter Harrison, 25 June 1964, Harrison papers, National Library of Australia, Canberra.

20. *New York Times*, 24 May 1912.

21. W B Griffin, 'Canberra: the architectural and development possibilities of Australia's capital city', *Building*, 12 November 1913, pp 65–66.

22. Louis Sullivan, *Kindergarten chats* (1901), reprinted, Dover, New York, p 106.

23. W B Griffin, letter to Edwin J James, 12 February 1913, University of Illinois Archives; 'Australia's capital city', *The Public*, vol 15, no 739, 31 May 1912, p 507; 'Walter B. Griffin: single taxer and social reformer', *Progress*, 1 September 1913, pp 1–2.

24. W B Griffin, 'Planning a federal capital city complete', *Improvement Bulletin*, vol 55, no 25, 6 November 1912, p 16.

25. Elwood Mead, 'What Australia can teach America', *The Independent*, vol 71, no 3272, 17 August 1911, pp 367–70.

26. Frank Brennan, *Canberra in crisis: a history of land tenure and leasehold administration*, Dalton, Canberra, 1971, pp 22–35.

27. W B Griffin, 'The Canberra plan', paper presented to the Australia and New Zealand Association for the Advancement of Science, Melbourne, 14 August 1914, p 3, unpublished ms, Mitchell Library, Sydney.

28. W B Griffin, letter to King O'Malley, 12 January 1913, Australia, Commonwealth Parliamentary Papers, 346/1914–1916, pp 5, 7.

29. This reading of the Canberra plan is based on the competition entry of 1911 and Griffin's first revision of the scheme, the preliminary plan of October 1913, see: W B Griffin, 'Federal capital design no 29: original report', (1911), in Australia, Senate, Report from the Select Committee to Inquire into and Report upon the Development of Canberra', *Senate Journal*, Session 1954–1955, vol 1, Appendix B, pp 93–102; W B Griffin, 'Report explanatory of the preliminary general plan' (1913), *CPP*, 346/1914–1916; W B Griffin, 'Canberra — III: the Federal city site and its architectural groupings', *Building*, 12 January 1914, pp 65–68.

30. W B Griffin, 'Report explanatory', p 3.

31. Michel Foucault, 'The eye of power', in Colin Gordon (ed), *Power/Knowledge: selected interviews and other writings, 1972–1977*, Pantheon, New York, p 152.

32. Ralph Waldo Emerson, 'Nature', (1836) in *Collected works*, Greystone Press, New York, 1941, p 347.

33. *Western Architect*, vol 18, no 9, September 1912, pp 93–94, plus 13 plates; the term 'Sullivan School' has been adopted instead of 'Prairie School' at the suggestion of Paul Sprague.

34. Alan Trachtenberg, *The incorporation of America*, Hill & Wang, New York, 1982.

35. Robert C Twombly, 'Saving the family: middle class attraction to Wright's Prairie house, 1901-1909', *American Quarterly*, vol 27, no 1, 1975, pp 57–72; Robert C Twombly, 'The Prairie School: design vision for the midwest', *Art Institute of Chicago Museum Studies*, vol 21, no 2, 1995, p 90.

36. Leonard K Eaton, *Two Chicago architects and their clients: Frank Lloyd Wright and Howard Van Doren Shaw*, MIT Press, Cambridge, Mass, 1969; H Allen Brooks, *The Prairie School: Frank Lloyd Wright and his midwest contemporaries*, University of Toronto Press, Toronto, 1972, pp 332–35.

37. T J Jackson Lears, *No place of grace: antimodernism and the transformation of American culture, 1880–1920*, Pantheon, New York, 1981, p 301.

38. The Griffin pencil drawing is located in the E M Nicholls collection; for the H V Peters house, see Mati Maldre and Paul Kruty, *Walter Burley Griffin in America*, University of Illinois Press, Urbana, 1996, pp 21–21, 50–53.

39. Alan Roberts, 'Memorials in the national capital: developing a sense of national identity', *Canberra Historical Journal*, ns no 26, September 1990, pp 2–16; C D Coulthard-Clark, *A heritage of spirit: a biography of Major-General Sir William Throsby Bridges KCB, CMG*, Melbourne University Press, Carlton, 1979, pp 181–182; Derham Groves, *Feng-shui and western building ceremonies*, Brash, Singapore, 1991, pp 52, 57–58; Anne Watson, 'Walter Burley Griffin's "other" Canberra legacy', *Australiana*, vol 19, no 4, pp 99–102, 112; Jim Gibbney, *Canberra, 1913–1953*, AGPS, Canberra, 1988 pp 85–87.

40. *A century of achievement: Stuart Bros, 1886–1986*, Toghill, Mosman, 1986, pp 15–16, 68; I am indebted to Cath Rush and Michael Wright for bringing the Stuart tomb to my attention; the lettering and some half-round moulding suggest that the tomb was completed by J Burcham Clamp.

41. Durrell, *Tunc*, p 77.

42. W B Griffin, 'Town planning and its architectural essentials', p 52; W B Griffin, 'Architecture and democracy', p 64d.

43. George Taylor, *There! A pilgrimage of pleasure*, Building Publishing, Sydney, 1916, pp 226–27.

44. George Taylor, 'American and German town planners', *Town Planning and Housing Review*, 31 May 1915, p 19; 'Town planning: Governor-General speaks', Brisbane *Daily Mail*, 1 August 1918.

45. M M Griffin, 'The magic of America', vol 2: 'The Federal Battle', p 309, unpublished manuscript, New York Historical Society, New York.

46. W B Griffin, 'The menace of governments', *Progress*, 1 May 1924, p 3.

47. W B Griffin, 'The modern architect's field: its limits and discouragements', *Australian Home Builder*, ns, no 6, November 1923, p 38.

48. For the Griffins' enthusiasm for *The Freeman* see Marion Griffin, letter to Susannah Franklin 16 March 1924, Miles Franklin papers, Mitchell Library, Sydney.

49. Bruno Taut, *Die Stadtkrone*, Eugen Diederichs, Jena, 1919, pl 64; Herman George Scheffauer, 'The architecture of aspiration', *The Freeman*, vol 2, no 43, 5 January 1921, p 400; see also, Herman George Scheffauer, 'Bruno Taut: a visionary', *Architectural Review*, vol 52, no 313, December 1922, pp 155–65; Herman George Scheffauer, 'Hans Poelzig', *Architectural Review*, vol 54, no 323, October 1923, pp 122–27; Herman George Scheffauer, *The new vision in the German arts*, Huebsch, New York, 1924.

50. 'Mrs W.B. Griffin farewelled', unidentified press clipping, Melbourne, about November 1924, Hamilton-Moore scrapbook, copy courtesy of the late Eldred Hamilton-Moore.

51. Interview with Ula Baracchi (Ula Maddocks), Clifton Gardens, 9 December 1969; see also E I Horder, 'Chatswood Lodge', *Theosophy in Australia*, vol 32, no 3, 1926, pp 85–86; there is a quote from J J P Oud, 'The influence of Frank Lloyd Wright on the architecture of Europe', *Wendingen*, no 4, 1925, pp 85–89 in Griffin's 1928 address to the Theosophical Convention in Sydney, W B Griffin, 'The outdoor arts in Australia', *Advance! Australia*, vol 4, no 5, 1 May 1928, p 210.

52. *Advance! Australia*, vol 1, no 1, July 1926, p 46; see also I Anson 'Building for the future', *Advance! Australia*, vol 3, no 3, 1 September 1927, pp 116–19.

53. J J van der Leeuw, letter to J N van der Ley, 4 August 1926, copy courtesy of the van der Ley family.

54. C H van der Leeuw (1890-1973) commissioned the Van Nelle factory, Rotterdam from Brinkman and van der Vlugt (design architect, Mart Stam), 1926–1930; and from the same firm at least two other buildings for Van Nelle N V; two major houses; the Theosophical Society Headquarters, Amsterdam and another building for the 'TS' at Ommen. He also funded Richard Neutra's VDL Research house in Los Angeles, 1930–1931, see Giovanni Fanelli, *Architettura moderna in Olanda*, Marchi & Bertolli, Firenze, 1968, pp 229–31, 360–62; Richard Neutra, *Life and shape*, Appleton-Century-Crofts, New York, 1962, pp 255–56, 263–68; *Van Nelle Nieuws*, vol 26, no 10, 23 May 1973, p 4.

55. Dr E W Rivett was not a theosophist, however he was affiliated with the Liberal Catholic Church from the mid 1920s, Martha Rutledge, 'Edward William Rivett (1894–1962), Geoffrey Serle (gen ed), *Australian dictionary of biography*, vol 11, Melbourne University Press, Carlton, 1988, p 401.

56. Victor E Cromer, 'The Vrillic force: a wonderful healing power', *Federal Independent*, vol 27, no 2, 1 February 1927, pp 13–14; Victor E Cromer, 'The re-discovery of Vril', *Theosophy in Australia*, 1 February 1926, pp 330–32. I am indebted to **Samara Rivett** for bringing the New Renascence Society and the *Federal Independent* to my attention.

57. Mary Rivett, 'The healing work of Victor E. Cromer: is it based upon a discovery of scientific value?' *Federal Independent*, 1 August 1929, pp 4–5.

58. The perspective and working drawings of the Cromer Sanitorium [*sic*] are located in the Block Museum of Art, Northwestern University, Evanston, Illinois; for a discussion of Griffin's concrete block system, see James Weirick, 'Griffin and Knitlock', *Content*, no 1, 1994, pp 102–17.

59. *The Sydney Morning Herald*, 4 April 1928.

60. W B Griffin, 'The outdoor arts in Australia', *Advance! Australia*, vol 4, no 5, 1 May 1928, pp 207–11; W B Griffin, 'Building for nature', *Advance! Australia*, vol 4, no 3, 1 March 1928, pp 123–27; W B Griffin, 'Architecture and the economic impasse', *The Theosophist*, November 1932, pp 186–91.

61. Gregory Tillett, *The elder brother: a biography of Charles Webster Leadbeater*, Routledge & Kegan Paul, London, 1982; Peter F. Anson, *Bishops at large*, October House, New York, 1964, pp 342–366.

62. 'New Renascence Society', *Federal Independent*, August 1928, Supplement p iv; 1 February 1929, p 15; 1 November 1929, p 14; Victor E Cromer, 'Practical Christian mysticism', *Federal Independent*, 1 June 1929, pp 1–3.

63. Jill Roe, 'The magical world of Marion Mahony Griffin: culture and community at Castlecrag in the interwar years'; Shirley Fitzgerald and Garry Wotherspoon, eds, *Minorities: cultural diversity in Australia*, State Library of NSW Press, Sydney, pp 94–100.

64. Rudolf Steiner, *Anthroposophical leading thoughts*, (1924), trans by G & M Adams, Rudolf Steiner Press, London, 1973, p 13.

65. Rudolf Steiner, *Knowledge of higher worlds and its attainment*, trans by H Collison, Anthroposophic Press, New York, 1910; Rudolf Steiner, *The gates of knowledge*, trans by M Gysi, Putnam's, New York, 1912. Another important aspect of Steiner's appeal to the Griffins was his spiritual approach to socio-political issues, see Rudolf Steiner, *The threefold Commonwealth*, trans by E Bowen-Wedgwood, Anthroposophical Publishing, London, 1923.

66. W B Griffin, 'Traditional v. modern contemporary architecture: a discussion', *Architecture*, vol 19, no 12, December 1930, pp 567–68.

67. W B Griffin, 'Toward simpler homes', *Architecture*, vol 20, no 8, August 1931, p 171; W B Griffin, 'Canberra in occupation: recapitulation and projection of the plan', *Canberra Annual*, 1934, p 6; W B Griffin, 'Architecture in India', unpublished ms, about December 1936, M M Griffin, 'The magic of America', 'I: The Empirial Battle', pp 174–85.

68. Guenther Wachsmuth, *The etheric formative forces in Cosmos, Earth and Man: a path of investigation into the world of the living*, vol 1, trans by O D Wannamaker, Anthroposophic Press, New York, pp 40–44; W B Griffin's handwritten notes and schematic diagrams from this book are in the E M Nicholls collection.

69. W B Griffin, 'Canberra — II: the Federal city site and its architectural possibilities', *Building*, 12 December 1913, p 68.

70. Rudolf Steiner, 'Concerning the lost temple and how it is to be restored', lecture given in Berlin, 15 May 1905, *The temple legend*, trans by J M Wood, Rudolf Steiner Press, London, 1985, pp 150–51.

71. A photograph of the pen-and-ink perspective of this scheme is in the E M Nicholls collection; Eric Nicholls joined the Anthroposophical Society on 10 September 1935, Membership file 89/1935; he served as General Secretary of the Anthroposophical Society in Australia from 1948 to 1965.

72. Paul Kruty and Paul E Sprague, *Two American architects in India: Walter B. Griffin and Marion M. Griffin, 1935–1937*, School of Architecture, University of Illinois, Urbana-Champaign, 1997, pp 12, 32, 36–37, 58–59.

73. W B Griffin, 'The modern architect's field', p 38.

74. Lawrence Durrell, *Nunquam*, Faber & Faber, London, 1970, pp 66, 194. R W Dasenbrock, 'Lawrence Durrell and the modes of modernism', *Twentieth century literature*, vol 33, no 4, Winter 1987, p 523.

75. Emerson, 'Nature', p 347.

THE LANDSCAPE ART OF WALTER BUR

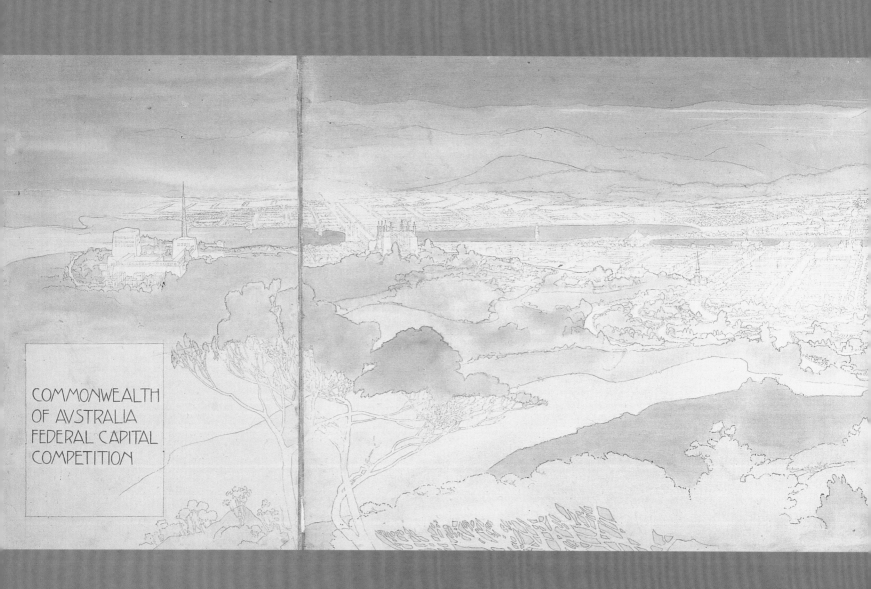

COMMONWEALTH
OF AVSTRALIA
FEDERAL CAPITAL
COMPETITION

VIEW FROM
SVMMIT OF
MOVNT AINSLIE

In his native United States of America, Walter Burley Griffin[1] until only recently was remembered as an obscure protégé of that nation's most celebrated architect, Frank Lloyd Wright. In Australia, however, Griffin has consistently received far greater professional and popular attention, stemming from his renown as the designer of its federal capital city, Canberra. Common to both nations is the popular perception of Griffin as an architect and, to a lesser extent, a town planner. This perception is far too restrictive and diverges significantly from fact: Griffin, in complement with and parallel to architecture, was educated in and practised *landscape* architecture. This essay overviews his ideas and a selection of his works within this lesser known discipline. Crucially, some of these works were informed by Marion Mahony Griffin's ideas. While the essay recognises her contribution, further research is required to document and clarify its scope. Lastly, the essay emphasises the initial five years of the Griffins' Australian residence: their first impressions and reactions to the Australian landscape were formative ones, setting the trajectory for the remainder of their careers.

In order to gain insight into the Griffins' Australian work, it is necessary first to situate Walter Burley Griffin within the American context which fundamentally shaped his, and subsequently Marion's, approach to landscape architecture. Educated in both architecture and landscape architecture at the University of Illinois (1895–1899), Griffin early and importantly worked with Frank Lloyd Wright from 1901 until early 1906. This period, during which Marion Mahony also was in Wright's employ, saw the emergence of Wright's Prairie house, a type named for and inspired by the Chicago region's indigenous landscape. Among other roles, Griffin served as Wright's landscape architect. Theirs was a collaborative relationship: upon receipt of a new commission, Wright first conceived the general site organisation and Griffin next prepared detailed landscape designs.

Wright and Griffin's relationship eventuated in a mutual landscape design approach. Seeking to unite and equally value house and garden or architecture and nature, Wright typically organised grounds by extending the plan geometry of the house outward into its larger surrounds, engaging the full extent of the block. This geometric order was often expressed in the design of pergolas, courtyards, low terrace projections, and pools. However, the seeming irregularity of the natural landscape was never completely absent. Dwellings, for example, were carefully inserted into any extant groves, preserving mature trees within the precincts of attendant gardens. 'Naturalistic' or irregular plantings predominated at the block perimeters, providing the larger frame to contain and effectively foil the geometric matrix of house and garden. Opportunities for extensive garden designs, however, were infrequent. The celebrated intimacy between Wright's Prairie houses and their setting was achieved more often by analogous architectural means, such as out-reaching walls and terraces, than by the literal use of lavish garden treatments. Following his departure from Wright's office, Griffin initiated a period of design experimentation; a search for his own voice, independent of Wright's.

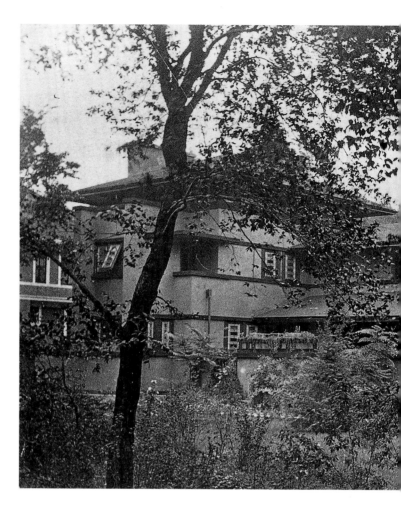

The concept of nature was the emphatic, shaping force underpinning Griffin's landscape architecture; his childhood experiences and those while practising in Chicago being amongst its greater stimuli. Accelerating, largely unregulated urban and suburban expansion transformed late nineteenth and early twentieth-century Chicago. The city's formerly open natural and agricultural surrounds quickly metamorphosed into speculatively motivated city extensions and new suburbs. Griffin witnessed this abrupt transformation, reflecting on the loss: 'When I was a child there was plenty of open ground to play in, about ten allotments to each boy'. 'Now', he continued, 'it is ten boys to each allotment'.[2] Griffin's preoccupation with nature also constituted his impassioned response to the dynamics of modernity: the rapidity of landscape transformation stimulated not only his design interest in permanency, but also punctuated the need to reconnect with or re-acculturate nature. Griffin's designs, although in themselves instruments of suburbanisation, were envisaged as alternative Arcadian venues for this reconnection and quiet communion.

In concert with his design response, Griffin's witness to the destruction of the primeval compelled his direct participation in efforts to conserve the remnants. Beginning in

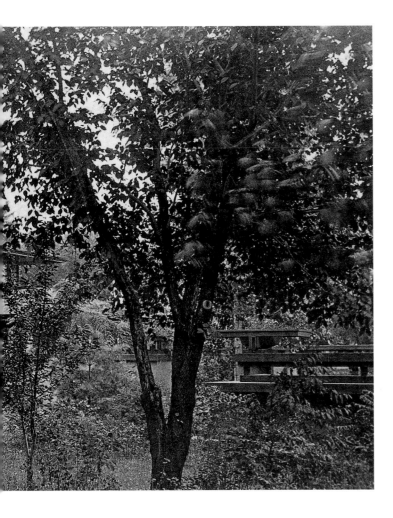 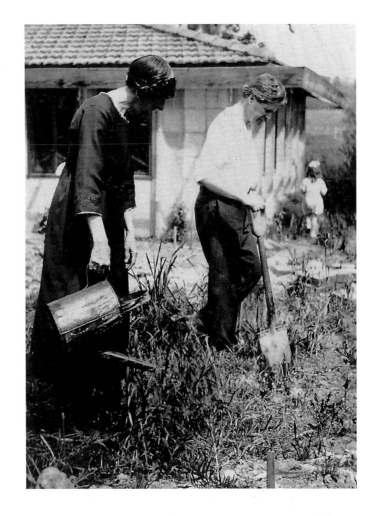

Above: William Martin house (1903) and garden (designed about 1904 and re-designed in about 1910) at Oak Park, near Chicago, Illinois; Frank Lloyd Wright, architect and Walter Burley Griffin, landscape architect. Photographed in about 1910. 'Naturalistic' plantings dominated the perimeter of the Martin block, providing the larger frame to contain the geometric matrix of house and garden.

Courtesy William Martin family collection.

Above right: Marion and Walter in the garden of *Pholiota*, the one-room, Knitlock tile house they built at Heidelberg, Melbourne, in 1922.

Courtesy National Library of Australia, Canberra (P480/1–5).

Previous page: 'View from the Summit of Mt Ainslie', Canberra, 1911, ink, watercolour and gouache on linen, 76 × 305 cm. One of thirteen renderings submitted by Marion and Walter for Australia's Federal Capital competition. Griffin's Land Axis was determined by the alignments of Mount Ainslie and the distant Mount Bimberi.

Courtesy National Archives of Australia, Canberra (CRS A710, item 48–50).

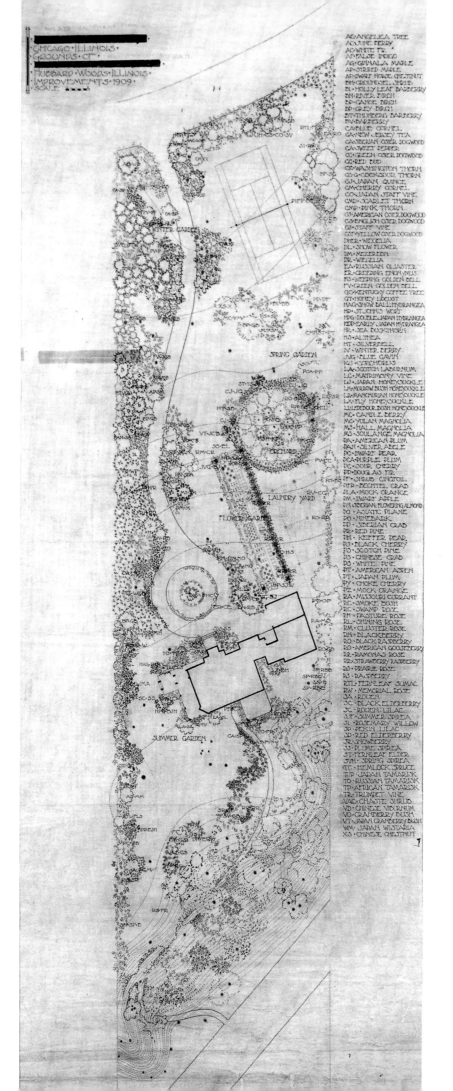

Garden plan for Mrs J W Bolte, Hubbard's Woods, near Chicago, 1909, ink on linen, 109 × 50 cm. Walter Burley Griffin, landscape architect; drawing by Marion Mahony (?). Griffin created separate, distinct gardens for each season, animating the cycle of the year.

Courtesy the Mary and Leigh Block Museum of Art, Northwestern University, Illinois, (1985.1.73).

1908, Griffin and others, under the auspices of the Playground Association of Chicago, led public walks to the region's indigenous landscape remnants with the aim of stimulating interest in their conservation. Griffin supplemented these excursions with individual field study, cultivating a 'command of geography which was his by instinct and industry' and a detailed knowledge of the native flora.[3]

Griffin's participation in the Playground Association walks facilitated his contact with Chicago's scientific community, particularly its geographers and botanists.[4] Through this association (and other sources), Griffin undoubtedly gained insights into developments in these natural sciences. Ecological and geomorphological knowledge, for example, collectively revealed the structure of the land and the inter-relationships of its functioning component parts: vegetation, soil, topography, and climate.[5] Synthesising science with the theoretical discourses of architecture and landscape architecture, Griffin now conceived of land as the dynamic product of geomorphic processes and as a system of inter-related, less pictographic components. As a result, Griffin's landscape architecture sought to interpret and accentuate this otherwise latent order.

In Griffin's 1909 landscape design for Mrs J W Bolte his knowledge of natural processes was more conceptual than literal in its application and expression. In this design, the planting merits special consideration. Rather than creating a conventional mosaic of floral colour uniformly distributed throughout a planting composition, Griffin created separate, distinct gardens for each season, coordinated by colour.[6] Not only could landscape colour complement related architectural and interior colour schemes, it also could now animate natural processes, the cycle of the seasons.

Of all his American works, this approach is most comprehensively exemplified by his community design for Rock Crest–Rock Glen at Mason City, Iowa, about 1912. The 7-hectare site, situated at varying levels below the surrounding streets, encompassed a sweeping bend of Willow Creek and its limestone bluff embankments. Located in the city centre, the site had been neglected owing to the building difficulties posed by its comparatively steep topography. Formerly quarried and partly used as a rubbish tip, the site, moreover, was in a state of dereliction at the time of Griffin's commission. The clarity of his design vision was unblurred by the evidence of previous use, if not consumption, and he sought to rehabilitate and conserve the creek valley as a place for human habitation. Importantly, however, he did not seek to recapture a sense of pristine, primeval nature. Instead, the future residents of Rock Crest–Rock Glen were to dwell in an idealised, cultivated nature.

In order to accommodate dwellings (also of his design) at the site perimeters, Griffin's redemptive vision entailed corrective manipulation of the landforms, disturbed by earlier quarrying. The dwellings, individually oriented in response to water and other views within the site, were then cut and terraced into the perimeter bluffs. This strategic dwelling placement in itself architecturally reinscribed the site's topographic structure, at once revealing and articulating geomorphic process. Moreover, by positioning the dwellings at the road-bounded site perimeters, Griffin maintained the open quality of its waterside centre. Willow Creek was widened and its margins held in reserve as a community park. The creek was made the quiet, luminescent focus of his visually and spatially self-contained enclave. At the larger scale, Griffin's compact, cubic architecture became but incidents in and subordinate to his larger landscape composition.

The increasing primacy Griffin awarded nature was profoundly expressed in his 1911 prize-winning Canberra design, prepared at a distance in Chicago. The majority of the international competitors essentially responded to the Canberra site as though it were a sort of isomorphic plane, distorting it into conformity with various aesthetic formulae. Alternatively, through his fundamental reliance upon the native topography to organise his plan, Griffin appropriated the physical site itself as the new Australian nation's primal monument. Mount Ainslie, for example, was ennobled by Griffin's monumentalising use of it as the focus of one end of his heroically-scaled 'Land Axis'; Mount Bimberi, some 25 kilometres away, terminated the opposite end. In this monumentalisation of the land, Griffin's design also drew upon a seminal American source: the spatial and symbolic concerns of Washington DC as envisaged by Pierre Charles L'Enfant. In L'Enfant's 1791 plan, the vast interior continental landscape, then perceived as an unspoilt wilderness, was made symbolic of the fledgling nation's potential and development westward through his use of it as the western focus of the capital city's axial Mall, anchored to the east by the Capitol building. A cross-axis extended southward some 11 kilometres from the White House, encompassing in its prospect the Potomac River. L'Enfant's powerful landscape effects, however, were destroyed in the opening decades of the twentieth century.[7] In Canberra, Griffin archaically revalued the potency of landscape as a container and bearer of meaning, evoking and transforming L'Enfant's eighteenth-century ideals. As had been the design aspiration in America, so it was with Canberra: cultural history was made from natural history.[8]

By the time of his departure from the United States, Griffin's landscape design approach was typified by his fusion of geometric reason with picturesque naturalism.[9] In transformation of Wright's architecturally-derived geometric site templates, Griffin turned to a supplemental, primordial source of geometry: 'the architecture of plants and of the animals', even adapting biological forms as garden plans. For him, geometry was the language or 'aesthetic skeleton' of nature, as evidenced in the cells of a beehive or in crystal formation. Landscape architecture ultimately was both process — the holistic design of architecture plus landscape — and result.

After accepting the Commonwealth invitation, Walter Burley Griffin first travelled to Australia in 1913. On 19 August 1913 *The Sydney Morning Herald* included an interview with the designer a day after his arrival. Perhaps it was indicative of landscape architecture's professional obscurity in Australia that the reporter queried Griffin as to whether 'landscape work' was amongst his 'hobbies'. Griffin affirmatively replied and explained, politely correcting the reporter by inference, that landscape architecture was an 'art that is dragging along at the heels of architecture, but it is coming into its own'.

Griffin soon developed what would prove to be a deep and abiding passion for Australian flora. His first, enthusiastically favourable response to it appeared in the 2 October 1913 *Herald*. Therein, Griffin revealed and admonished that the 'gum tree, instead of being one big continual monotony, has strongly appealed to me' and it 'ought to have a more dignified name'. Griffin's reference to the 'monotony' of the gums suggests he was aware that his favourable regard for them was not necessarily a popular one. For him, the appeal of gum trees was profoundly aesthetic: identifying them as 'decorator's trees', Griffin contended that the gum's 'foliage is beautiful, and varies a great deal, its bark and twigs have a beauty all their own'. As well as discerning their aesthetic appeal, Griffin advocated their use in landscape design, judging that 'no tree equals the eucalyptus for embellishing the landscape'. Moreover, Griffin crucially asserted that 'foreign trees' were 'not so suitable' and 'not so beautiful'. In this context, 'suitability' reflected his nascent identification of eucalypts as central to the visual character of the larger Australian landscape.

Griffin's visit of nearly three months culminated with his appointment as Canberra's Federal Capital Director of Design and Construction. Given six months leave of absence to settle his American affairs, Griffin departed Australia in November 1913. He returned the following May, accompanied by Marion Mahony Griffin.[10]

The offer of the position as Federal Capital Director of Design and Construction, which Griffin perceived to be the opportunity to realise his design for an entire ideal city, was the catalyst for his move to Australia. For Griffin, Australia was the last 'new frontier' and 'new world'. Not unlike D H Lawrence's later contention that the country was 'the land that as yet has made no great mistake, humanly',[11] Griffin saw Australia as presenting alluring opportunities to perfect and apply lessons learnt from the failings of the immediate American past.

Once in Australia, Griffin was soon enraptured by its flora, believing it crucial to the country's landscape distinctiveness and, more symbolically and at the larger scale, of Australia as place. Sparsely populated, compared to Chicago's increasingly urbanised hinterland, Australia was the place where, as Lawrence asserted, 'people mattered so little'.[12] Partly owing to the relative invisibility or spatial insignificance of the human occupation, it was the indigenous bush, both real and imagined, that was more prevailing. In contrast to Chicago's offering of fragmented 'beauty spots', vestiges of a rapidly consumed, spent nature, Australia provided a natural landscape much less occupied. Equally fundamental to Griffin's favourable reaction to the Australian environment was its salubrious climate. Unlike Chicago's 'six months of generally dull' winter landscape,

Right: Plan of Rock Crest–Rock Glen, Mason City, Iowa, about 1912, ink on paper, 40 × 30 cm. Walter Burley Griffin, architect and landscape architect; drawing by Marion Mahony Griffin. Griffin rehabilitated the community site, a former quarry and rubbish tip, transforming it into a prairie Arcadia.

Courtesy Nicholls collection, Sydney.

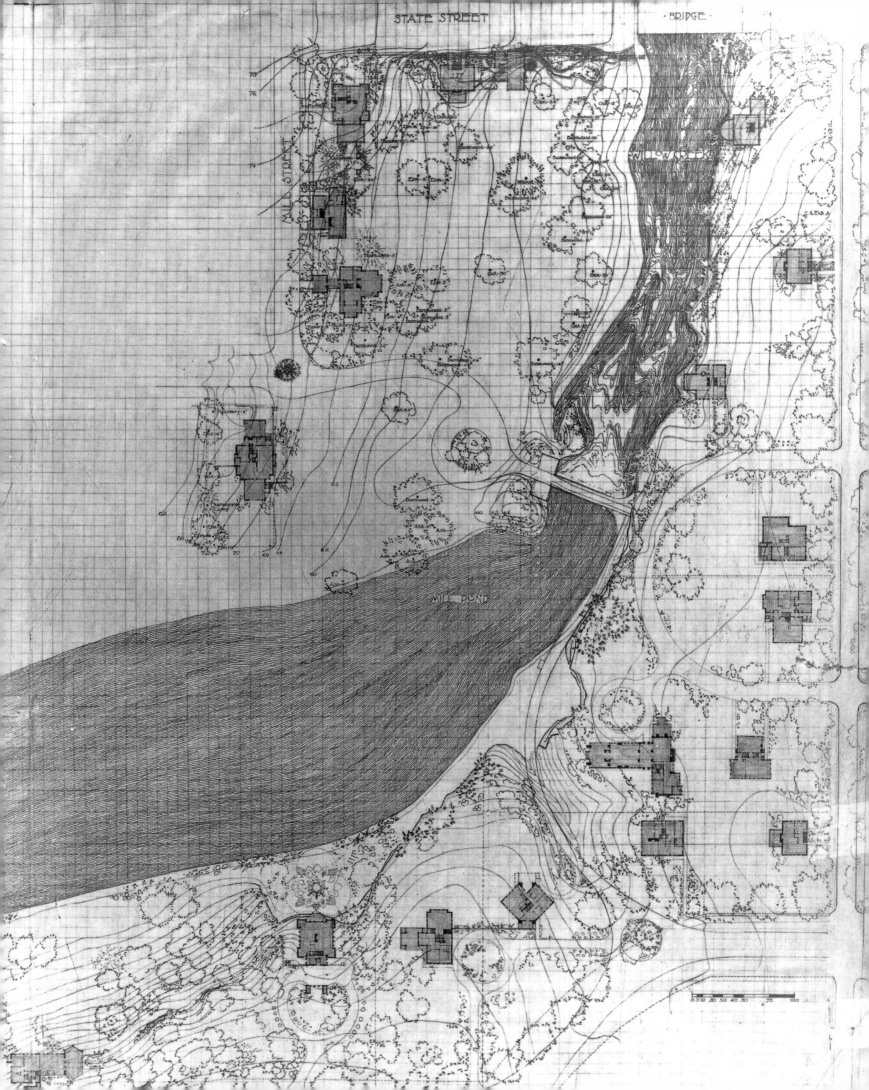

STATE STREET · BRIDGE ·

MILL POND

Australia's year-round gardens lacked the climatic deprivation and became a 'requisite in the subtropical evergreen Australian setting'.[13]

After the Griffins settled in Sydney, that city and other state capitals became venues for one of Australia's most notable scientific events held up to that time, the eighty-fourth meeting of the British Association for the Advancement of Science (28 July – 31 August 1914). The meeting attracted 300 overseas scientists and, importantly, the local participants included the Griffins.[14] Their attendance not only served to immerse them in a cross-section of the latest scientific discourses, but also marked Walter's continuing interest in synthesising the aesthetic with the scientific in landscape design.

Following the association meetings, the Griffins furthered their now mutual interest in Australian flora. In August 1914, Marion Mahony Griffin joined the Naturalists' Society of New South Wales; Walter in the following month.[15] Membership provided them opportunity for organised bushwalking and field study, and also facilitated their contact with the local scientific community, especially botanists. As they had done in Chicago, the Griffins supplemented organised excursions with their own, using 'every possible opportunity for learning the points of the wonderfully rich native flora'.[16] The Botanic Gardens in Sydney, and later those in Melbourne, became an early locus of their studies. Further afield, Mahony Griffin recollected that 'Saturday was always kept free for walks in the outlying districts of Sydney, anything up to 20 miles, with [Constance] LePlastrier, the botanist'.[17] Other botanists also accompanied the Griffins, including Alexander G Hamilton and Edwin Cheel.[18] While in their company, Griffin solicited 'seven and eight hour' lectures 'on relationships and soil conditions and habit' which, Mahony Griffin explained, they 'never resented'. By the end of 1914, she believed that Griffin 'knew more than anyone in Australia of what was significant for a landscape architect'.

Griffin's passion for Australian flora found early design application and expression in his 1914 town plan for Leeton, New South Wales, in the Murrumbidgee Irrigation

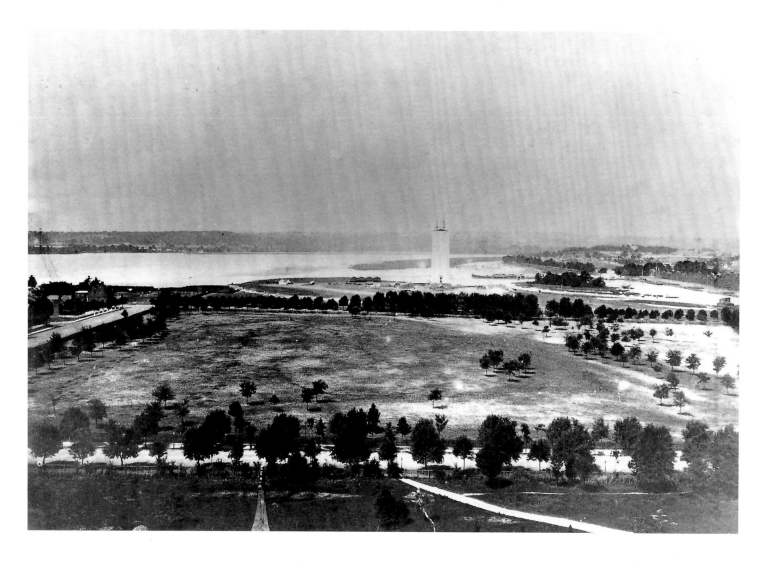

Area. *The Irrigation Record* prefaced its publication of the plan by noting that not only did Griffin have 'a very high opinion indeed of the decorative value of Australian flora', but also that he believed it was 'all too little appreciated by Australians generally'.[19] Echoing sentiments expressed during his first Australian visit, he explained in his Leeton report that the reason why the 'Australian sylva is unsurpassed for home embellishment' was owing to its aesthetic attributes, its 'open lacelike delicacy, half concealing, half revealing, also in its subtle and quiet colourings of bark and stem as well as foliage and often profuse flowering'. The Leeton town plan may have been the first design in which Griffin sought to use native vegetation, however, this planting ideal apparently was not realised.

Griffin was not alone in his passion for the Australian flora; it also held great appeal for Marion. The 12 January 1915 issue of *Building* announced that 'Marion Mahony Griffin, Landscape Architect' had served as the adjudicator of the magazine's design competition for 'a garden of one acre'.[20] Marion's assessment of the winning entries offers

Left: A rare photographic view, taken in about 1855, of the original western landscape focus of Washington's Mall (USA) (the partially constructed Washington Monument is visible to the right of centre). The Mall's landscape focus was destroyed in the early twentieth century through the completion of the monument, extensive filling of the Potomac River, and the construction of the Lincoln Memorial.
Courtesy Library of Congress.

Below: Aerial view from Parliament House toward Mount Ainslie, 1993. Griffin appropriated Canberra's site itself as the new nation's primal monument.
Courtesy Christopher Vernon.

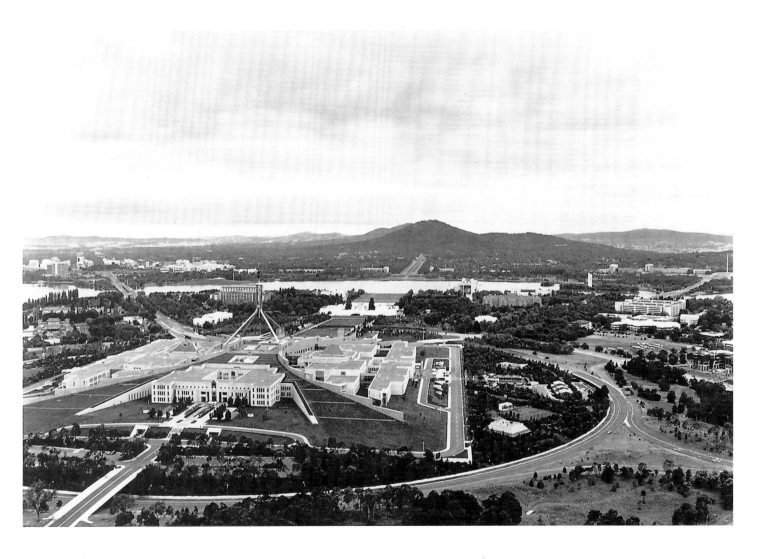

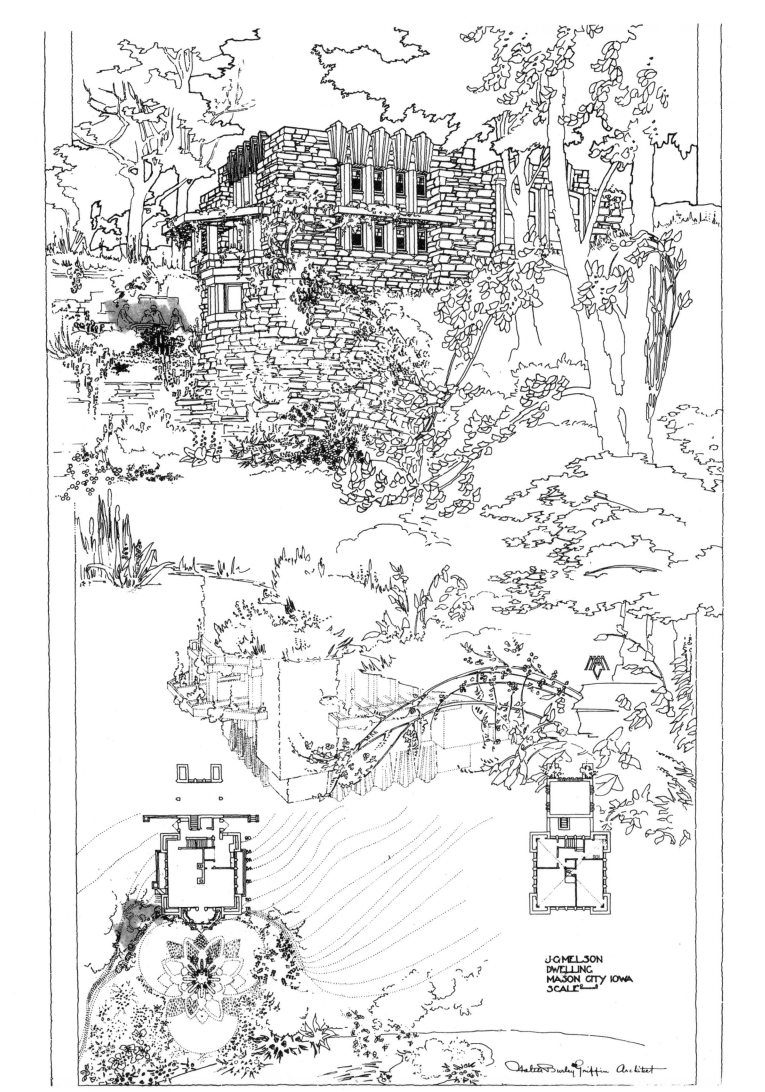

J·G·MELSON
DWELLING
MASON CITY IOWA
SCALE

Walter Burley Griffin Architect

insight into her own seldom-published views on garden design. 'Flower beds', for example, were only 'tolerable' in 'closely circumscribed recesses, where they do not interfere with the integrity of a quiet stretch of green, and where their marked individuality will not conflict with the simplicity of the whole scheme'. Marion's design interest in 'quiet' and 'simplicity' was compatible with Walter's view. Curiously, however, Marion neither was commonly known as a landscape architect in the United States nor did she inscribe her drawings with the title (unlike Walter). Perhaps her enchantment with the landscape and the possibility of 'year round' gardens became catalysts for her more comprehensive pursuit of landscape architecture once in the Antipodes. As this announcement also was one of the first in the professional press to focus upon Marion and her own expertise, that she chose to be titled 'Landscape Architect' suggests the increasing, if not new, importance she awarded the pursuit.

Walter Burley Griffin's own botanical passion was expressed in his 1915 design for Canberra's 'Botanical Reserve', a national arboretum. The arboretum's systematic organisation by continents was at the suggestion of Griffin's bushwalking companion Edwin Cheel.[21] Cheel's advocacy of a continental or geographical classification scheme in itself is not unusual. However, Griffin's composition and arrangement of the continental representations is. Intriguingly, their juxtaposition suggests his knowledge of the prehistoric unification of continents into a larger land mass, Gondwanaland; a concept discussed in the previous year's British Association meetings.[22] Griffin's arboretum design evoked this antique 'inter-connectedness', attempting to symbolically imbue Canberra with a sense of 'permanence' and redress antipodal isolation. The arboretum, however, would remain an unrealised vision.

That Griffin then saw native vegetation as definitive and resonant of place, as initially alluded to in his 1913 newspaper interview, is confirmed by his 1916 selection of Australian floral names as place-names for Canberra's new suburbs and streets, such as Grevillea Place, Telopea Park, Clianthus Circle and Blandfordia.[23] This symbolism was more explicit and legible than that of his earlier arboretum, however, it would prove short lived: Griffin's successors excised most of his botanically-derived names in the 1920s, believing them 'not in keeping with Australian sentiment'.

In 1917, Griffin received an opportunity to comprehensively use native vegetation in landscape design. However, the genesis of the opportunity actually came two years earlier. In 1915 he was commissioned to design the buildings for the new 'Catholic College at the University of Melbourne'. Griffin included, in complement to his building design and as had been his custom in America, a 'plot plan' for the larger campus. The plot plan delineated mass plantings of Australian flora, organised by seasonal floral colours and combinations thereof, including 'orange, scarlet and yellow', 'salmon and copper' and 'silver, pink and blue':[24] a botanical colour symphony in keeping with 'Griffin's method of planting together according to colour'.[25]

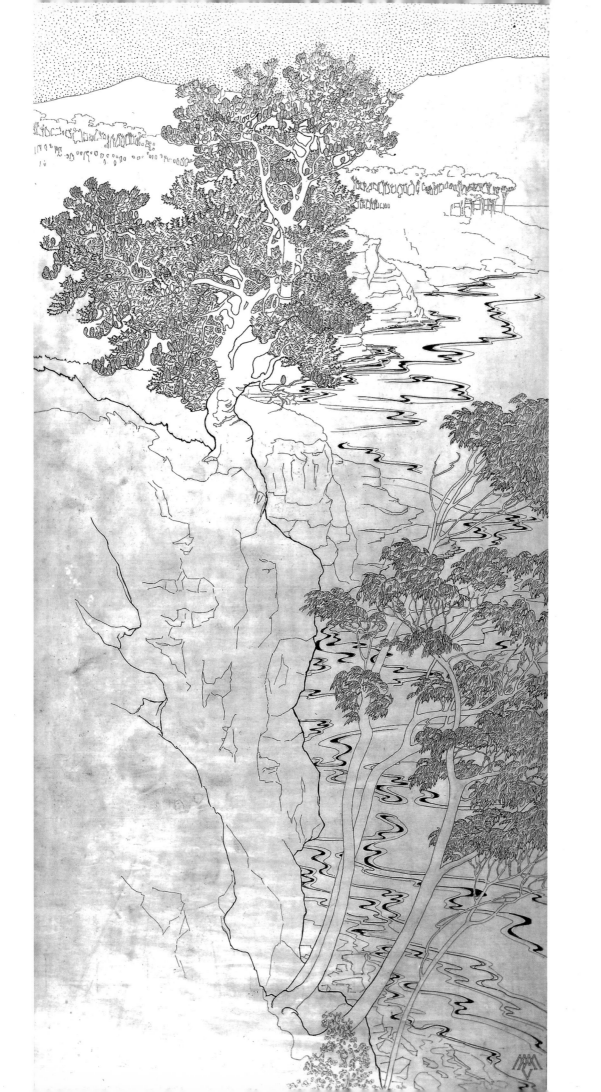

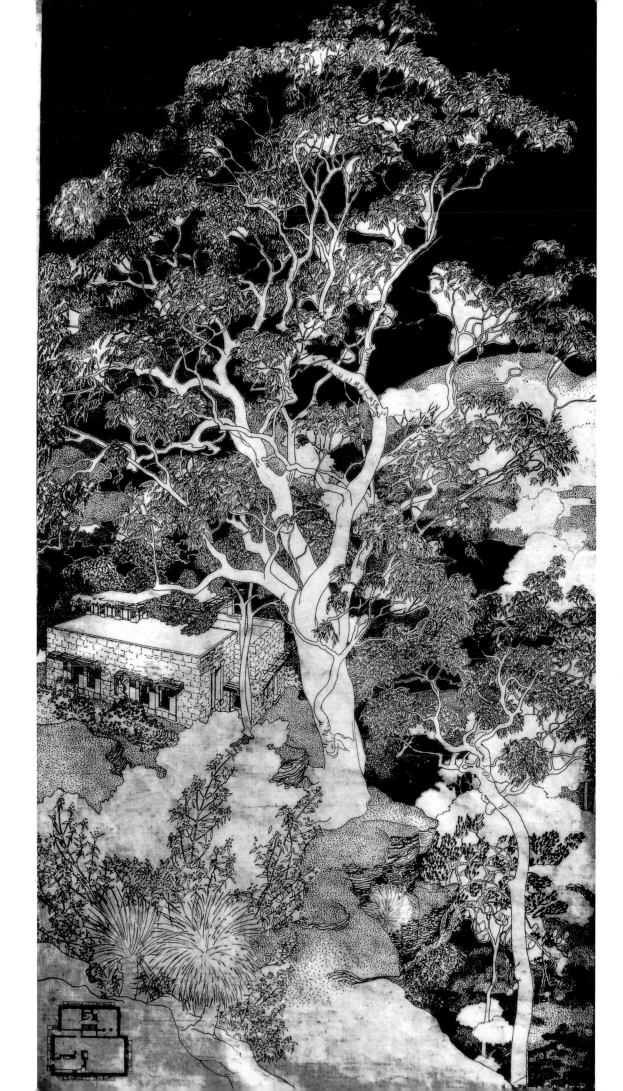

When Griffin developed this method in America, it was executed with native as well as exotic plants. In Australia, however, he sought to realise it almost exclusively with native flora. The plan also is evidence that his parallel landscape design concern for the larger campus was integral to his architectural vision. A year later, Griffin prepared a detailed design derived from his earlier, more schematic, plot plan for the now named Newman College. It was a remarkable garden design, composed predominantly of native vegetation. Recorded on ten 50 cm by 153 cm Chinese scroll-like blueprints,[26] replete with vegetation individually identified by botanical name, the Newman College garden is one of the first examples of an Australian flora garden designed by a landscape architect.

Of equal significance is that the Newman garden design undoubtedly was a collaborative one; Marion herself recorded that she worked on the plans. As well, despite Walter Burley Griffin's signature, it is probable that Marion's involvement was substantial, because at this time Walter was increasingly preoccupied with work demands in Canberra. While Newman College 'was already on the draughting boards', Mahony Griffin began a project that would take many years to complete: compiling a list of native plants 'for use in any and all planting schemes [;] tabulated to show different growth requirements, as soil, moisture [etc]; heights and shapes of growths; colour of flowers, foliage, berries and barks'.[27] For this, she made a series of stunning botanical illustrations or studies. Marion also shared Walter's advocacy of using native flora in landscape design. For example, shortly after the Newman design, the 23 March 1918 *Australasian* reported that Marion, in her lecture 'Community planning and planting', 'emphasised the beauties of the Australian flora'. Beyond this aesthetic rationale, she asserted that use of native plants would result in 'maximum beauty', 'attained in the shortest time' and 'with the least expenditure'. Most important was her specificity in urging that more be used, 'at least nine-tenths of native flora to one-tenth of foreign material': neither of the Griffins were purists in their advocacy of Australian flora. She later reported that Griffin, for example, 'supplemented the flora somewhat, especially with South African plants whose local conditions closely resemble those of Australia'.[28] The nature of the potential deficiency in the native flora which apparently was redressed by the use of South African or other exotic species, however, remains unclear.

By 1919, Griffin's efforts to realise his ideal Canberra had been consistently undermined by calculated political and other antagonisms, culminating in the 1920 abolition of his position. Unwilling to serve in a much diminished capacity as a member of an advisory design committee and no doubt deeply demoralised, Griffin disassociated himself from the still embryonic city.

Fourteen years after the Griffins' arrival, landscape architecture remained a nascent profession in Australia.[29] 'Landscape architecture', Griffin contended in 1928, was 'a term as yet unused here'; asserting as well that there then was only 'a handful' of 'landscape gardeners, professionally trained abroad, whose opportunities are confined to the narrow scope of domestic plantations'.[30] However, the Griffins themselves already had contributed to local professional education: Emily Gibson entered their employ in 1917 as an apprentice *landscape* architect, most likely assisting with the Newman College garden.[31] Gibson perhaps was the first person, in either America or Australia, to apprentice to the Griffins to pursue a career explicitly in landscape architecture.

As in America, Griffin soon became an advocate of conservation in Australia. This concern, which also became characteristic of his Australian work, was early displayed in his community design for Eaglemont, about 1915, in increasingly suburban Melbourne. Here he joined development with conservation, including reserves situated so as 'to conserve ancient Red gum trees'.[32] Eaglemont's conserved gum trees not only layered a patina of relative antiquity over the otherwise rawness of Griffin's community, but they also acknowledged his conviction that such flora was central to Australia's distinctiveness. Griffin later made this explicit, believing that: '[the] landscape gardener with appreciation for and equipped with the unique technique of Australian flora is the great desideratum for a legitimate art that can be distinctive of Australia and Australia alone. May he [*sic*] come before his medium is destroyed'.[33]

The Griffins' later (1920–1935) writings not only see their ecological knowledge become increasingly sophisticated, but also document an emerging environmental concern. In 1935, writing in the journal of the Wildlife Preservation Society of Australia (of which he was a member), Griffin urged that land be 'accorded the respect due to a highly developed and perfected living organism not to be exterminated nor treated as dead material, or as a mere section of the map'.[34] The Griffins' increasing environmental concern led to their landscape rehabilitation and conservation work at Castlecrag, an object-lesson begun in the 1920s and continuing until Walter Griffin's 1935 departure for India.

Griffin's movement across the prairies to the Antipodes resulted in the transference and transformation of the ideas and design approach borne of his American experience. Beginning with his envisaged object-lesson Canberra, Griffin set out to define Australia by an idealised articulation of its indigenous landscape. Through holistic, comprehensive design, he hoped, more fundamentally, to create a habitable 'second nature' — one referential to its increasingly more remote, primeval counterpart — and resolve a perceived dialectic between nature and culture. Rejected at Canberra, this was later achieved at Castlecrag in suburban Sydney. There, architecture receded in deference to his cultivated, rehabilitated nature and landscape was given primacy: Griffin realised, if only fleetingly, the ideal of a more fertile Arcadia, which America was losing.

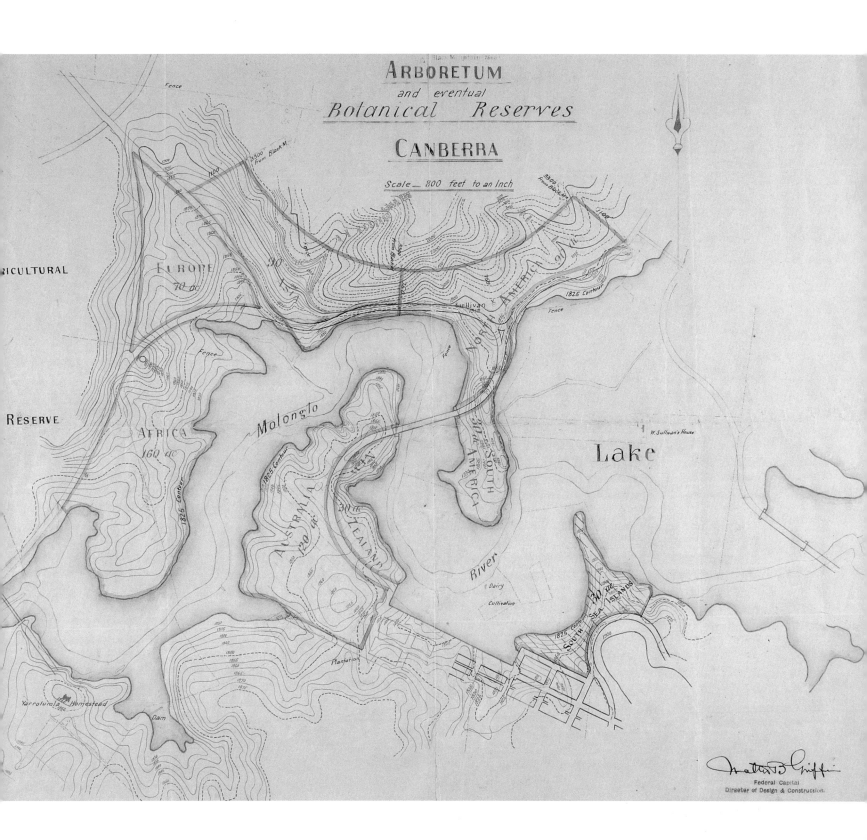

Proposed 'Arboretum' and 'Botanical Reserves', Canberra,
1915, dyeline print, 25 × 30 cm. Walter Burley Griffin,
landscape architect. Griffin's juxtapositions of the
arboretum's continental organisation evoked the antique
'inter-connectedness' of Gondwanaland.

Courtesy National Archives of Australia, Canberra, (AA 1966/33).

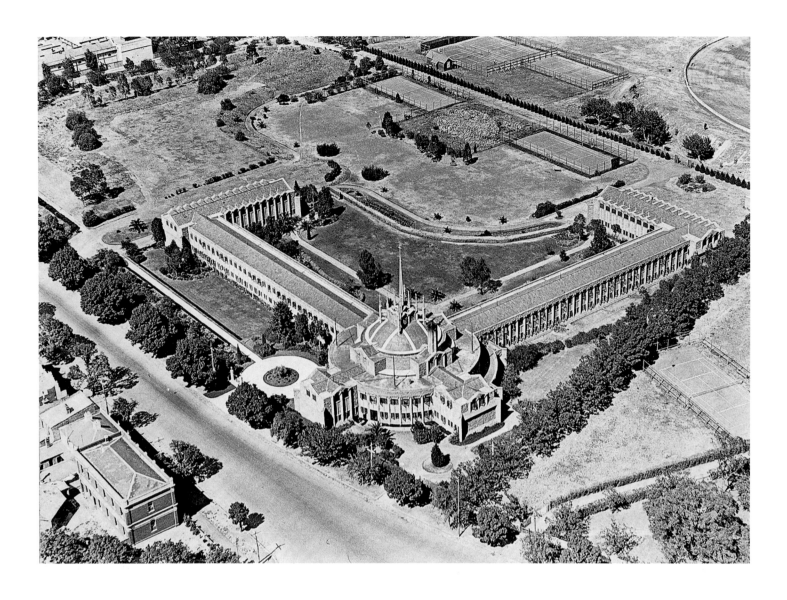

Above: Aerial view of Newman College and garden, Melbourne, 1929. Walter and Marion's design was one of the first Australian native flora gardens by landscape architects.

Photograph courtesy of Newman College collection.

Notes

This chapter is partly extracted with permission from the author's ' "A legitimate art distinctive of Australia and Australia alone": the Griffins' contribution to the formation of an Australian landscape design ethos', first published in *Landscape Review*, vol 3, no 1, 1997, pp 2–27. Readers seeking more on the American context, later Australian reception and transformation of Griffin's ideas, and full annotations are referred to this piece.

1. Griffin is known as Burley Griffin (for example, Lake Burley Griffin in Canberra) apparently only in Australia and is not known to have referred to himself by this shortened form of his name. In the United States he was and remains consistently known as Walter Burley Griffin or Walter Griffin.

2. [Griffin, Walter Burley] 'Mr. W. B. Griffin's view: architect and social student', *The Salon*, vol 2, no 2, 1913, p 112.

3. Marion Mahony Griffin, 'The magic of America', unpublished manuscript, about 1949, pp 280 and 283. These quotations (as well as others elsewhere in the text) are from 'The magic of America'. Pagination refers to the typescript in the collection of the Burnham Library of Architecture at the Art Institute of Chicago. For more on this invaluable document see James Weirick, '*The magic of America*: vision and text', in J Duncan and M Gates, eds, *Walter Burley Griffin: a re-view*, Monash

University Gallery, Victoria, 1988; and the exceedingly well-considered account of Mahony and her work: James Weirick, 'Marion Mahony at M.I.T.', *Transition: discourse on architecture*, vol 25, 1988, pp 49–54.

4. Other members included, for example, the University of Chicago's pioneering plant ecologist Henry Chandler Cowles and geographer Rollin D Salisbury. For more on the Playground Association walks see Emma Doeserich, ed, *Outdoors with the Prairie Club*, Paquin, Chicago, 1941.

5. For example, in his description of the site for his proposed 'Ridge Quadrangles' community in suburban Chicago, Griffin explained that the site embraced a 'sand spit or bar [the community's namesake 'ridge'] that mark[ed] the former existence of lake or sea over the Chicago district, in this case some 20 feet above the general level about it'; see Walter Burley Griffin, 'Ridge quadrangles', *The Western Architect*, vol 19, no 8, 1913, pp 71–72.

6. Griffin's interest in colour was informed by British (for example, the work and writings of William Robinson and Gertrude Jekyll) and German sources; see Christopher Vernon, '"Expressing natural conditions with maximum possibility": the American landscape art (1901–c.1912) of Walter Burley Griffin', *Journal of Garden History*, vol 15, no 1, 1995, pp 19–47. Reprinted in *Landscape Australia*, vol 17, nos 2/3, pp 130–37 and 146–52, 214–16; Christopher Vernon, 'Wilhelm Miller and the prairie spirit in landscape gardening' in T O'Malley and M Treib, eds, *Regional garden design in the United States*, Washington DC, Dumbarton Oaks Research Library and Collection, 1995. Also includes reprint of Miller, 1915; Christopher Vernon, 'Frank Lloyd Wright, Walter Burley Griffin, Jens Jensen and the Jugendstil garden in America', *Die Gartenkunst*, vol 7, no 2, 1995, pp 232–46.

7. It was at this time that Washington was redesigned in accordance with the landscape de-valuing views of D H Burnham and the Senate Park Commission. For example, architectural objects, such as the Lincoln Memorial, supplanted the landscape focii of L'Enfant's axes.

8. This, of course, reflected an implicit blindness not only to indigenous Aboriginal culture but also to the country's British colonial past.

9. It is important to note that, transferred from its British source, picturesque naturalism, too, already had been transformed by and ideologically adapted to American conditions.

10. The Griffins also were accompanied by Walter's sister Genevieve and her architect husband Roy A Lippincott.

11. D H Lawrence, *Kangaroo*, HarperCollins Publishers, Sydney, 1995 (original, 1923), p 405.

12. Ibid, p 402.

13. W B Griffin, 'Ridge quadrangles', 1913, p 72, and W B Griffin, 'The factors in the design of this building...', typescript, Newman College archives, October 1915.

14. British Association for the Advancement of Science, *Report of the eighty-fourth meeting of the British Association for the Advancement of Science*, Australia: 1914, John Murray, London, 1915, pp 112, 144. Griffin also presented an explanatory paper, 'The Canberra Plan', to the delegates at the Melbourne session on 14 August.

15. Notice of the Griffins' memberships was included in the 6 October 1914 issue of *The Australian Naturalist*, vol 3, no 4, pp 37–38. Information on the society's membership was derived from a review of this journal during the 1914–20 period.

16. M M Griffin, 'The magic of America', p 200.

17. Ibid, p 335. C LePlastrier, with Agnes A Brewster (also members of the Naturalists' Society), published *Botany for Australian students* in about 1916 (no date was included in the edition consulted by the author at the National Library of Australia. However, this copy bears the imprint: 'Commonwealth of Australia; Library of the Parliament; 21 July 1916'). Important to this essay is that the book included a chapter, 'The plant, a member of a community', which outlined the ecological concept of a plant association, as Cowles earlier had defined in America. The Griffins may have met LePlastrier during the formative stages of this book.

Moreover, the fourth edition (1930) included a chapter, 'Plant ecology', and was accompanied by an 'Ecological map of New South Wales'. As the author only has been able to consult these two editions, he is unable to ascertain the date in which the ecology chapter first appeared.

18. Hamilton and Cheel also were members of the Naturalists' Society (then serving as vice-president and honorary secretary, respectively) and contributors to A Brewster and C LePlastrier, *Botany for Australian students*. See their biographical entries in Ray Desmond, *Dictionary of British and Irish botanists and horticulturists*, Taylor and Francis and the Natural History Museum, London, 1994, and Bede Nairn and Geoffrey Serle, eds, *Australian dictionary of biography*, Melbourne University Press, Melbourne, 1983. Another entry on Cheel is to be found in Norman Hall, *Botanists of the eucalypts*, Commonwealth Scientific and Industrial Research Organisation, Melbourne, 1978.

19. Walter Burley Griffin, 'The town plan of Leeton', *The Irrigation Record*, vol 3, nos 4 and 5, 1915, p 65.

20. The competition first was announced in the 12 June 1914 issue of *Building*, p 116. Apparently organised at a later date, Marion's role as adjudicator was not published until the 12 January 1915 issue, p 103. The announcement elaborated that Marion Mahony Griffin, an 'acknowledged expert', was 'now with her husband (Walter Burley Griffin) resident in Australia'. The author is grateful to Mr David Nichols for calling this reference to his attention.

21. Griffin (18 December 1915), letter to Edwin Cheel, National Archives of Australia.

22. See, for example, 'The vegetation of Gondwana Land' in *British Association for the Advancement of Science* (1915), pp 584–85.

23. W B Griffin, 'Canberra plan of city and environs', National Archives of Australia, 14 August 1916.

24. W B Griffin, 'The factors in the design of this building ...'; this report confirms that native flora was to be planted on the campus; the author is grateful to Peter Navaretti and Jeff Turnbull for calling this source to his attention. A reproduction of this plan [dated 15 February 1916] is included in The Burnham Library of Architecture — University of Illinois Microfilming Project micro-film of a selection of Griffin's drawings (frame 98); copy at National Library of Australia.

25. M M Griffin, 'The magic of America', p 341.

26. Newman College archives. The drawings are signed 'W B Griffin, Landscape Architect'.

27. M M Griffin, 'The magic of America', p 335.

28. Ibid, p 341.

29. For example, the Australian Institute of Landscape Architects was not founded until 1966.

30. W B Griffin, 'The outdoor arts in Australia', *Advance! Australia*, 1 May 1928, p 210.

31. Jane Shepherd, 'Early women landscape architects: Olive Mellor and Emily Gibson', *Transition: discourse on architecture*, vol 25, 1988, pp 61–63.

32. Nancy E Price, 'Walter Burley Griffin', BArch thesis, University of Sydney, Sydney, 1933, p 12.

33. W B Griffin, 'The outdoor arts in Australia', 1928, p 210.

34. W B Griffin, 'Occupational conservation', *Australian Wildlife*, vol 1, no 2, 1935, p 24.

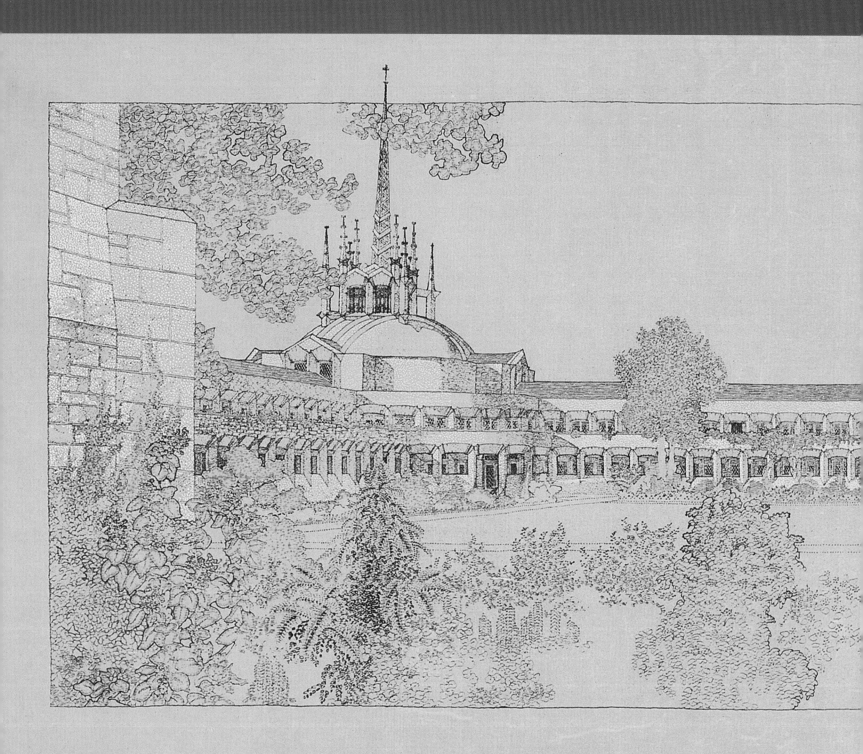

JEFFREY TURNBULL

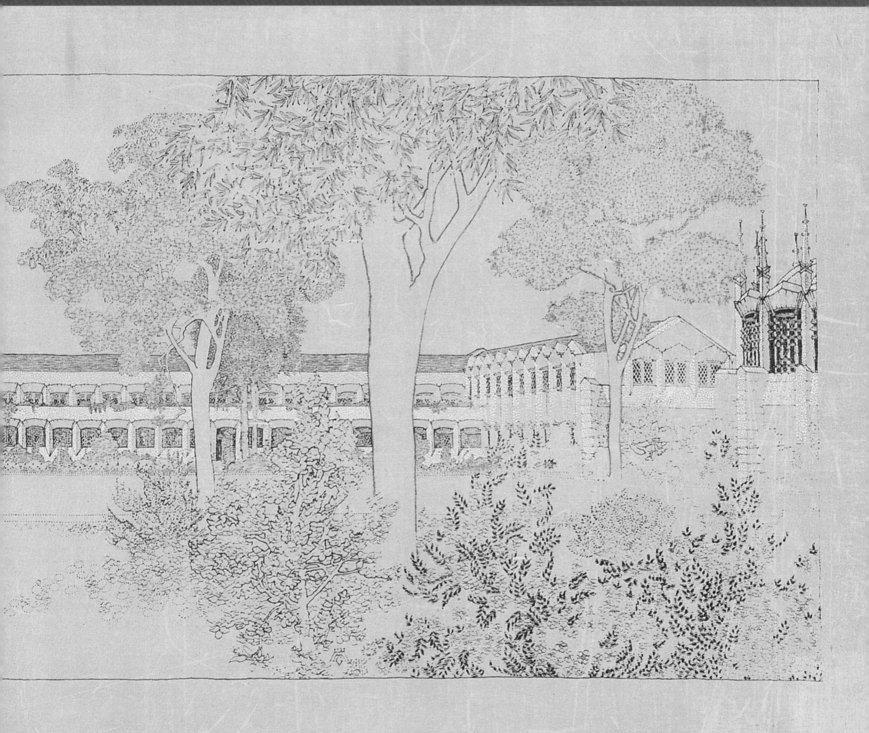

Marion Mahony Griffin's unpublished manuscript, 'The magic of America' (1939–1949), was a reverie, reflecting upon career and life successes and conflicts that she and Walter had experienced or endured together.[1] As a reverie, 'Magic' was written in the manner of a memoir, rather than as a logical, linear, chronologically driven history. It was arranged in four sections, differing in subject and locality: India (1935–1937); the Canberra plan (1911–1920); the Castlecrag settlement (1920–1935); and biographical sketches of herself and Walter.

Reminiscences about the Griffins' major Melbourne works and their clients, (1914–1924), were scattered throughout 'Magic', and this essay attempts in part to consolidate that story. But Marion had a greater aspiration: to record their professional and philosophical ideas and attitudes, and to be understood through reading their buildings and written thoughts. Accordingly, there are four themes in this essay, which emphasise the Griffins' position: equity and democracy; the Canberra plan idea; the community and land settlement; and, the origins of their philosophical allegiances.

Equity: universality, equity, and democracy — being the magic of America

Ideals of equity, and the oneness of universality, were paramount to the Griffins in creating their works and projects. They also desired to express their ideas about a universal democracy, for example, through the Canberra plan, and by the provision of non-hierarchical spaces, where appropriate, in their building plans.[2] Universal modernity was also reflected in their building forms, by including the latest constructional techniques in reinforced concrete, and by installing inside these buildings the most modern furnishings, plumbing and heating services.[3]

Universality was an aim that can be identified through a visual analysis of the forms of the architectural elements seen in their buildings. A visual analysis of a building can involve identifying the shape of architectural elements, such as a roof construction, or a window fenestration, etc, and researching the origin of that roof or window form in previously constructed contemporary or historical buildings. The origins of the forms chosen by the Griffins were culturally various and diverse, befitting the Griffins' aspirations for creating a universal architecture from worldwide sources.[4]

Equity was a principle that Marion often propounded in 'Magic'. She believed that fairness and the application of the principles of justice, on a person to person basis, should balance or supplement the laws of society. The Griffins always strove for equity, evident in their dedicated work on behalf of their clients, and the friendships they had with them. Equity was an ideal in their communal land settlements. Of course, equity would be enhanced in the context of a democratic state. Marion fervently believed that America had equity and democracy, nourished by its lifestyle, constitution and form of government. But she found Australia sometimes wanting in these regards. She found life here too dominated by bureaucrats.

Marion was perhaps a harsh judge of Australia in 'Magic'. The Griffins' dream of finding equity and democracy in Australia was first shattered by bureaucratic obstruction to the implementation of the Canberra plan. She therefore despaired of the Westminster System. While she and Walter could enthusiastically enjoy the company of their private clients and other individual Australian friends, she reckoned that there was no universal equity and democracy in this country.

Marion's criteria for evaluating Australian social and political conditions were set by the standards the Griffins found and admired in the writings of the leading Chicago architect, Louis Henry Sullivan. But ironically, American society, by his own standards, Sullivan described as largely feudal, rather than modern and democratic.[5] The general context for the Griffins' ideology concerning equity and democracy can be identified in American transcendentalism, which had informed Sullivan's points of view,[6] sharing ideas that emphasised individuality, the intuitive mind and soul as one with nature, and eschewing political and social subjugation.

The ideal of democracy for Sullivan was that the individual should stand self-centred and self-governing, an individual sovereign, an individual god. In one of his essays,[7] 'Sullivan repeated his conviction that architecture reflected social values, that nature was the best teacher, that contemporary design was misdirected into commercial pursuit and not into its proper role as art, and that the individual was paramount'.[8]

As with the English architectural critic John Ruskin, the American transcendentalists believed that democratic life could be empowered and illuminated by literature, art and architecture.

Griffin in October 1913, during a lone four-month visit to Australia, spoke to Melbourne architects on the subject of 'Architecture and democracy'. He suggested that the principles enunciated by Louis Henry Sullivan recommended themselves to close scrutiny and attention.[9] Griffin also noted that the architect Frank Lloyd Wright had been able to find forms which well expressed Sullivan's principles.[10] Sullivan, said Griffin, gave emphasis to the idea that form follows function, analogous to organisms in nature.[11]

Idea: the Canberra plan, 1911[12]

The Griffins' Canberra plan was formed from strongly articulated and recognisable parts. The organic whole essentially was the central triangular frame spanning the lake, knitted together with a fabric of natural and artificial elements. The Griffins layered a geometry of roads and vistas over the landscape. The geometry coincided with the lines that could be drawn through the Molonglo River valley between the landforms of hills within the city area and the distant mountains. The city and the landscape were to act transcendentally or organically together, in a conjunction that rendered the landscape monumental.

The Canberra plan, too, reflected the value of the individual within the city community and the nation. The

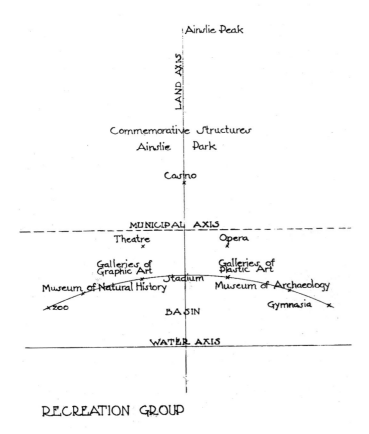

RECREATION GROUP

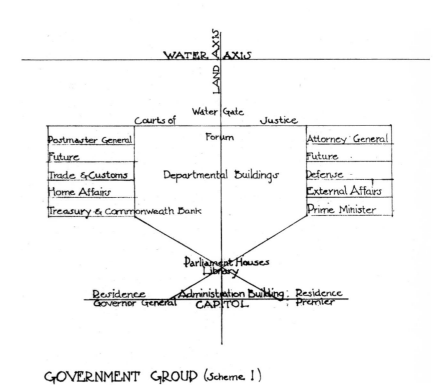

GOVERNMENT GROUP (Scheme 1)

Griffins assigned cultural institutions for the people to the tops of the city's hills, which were cradled in the river valley between the mountain ranges. Here was no physical and hierarchical subjugation on behalf of those who administer the community or the nation, and pass its laws. From all vistas within the plan, the individual was to see either a friendly communal facility or nature's mountain peaks.

The planning arrangements and form of the Canberra design as a diagram of a 'classic Utopian democracy' has been effectively made by James Weirick.[13] The Griffins' Canberra plan reflected a generally enthusiastic turn-of-the-century American perception of the growth and establishment of Australian democratic institutions and freedoms. Democracy in Australia, it was thought, was manifested in the act of Federation in 1901, and in measures such as universal suffrage and economic and political equality.

According to diagrams prepared by the Griffins to explain their Canberra plan, the area north of the lake was to act as a people's domain, with a government and administrative domain being on the south side of the lake system. The Capitol was on the government side, with the Civic and Market Centres on the people's side. The sports and recreation casino was to nestle on the Land Axis below Mount Ainslie.[14] Also on the people's side, against the lake's northern edge, the Griffins envisaged facilities for the arts.

Above: Two diagrams prepared by the Griffins to explain the Government Group and the Recreation Group appearing in 'The magic of America', vol 2, pp 134 and 136.
Reproduced from David Van Zanten, *Drawings of Walter Burley Griffin architect*, Prairie School Press, Palos Park, Illinios, 1970, pp 10–11. © Collection of the New–York Historical Society

Previous pages: Perspective view of Newman College courtyard, University of Melbourne, 1915–1918, drawn by Marion Mahony Griffin, lithograph and gouache on silk sateen, 47.5 × 118 cm.
Courtesy Art Institute of Chicago, gift of Marion Mahony Griffin through Eric Nicholls (1996.24.2).

COMMONWEALTH OF AVSTRALIA
FEDERAL CAPITAL COMPETITION

CITY AND ENVIRONS.

SCALE

Left: 'City and environs', plan of Canberra submitted by the Griffins in the Federal Capital competition, 1911, ink, water-colour, gouache and gold oil paint on linen, 152 × 76 cm. Courtesy National Archives of Australia, Canberra, (CRS A710, item 38).

Right: Section rendering of Canberra showing the Capital Hill Archive building, submitted in the Federal Capital competition, 1911, ink, watercolour, gouache and gold oil paint on linen, 76 × 152.5 cm. Courtesy National Archives of Australia, Canberra (CRS A710, item 43).

Following pages: Photograph of the interior of the Capitol Theatre auditorium, Melbourne, 1921–1924. Courtesy Dorothea Irving, youngest daughter of AJJ Lucas, Melbourne.

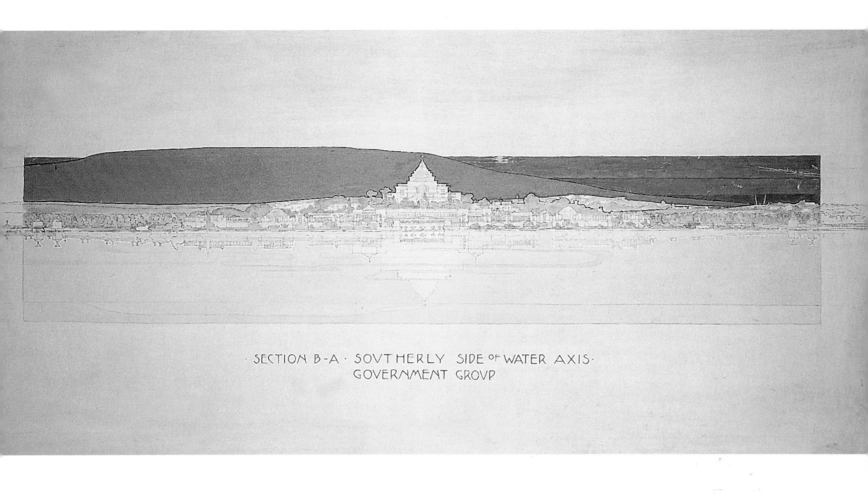

· SECTION B-A · SOVTHERLY SIDE of WATER AXIS ·
GOVERNMENT GROVP

The people's Capitol, crowning the natural hill at the apex of the triangle of avenues on the government side, was intended to be a place of national assembly, and an archive of Australian culture. Capital Hill was not to be the site of a parliament building, which nowadays occupies this site, nor was it to be the site for any other kind of government administrative facility. The Griffins' proposed Capitol building would have looked like a great Oriental masonry pagoda, apparently their gesture to this region of the world.

Although the Griffins were awarded first prize for their Canberra plan, the competition conditions had not provided that the winning design would actually be constructed. Instead the infamous Departmental Board Plan was devised, a bureaucratic pastiche of bits from all the premiated competition designs. The Departmental Board plan was being implemented when Griffin visited Canberra in 1913 to advise on these new works. Griffin accepted then a directorship for establishing his own Canberra plan, but consequently he was constantly thwarted in achieving that end by a rapid succession of government ministers and by a hostile bureaucracy.

The Griffins' Canberra plan has never been fully realised. For example, the institutions that the Griffins envisaged for the prominent sites in the topography were substituted for others. Their casino site was eventually

chosen for the Australian War Memorial. Their Market Centre at the northeast apex of the triangle of avenues was never built. The Defence offices and the American War Memorial now dominate this area. Instead of the Griffins' Civic Hall being placed on top of the Civic Centre knoll, there is now a void of shadowed lawn and dark cypress trees. As already observed, the Capital Hill has been occupied since 1988 by the new Parliament House. This building at least restores the site for occupation by the people, by providing pedestrian access to the top of the hill, enabling the public a view downward into the politicians' skylit members hall.[15]

Community and land settlement: Henry George and the Griffins' Melbourne clients

In 1913, Walter Burley Griffin was invited to address the Henry George League in Melbourne, and to have a celebratory dinner with the Georgists in Sydney. During the Melbourne lecture Griffin claimed that from the age of fourteen years he had been an ardent supporter of Henry George, when he read *Social problems* (1884). A resident of California, Henry George was disturbed by the plight of the poor in their slum habitations, and of conspicuous consumption by the rich, which he saw when visiting cities such as New York. He deplored the waste caused by speculation on vacant unimproved lots.

Desiring to modify the extremes of capitalism, George advocated that everyone should pay a single tax only, on land improvement exclusively, a 100 percent tax on what he called the annual economic rent of land. The difference between the value of the production of any given piece of land, and the value of the production of the least productive land in actual use, was considered by George to be an unearned economic rent, and should be handed over as tax for community benefits. Land was indispensable to production, George believed, thus land should be a free gift to all.

For Georgists, land settlement for everyone became a theoretical necessity for a healthy, equitable society. The Griffins were delighted with the federal government's policy of providing only leasehold land in the new city of Canberra, thereby avoiding the social and economic pitfalls of land speculation and profit-taking.[16] Griffin had been an active member of the Chicago Single Tax Club, and he boasted to the Georgists of Melbourne and Sydney that he always talked about single tax with those he met, or about community land settlement. The Griffins proposed in about 1912 to build such a settlement in Winnetka, north of central Chicago, but they moved to Australia instead. From about 1920, Castlecrag became the site for the Griffins' dream of community land settlement.

The Griffins' Melbourne buildings, 1914–1924, involved clients from a remarkably diverse range of ethnic and cultural backgrounds. The buildings and their clients in the major Melbourne commissions were: Newman College, 1915–1918, the Roman Catholic college at the University of Melbourne, with a building committee led by the Irish clergyman, Dr Daniel Mannix; Cafe Australia, 1916, in Collins Street, and Capitol House and Theatre, 1921–1924, in Swanston Street, both projects predominantly involving the Greek Consul General and businessman, A J J Lucas; the Kuomintang Club, 1922, premises in Little Bourke Street for the Chinese Nationalist Party in Melbourne, with the club president, Reverend Cheong Cheok Hong of the Chinese Methodist Church, and businessman, Philip Ching Lee, as the clients; and Leonard House, 1922–1923, the client being Nisson Leonard-Kanevsky, a successful businessman in the clothing trade in Melbourne who had been a Jewish refugee, having fled from pogroms in the city of Kiev in the Ukraine.

The somewhat beleaguered Roman Catholic community in Melbourne was predominantly of Irish background, and the clergy who served it were usually appointed from Ireland. There was solid support in Melbourne for Irish nationalism, and for the pursuit of land rights for the Irish in Ireland. The Roman Catholics of Victoria had created a primary and secondary school system, after state legislation in the last quarter of the nineteenth century ended funding of all church schools. During the second decade of the twentieth century the Roman Catholic community was ready to finance tertiary education for its young men and women.

Why would the Irish Roman Catholics of Melbourne choose the office of Walter Burley Griffin to be involved in the procurement of a Catholic college at the University of

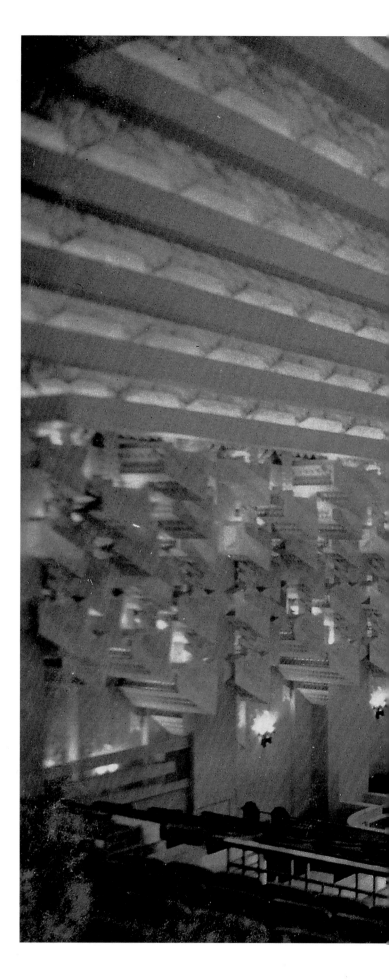

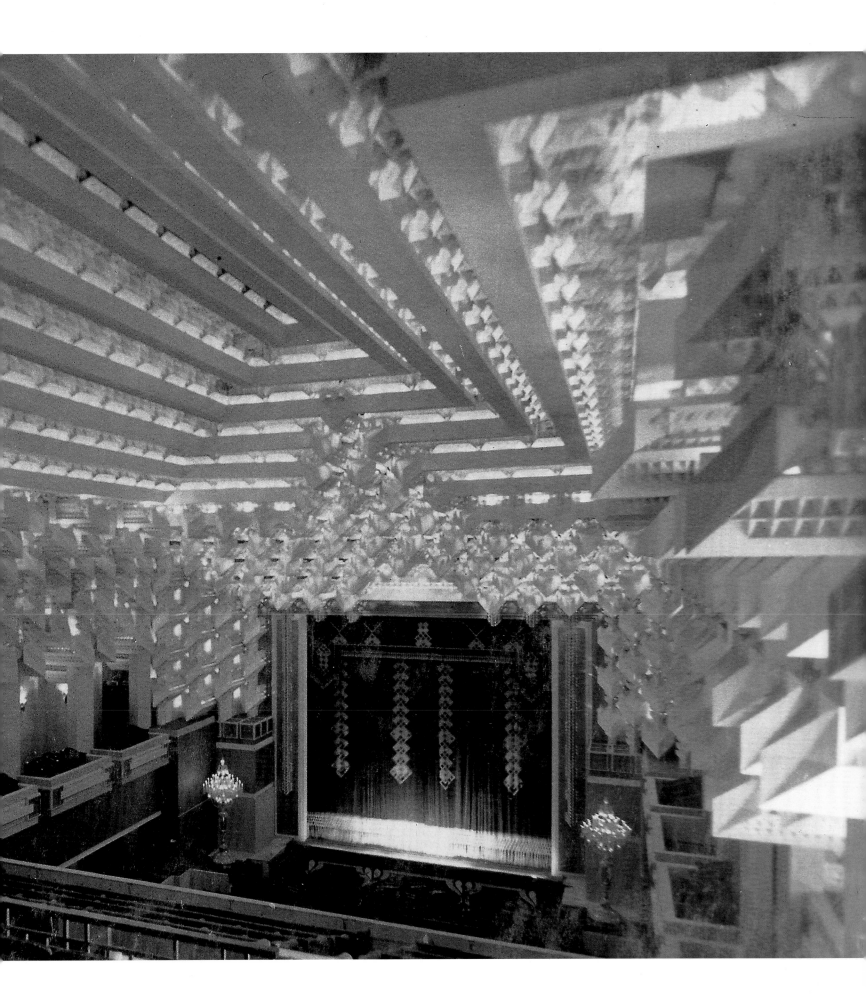

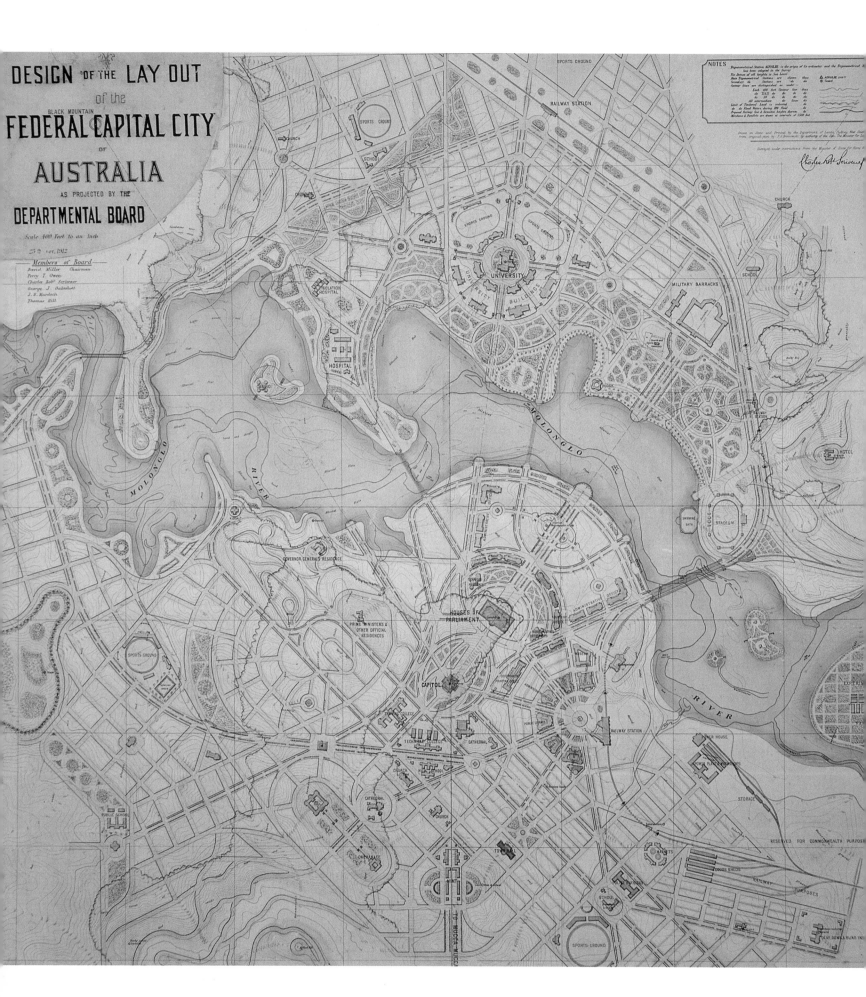

Melbourne? The Henry George League meetings in Melbourne provided a network of people who became the Griffins' friends, and some became their clients. Frank Brennan MHR, and his barrister brother, Thomas, were both involved in lecturing for the Melbourne Henry George League in early 1914, before Walter returned to Australia with Marion in May that year.

Frank Brennan was one of King O'Malley's Labor circle, O'Malley having been the minister responsible for the conduct of the 1911 Canberra competition. The Brennan brothers were members of the inaugural general committee for the new college. Thomas was appointed a joint secretary of the executive committee, together with medico Dr Augustus Leo Kenny. Before being commissioned for the college work, many other connections may have already existed between the Griffins and executive committee members, such as with Cornelius J Ahern MHR. Both Ahern and the Griffins had their offices at 395 Collins Street.

Marion's father had been Irish-born and was a Roman Catholic. That the Roman Catholic church in Melbourne had felt comfortable with a pair of Georgists could be explained by the fact that Henry George and his 1880s involvement with the Irish land rights movement, and his very well-attended public lectures delivered in the Melbourne Town Hall and the Royal Melbourne Exhibition Building during 1890, had been prominently reported in the local Roman Catholic newspaper, *The Advocate*.[17] George achieved the status of hero in this newspaper, which reported that on one of his visits to Dublin, the British had incarcerated him, while his baggage was searched for subversive material. Henry George married an Irishwoman, and their three children were brought up as Roman Catholics.

In July 1915, Walter Burley Griffin was commissioned to work on the college as an impartial outsider, in association with a successful local Roman Catholic architect, Augustus Andrew Fritsch. A costed brief for the college had already been prepared that was liberal, equitable, and generous in the accommodation required. When the first sketch design for the college appeared in August 1915, Thomas Donovan wrote vehement letters, hostile to the facilities and form proposed. Donovan, a Sydney lawyer, had in 1914 precipitated the whole college project by offering to donate money for student bursaries if the Church raised enough money for an adequate building fund. The Griffins' scheme responded imaginatively to the brief, providing a study-plus-bedroom suite for each student, standard furniture issue to each student and a circular non-hierarchical refectory, without high table. A billiards room and a swimming pool for recreation were provided, as well as a library, laboratories and classrooms.

The Griffins' major aims for the college design were for a modern expression, and for well-built sunlit and airy spaces. They intended that some of the details, such as the finials on the refectory dome, would provide a reminiscence of the gothic in Italy and Spain. The suites of rooms for each of the college men, and the undifferentiated dining-room space, would provide for the freedoms of democratic life.

Donovan, however, demanded English gothic revival architecture, with dormitories for the students arranged around a closed quadrangle, and a square refectory. He believed that the Griffins' proposed form was alien and bizarre, that the accommodation would promote moral decay, and that the concrete dome construction would be grossly expensive. The omission of a high table, in his opinion, was unforgivable. A second scheme, and a third scheme (lost), were drawn up before the close of 1915, to satisfy Donovan. Griffin was able to effectively argue that these alternative schemes were too costly, were highly impractical fire traps, and were autocratic in expression. The first scheme for the college was thus finally built and opened in March 1918, a new architectural statement about equity and democracy.

Antony John Jereus Lucas, the Cafe Australia and Capitol House and Theatre client, had migrated when a young man to Melbourne from Greece.[18] The Vienna Cafe, one of three cafes he owned and operated, was badly damaged by soldiers in 1916, probably because the cafe bore the name of the Austrian capital. The Griffins were commissioned to refit the renamed Australia Cafe. A number of spaces, of different volume and shape with distinct furnishing in each, flowed through the long narrow building offering many choices of setting for the customer.

On the former Town Hall Cafe site was built the Griffin-designed Capitol House and Theatre, opened in 1924 for the business partnership of Lucas and the brothers Herman and Leon Phillips from California. The theatre stairways and foyers were ample and provided an intriguing and majestic passageway to the auditorium. Within the auditorium itself was performed a miraculous light show before the film was screened: coloured light globes were concealed behind the flat steps of the pyramidal ceiling and in a phased sequence of colour mixes, electric light played upon the stalactite plaster shapes so that the ceiling appeared to be filled with endlessly changing and pulsating crystals. Lucas was to invest in the Griffins' Castlecrag land settlement.[19]

The Reverend Cheong Cheok Hong was born on the Ballarat goldfields. His family moved to Melbourne and lived in the inner suburb of Fitzroy before they moved in 1900 to a large eastern suburban tract in Croydon. The Chinese at that time suffered as a result of the White Australia Policy. A mutual friend of Reverend Cheong, and of the Griffins, was the Federal parliamentarian King O'Malley. The great Chinese reformer, Sun Yat Sen, the Nationalists' political mentor, was an ardent Georgist, but it is more likely that the friendship between O'Malley and Cheong led to the relationship being formed with the Griffins. An existing shophouse was refurbished by the Griffins for the Kuomintang quarters. It became famous for its crystalline multifaceted exterior.[20] Cheong, like O'Malley, invested in the Griffins' Castlecrag development.

The client for Leonard House, 1922–1923, was Nisson Leonard-Kanevsky. During 1910 Kanevsky was working on the Flinders Street Railway Station construction project. A

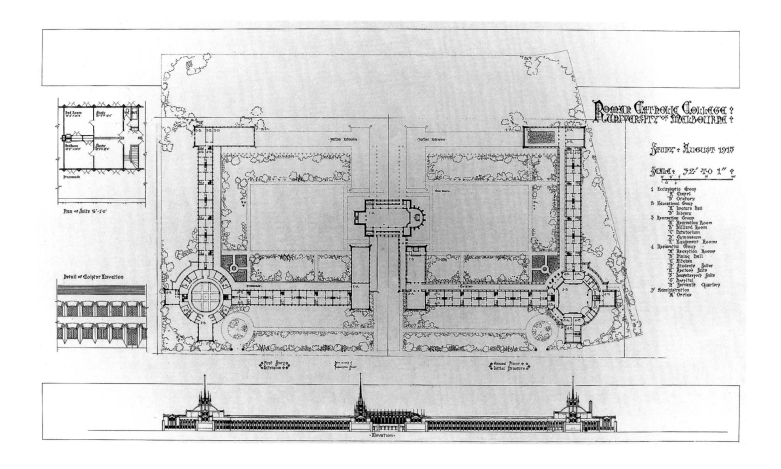

Above: First version of plan of Newman College, University of Melbourne, August 1915, ink on linen, 67 × 116.5 cm.
Courtesy Art Institute of Chicago, gift of Marion Mahony Griffin through Eric Nicholls (1996.24.6).

Right: Second version of plan of Newman College, University of Melbourne, November 1915, ink on linen, 56.7 × 92.3 cm.
Courtesy Art Institute of Chicago, gift of Marion Mahony Griffin through Eric Nicholls (1996.24.5).

Previous page: Plan of Canberra by the Departmental Board, 1912, ink and watercolour on paper, 135 × 135 cm.
Courtesy National Archives of Australia, (CRS A767, item 1).

brilliant entrepreneur, he quickly became prominent in the Flinders Lane clothing trade in central Melbourne. He engaged the Griffins to refurbish his premises in 1921 and then one year later to build the new multistorey office block in Elizabeth Street. Leonard House was an early and outstanding example of the use of curtain-wall construction, bringing natural light deep into the open office spaces. Kanevsky himself found the tenants for his building, including the Griffins, who fitted a new office for themselves on the fourth floor.

Perhaps the Griffins' enthusiasm for land settlement influenced Kanevsky to become involved in Jewish land settlement in Victoria.[21] In the late 1920s, Kanevsky and Trunof, with the former Melbourne City Council's sanitary engineer and inventor, John Boadle, formed the company that by 1929 became RIECo.[22] The Griffins in Sydney, with Eric Nicholls in the Griffins' Leonard House office in Melbourne, joined with RIECo in producing incinerator designs (1929–1937). When a RIECo office was opened in Sydney in about 1930 the Kanevsky family lived at the Griffin-designed Fishwick house, Castlecrag.

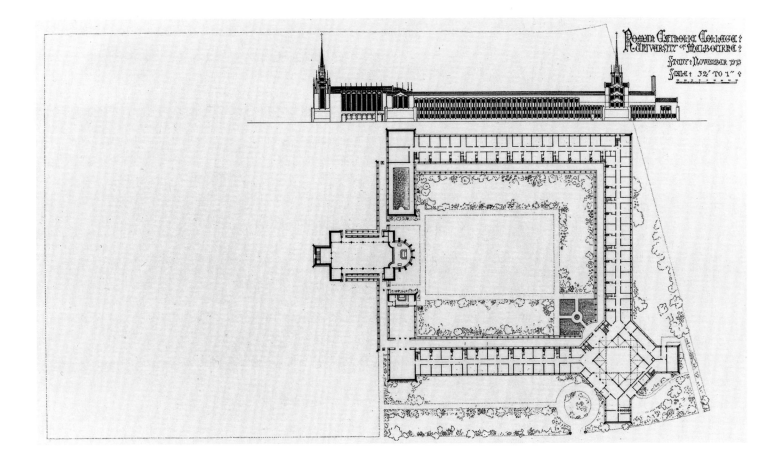

Origins: the Griffins' philosophical allegiances and commitments — the writings of Emerson, Thoreau, Whitman, Sullivan, Crosby and Carpenter

What was the disposition of the Griffins, that attracted and sustained such different clients from many countries of origin, in a city that for the Griffins was also a foreign place? The Melbourne clients would have been respected by the Griffins primarily for their individuality. Perhaps the Griffins recognised the societal forces that pressured each of these clients to deny their origins and to conform. By engaging them in an architectural enterprise, with forms that expressed a new universality, the Griffins could restore to each of them an ideal democratic status, to live as untrammelled individuals.

As already stated, the autonomy of the individual was the ideal for the Griffins. Their philosophy was thus aligned with the mid-nineteenth century American transcendentalists, such as the writer and public lecturer, Ralph Waldo Emerson, the naturalist, Henry David Thoreau, and the poet, Walt Whitman, as well as Sullivan. From the 1880s, Sullivan had published in Chicago architectural magazines and had spoken many times at conferences of architects on the topic of the essence and the constituent components of democracy.[23]

In summary of transcendentalist writings, an individual would act intuitively, as one with nature, and would also act with responsibility toward all in the community. The individual would be true to the self, would resist all the forces of subjugation and conformity, and be dedicated to the performance of duty to all humankind. Each person was unique, yet was a manifestation of the one overall human spirit.

Walt Whitman's prose poems in *Leaves of grass* were to leave an indelible impression upon Emerson and Sullivan. Whitman, the so-called Troubadour of Democracy, had forwarded a copy of his volume to Emerson in 1855. With great enthusiasm Emerson wrote that this was 'the best piece of American Buddhism that anyone has had the strength to write, American to the bone!'[24] Emerson called *Leaves of grass* a cross between the *Bhagavad Gita* and the *New York Herald*. American transcendentalism was drawn from a number of sources, including German and Scottish philosophy and letters, and included a profound knowledge of the great texts of India, China and Persia; the *Bhagavad Gita* was one of the better known inspirational texts. With such evidence of American culture's familiarity with Asia, it is therefore hardly surprising that, in 1911, the Griffins would find architectural precedent from Asia an appropriate reference for the Capitol for Canberra.

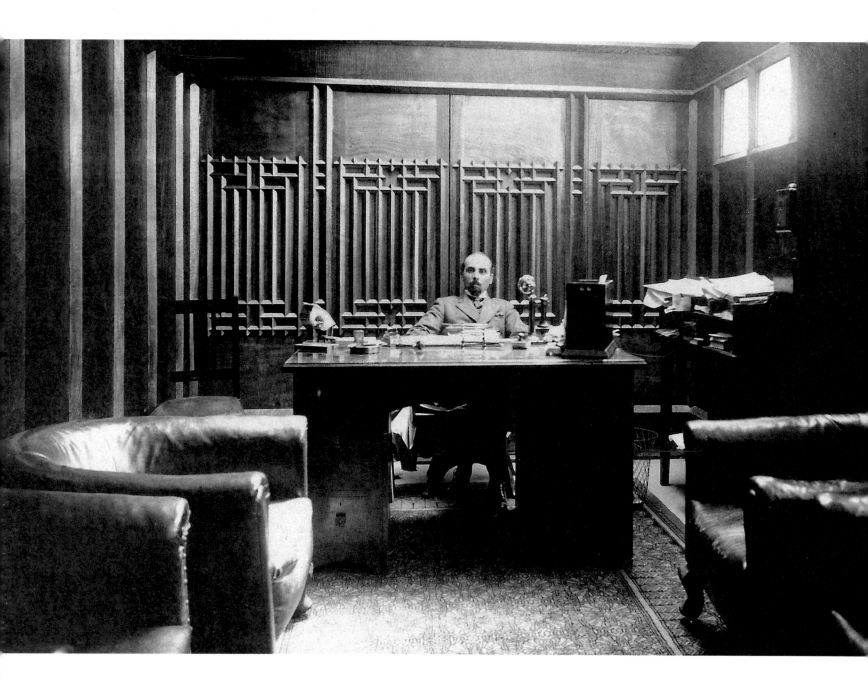

Above: Photograph of the interior of the office suite in
occupation by Nisson Leonard-Kanevsky, fifth floor,
Leonard House, Melbourne, 1922–1923.
Courtesy Dianne Betts, grand-daughter of Nisson Leonard-
Kanevsky, Melbourne.

Right: Leonard House, Melbourne, 1922–1923.
From Sands and Wilson, *Building a city*, Oxford University Press,
Melbourne, 1981.

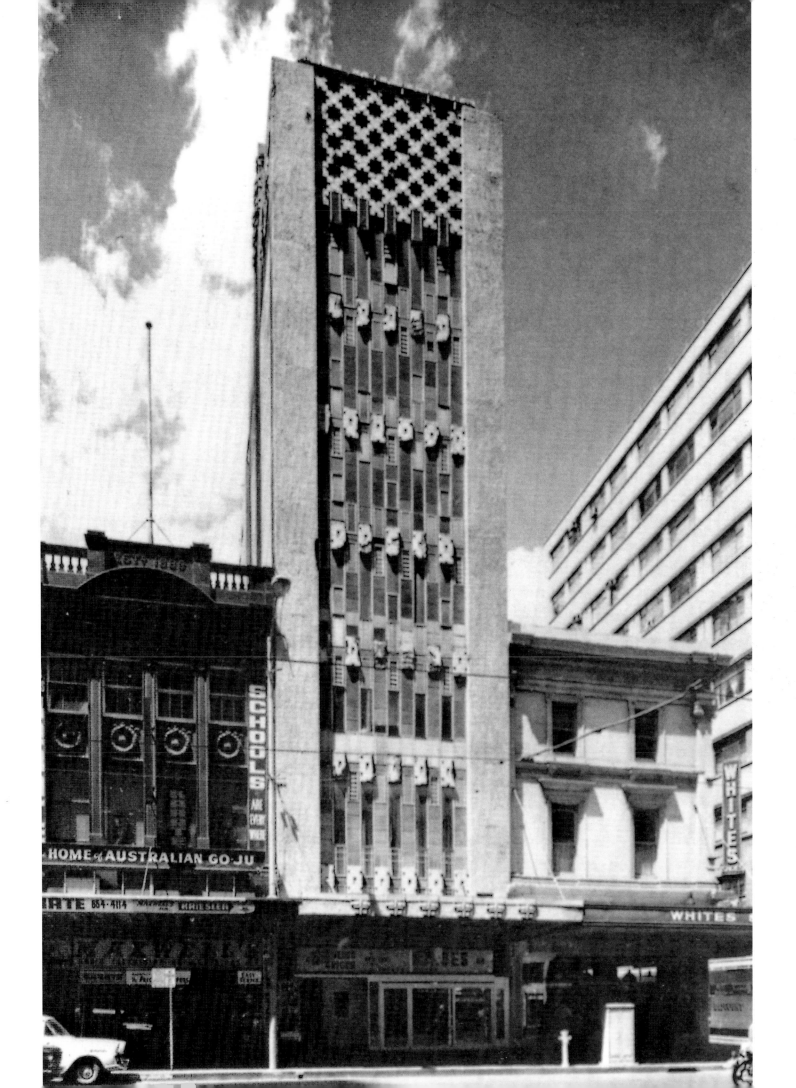

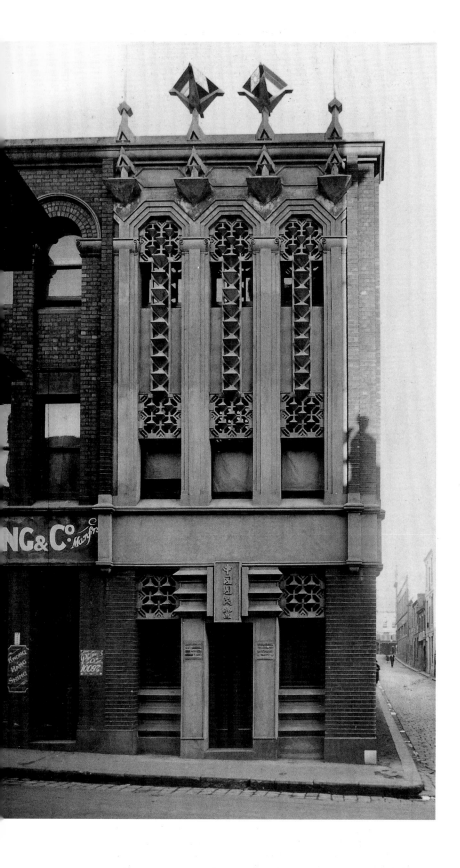

In March 1920, Walter Burley Griffin wrote a letter from Melbourne to his fellow architect and friend from Prairie School days in Chicago, William Gray Purcell, then living and practising in Portland, Oregon:

> The fight for a place in the sun was pretty definitely beaten, had I not read all of Edward Carpenter ten to twenty years ago [that is, about 1900–1910], my character might be much worse than it is. There are others I enjoy still more and probably my favorite of the lot is Earnest Crosley [*sic*] who died in 1907; if you can get his works read them, any of them. More later …[25]

After 1914, Emerson poems began to appear in the pages of the Melbourne Henry George League's newspaper, *Progress*. From the 1898 inception of the Chicago Georgist newspaper, *The Public*, there appeared not only Emerson poems but also the writings of Ernest Howard Crosby. Some years before, en route from Cairo to New York, after completing diplomatic duties in Egypt, Crosby visited Russia to seek out and meet the mystic and novelist, Leo Tolstoy. Crosby was advised by the Count to return immediately to America and to meet Henry George, whom the great Russian writer admired for his ideas on society and economics. After discussions with Henry George, Crosby became somewhat a crusader for single tax and for other causes typically allied to the predispositions of many Georgists.[26]

Significantly, Crosby published in 1901 the biography, *Edward Carpenter: poet and prophet*. Carpenter, like Emerson, was a public lecturer and prolific writer, but unlike Emerson, he lived with a younger working-class man on a market-gardening property on the outskirts of Sheffield, England. A vegetarian and socialist, Carpenter and his partner attempted an autonomous and self-sufficient lifestyle, growing their own food, and deriving income from hand-manufacturing leather sandals. William Morris, of arts and crafts fame, and Annie Besant, then leader of the theosophists, were amongst Carpenter's English friends. In 1877 and 1884, Carpenter visited Walt Whitman, a kindred spirit.[27] Having just read the *Bhagavad Gita*, translated for him by a Ceylonese friend, Edward Carpenter wrote a long prose poem entitled *Toward democracy*.[28]

This reverie has come full circle. In the *Bhagavad Gita*, Arjuna and Lord Krishna are in a chariot, galloping into battle against Arjuna's evil brothers, when a discussion ensues about God, the self and the community. The Lord advises that God must be loved and that duty to all must be served, without expectation of reward in this life, or in any future existence. This ethic clearly guided the lives of the Griffins,[29] unlike their former colleague, Frank Lloyd Wright.[30] When Marion wrote 'The magic of America' she told of their engagement in four 'Battles', the 'Empirial' [*sic*], 'Federal', 'Municipal', and the 'Individual', a metaphor for Walter and herself as Arjuna, going into life's battle with the human family, especially the bureaucrats.

Notes

1. One manuscript was lodged at the Art Institute of Chicago, and a second differently amended version was lodged with the New York Historical Society Library.

2. For example, the refectory at Newman College, University of Melbourne, 1915–18, was made circular in plan, and furnished with circular tables, so that no physical or spatial hierarchy was shaped.

3. Again, the refectory dome referred to one of the newest reinforced concrete dome construction systems, patented in 1889 by a French engineer. In 'Magic' Marion wrote proudly of the advanced plumbing and heating systems installed at Newman College.

4. The sources found for the Newman College refectory dome form, for example, referred to the Buddhist stupa and to Byzantium. The lantern ribs were inspired by a dome in Cordoba Mosque, and the finials outside derived also from Spain.

5. See, for example, Sullivan's essay, 'Is our art a betrayal rather than an expression of American life?', collected in Robert Twombly, ed, *Louis Sullivan: the public papers*, University of Chicago Press, 1988, pp 197–200. Twombly comments that Sullivan equated feudalism with authoritarianism that 'suppressed human creativity by restricting freedom. Democracy, on the other hand, was a liberating system encouraging individual expression as a means of seeking universal truths'.

6. See Narciso Menocal, *Architecture as nature: the transcendentalist idea of Louis Sullivan*, University of Wisconsin Press, Wisconsin, 1981.

7. Louis Henry Sullivan, 'What is architecture? A study in the American people of today', *American Contractor*, January, 1906.

8. Twombly, 1988, p 174.

9. The talk and consequent proceedings of this meeting were reported in *Building*, Sydney, 11 October 1913, pp 61–64i.

10. Sullivan's followers in the field of domestic architecture in Chicago have been identified as the Prairie School, which included the Griffins' colleague, Frank Lloyd Wright. Until 1909 Wright continued to compose in the manner of the 1880s American Shingle style, giving form to Sullivan's theories (and the formal characteristics of H H Richardson's style), by integrating elements through spatial and surface continuity. Griffin had his own tactics, and literally used the architectonic elements of pier, lintel and arch (that can generate the dome), as identified by Sullivan. Formal characteristics of these structural elements, chosen from a universal range of architectures from around the world, were assembled by Griffin in new compositions, as evident in the design of Newman College.

11. The American transcendentalist, Emerson, admired the sentiments of his New York sculptor friend, Horatio Greenough, writing in a letter in 1852, that an emphasis upon architectural features should be 'proportioned to their *gradated* importance in function', with the 'entire and immediate banishment of all make-shift and make-believe'. Emerson was thus prompted to deliberate upon the characteristics of beauty, saying in *Conduct of life*, 1860, that elegance of form and of structure are the same, and declaring that all beauty must be organic. Thus was the context set for the emergence of Sullivan's statement, that form follows function.

12. The period of the Griffins' early Australian work includes the creation in Chicago of a design for Canberra during the last months of 1911. In February 1914, the Griffins went to Europe, and Walter organised an international competition for a new parliament house in Canberra. The Griffins then arrived in Australia in May 1914. They established private practices in both Melbourne and Sydney, but their major commissions were in Melbourne until 1925, when they moved permanently to Castlecrag, NSW.

13. James Weirick, 'The Federal Battle' in an article, '*The magic of America*: vision and text', in J Duncan and M Gates, eds, *Walter Burley Griffin: a review*, Monash University Gallery, Victoria, 1988, pp 7–10.

14. The casino as a building type in 1911 was a residential or town recreation and sporting club, for example, the Newport, Rhode Island Casino, in the late nineteenth century, included a large open area with a number of lawn-tennis courts and lawn croquet fields. Gambling as a recreational aspect of the casino was to be emphasised about two decades later, with casino developments in Las Vegas.

15. The new Parliament House, 1980–88, was designed by Romaldo Giurgola, an Italian-American architect nowadays residing in Australia.

16. It is interesting to note that the municipal rating system in Australia has its roots in the successful adoption of the arguments put forward by local Georgists in the first quarter of the twentieth century. See *Progress*, Melbourne.

17. *The Advocate* has proven to be the only ready source of information about the fact that Henry George visited Melbourne, and of the involvement of George with the Irish people. The Church clergy could agree with George on his analysis of social and economic ills, but did not agree with the solution of a single land tax.

18. Antonios Ioannis Iereus Lekatsas, from the British-administered Greek island of Ithaki, changed his name in Melbourne to Antony John Jereus Lucas when he was 40 years of age in 1903. He had married Margaret Wilson ten years before, and they were to own and manage three very successful restaurants in Melbourne by 1908: the Town Hall Cafe in Swanston Street, and the Paris and Vienna cafes in Collins Street. Since 1898 Lucas had been a founder and leader of the Greek Orthodox community in Melbourne. It became necessary during World War I for him to align the community with the Allies, in defiance of pro-German, King Constantine of Greece. Lucas was involved then in the establishment of the pro-British Ulysses Club (mostly Ithacans).

19. Aged 72 years in 1928, Lucas retired from business, and occupied a nineteenth-century homestead, Yamala, in Mount Eliza, which had a new garden and building alterations by the Griffins.

20. O'Malley, himself a North American, owned a number of premises around eastern Lonsdale Street in central Melbourne, rented by Chinese cabinetmakers. O'Malley would regularly visit Cheong in Croydon for a supper of pancakes and maple syrup. The Griffins, too, designed a new subdivision for the Cheong estate in 1923.

21. Between 1925 and 1929 Kanevsky became involved in the Jewish Welfare Society, tendering to the needs at the dockside of swelling numbers of refugees from Russia, Poland and Germany. The society at this time also settled Jewish families on the land in Victoria — on orchards in Orrvale, Shepparton, and on market gardens in Berwick — under Kanevsky's direction. See Jeff Turnbull, 'From ghettoes to gardens', *Fabrications* (the Journal of the Society of Architectural Historians, Australia and New Zealand), vol 6, June 1995, pp 39–56, or a slightly expanded version in *Australian Jewish Historical Society Journal*, vol 8, November 1995, pp 25–37.

22. The Reverbatory Incinerator Engineering Company. See Peter Navaretti's essay in this book.

23. Ideas about democracy were numerous in an essay, 'The young man in architecture', which Sullivan delivered at the annual convention of the Architectural League of America, Chicago, June 1900. Walter Burley Griffin was in attendance and greatly admired its sentiments.

24. Robert D Richardson Jr, *Emerson: the mind on fire*, University of California Press, USA, 1995, p 527.

25. The letter had been signed on Griffin's behalf by N Mahady, apparently before Griffin could check the spelling. There is no author called Earnest Crosley who died in 1907. Various encyclopedias of biography have entries for Ernest Crosby, 1856–1907. This insight came courtesy of Paul Kruty.

26. Between 1899 and 1907, Crosby published two books of his own poetry, and volumes on the subjects of Tolstoy, the working class as conveyed by Shakespeare, vegetarianism (the Griffins were vegetarians), the absurdities of militarism, etc, and one about William Garrison, the activist abolitionist, a friend of the passivist anti-slavery advocates, the Concord (Massachusetts) Women's Anti-Slavery Group, in which the mothers and sisters of Emerson and Thoreau were so active. Emerson and Thoreau themselves wrote impassioned and telling essays on the topic of emancipation.

27. Carpenter's *Days with Walt Whitman* was published by George Allen, London, 1906. It also mentioned the acquaintance Carpenter made with Emerson.

28. First published in London in 1883, which enjoyed revision and enlargement and eighteen editions up to 1949. Carpenter visited his friend in Ceylon and also travelled with him in India and published in 1892, *From Adam's Peak to Elephanta*. In 1894, Carpenter published *Woman, and her place in a free society*, which stood for women's suffrage and equality. The arts and crafts Roycrofters in Aurora, New York, in 1898 printed on their handpress from handmade blocks, *Hand and brain*, essays from a symposium on socialism, including contributions from George Bernard Shaw, William Morris and Edward Carpenter. Two dramas, *Moses*, 1873, and *St George and the Dragon*, 1895, were also written by Carpenter.

29. Walter, on his way to India in 1935, having left Australia for the last time, wrote to Marion asking her to find his copy of the *Bhagavad Gita* amongst his things left behind in their home in Castlecrag, and to forward it to him in Lucknow.

30. See Brendan Gill, *Many masks: a life of Frank Lloyd Wright*, Heinemann, London, 1987.

THE INSIDE STORY:
FURNITURE AND LIGHTING

ANNE WATSON

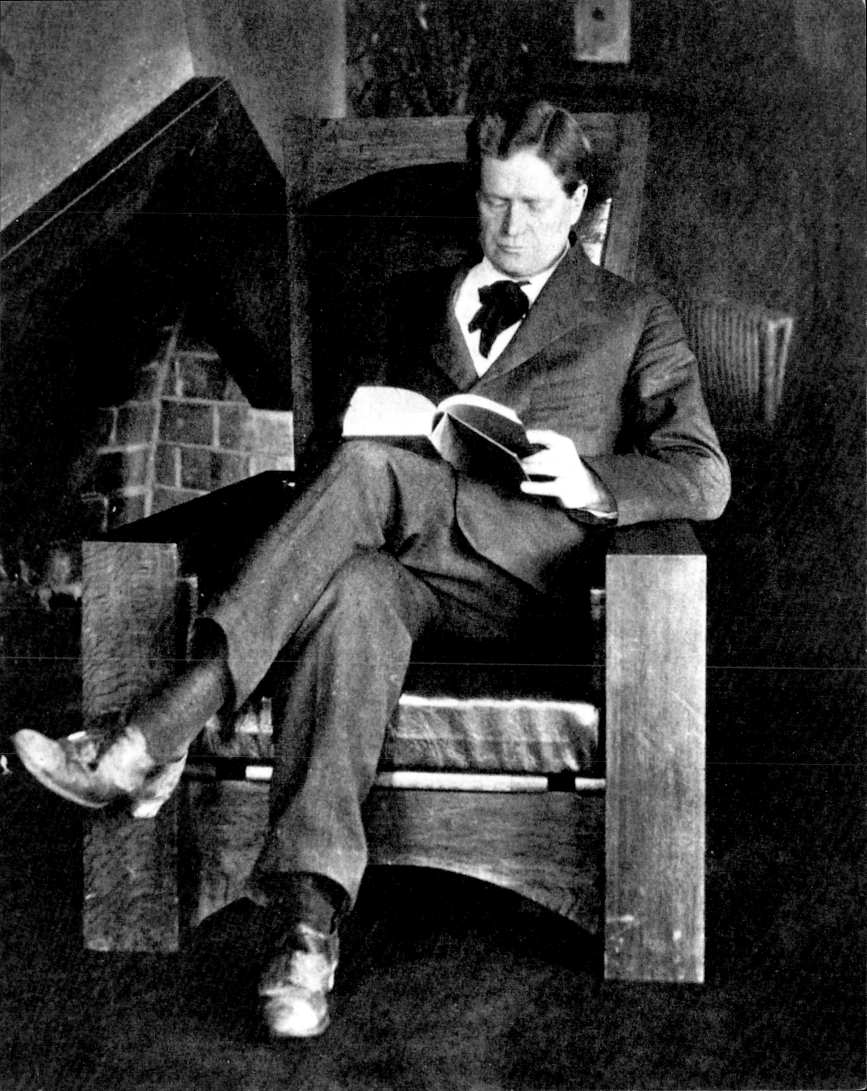

Individually and together, the Griffins and their architecture have provided an important research resource for North American and Australian scholars over several decades. Yet this research has largely omitted their interior design work, despite both architects' demonstrated insistence on the importance of integrating interior schemes within the architectural whole, and despite their execution of designs for many interior fittings and fixtures. This essay is intended to provide an introductory survey of one aspect of this interior work — the wide range of furniture and lighting designed by both Walter and Marion throughout their extremely productive professional lives.

Evidence of the Griffins' designs for furniture and lighting survive in a number of forms: photographs from contemporary periodicals, photographs and other documentation with a Griffin provenance (for example, the Nicholls collection, Sydney), Marion's autobiographical typescript 'The magic of America', (about 1949), presentation and documentation drawings for numerous projects and, of course, the objects themselves. The picture that emerges from this extensive resource is of two accomplished designers, assured in their philosophical approach and capable of creating a variety of highly imaginative design responses to the differing demands of individual projects.

The coincidence of the popularity of the arts and crafts movement in America with the first active decade of Marion and Walter's architectural careers had important consequences for their interior design work. Arts and crafts production furniture and lighting was readily available, either for direct use or as inspiration, from a number of sources. 'Craftsman' furniture from the Syracuse, New York, workshops of Gustav Stickley,[1] for example, is identifiable in a number of Marion and Walter's American interiors.[2] Whether this furniture, or the numerous examples of canework chairs that feature in contemporary interior photographs, was specified by the Griffins or reflects the taste of the client is usually impossible to determine. Suffice to say that the use of production arts and crafts furniture, such as Stickley's, was entirely compatible and consistent with the Griffins' own design and social philosophies, and a use they would no doubt have encouraged. Stickley's much-publicised belief in the ability of furniture and furnishings to affect the well-being of its users was closely aligned with the Griffins' own position: 'The confusion to which we doom ourselves when we use figured wall papers, figured rugs, figured curtains, figured upholstery, is responsible for much of the weariness of the women who spend so much of their time in the house, for peevishness of children … and for [the] grouchiness of men who need rest when they come home from a day's work …'[3]

The potential of functional design and sound construction to 'improve' the human lot was a fundamental arts and crafts principle and one that the Griffins adhered to long after the movement ceased to be fashionable. Considering the enduring centrality of a humanist philosophy to their work and lives one suspects they would have arrived at the same ideological position with or without the precedent of this movement.

Just as crucial as the availability of arts and crafts furniture were the coverage and promotion given the movement through books, articles, lectures and the creation of numerous arts and crafts societies throughout America. The Chicago Arts and Crafts Society, of which Marion was a founding member, was established in 1897, and Marion and Walter would have been familiar with the Chicago-based periodicals *The House Beautiful* and *The Western Architect*, both of which carried numerous articles on arts and crafts subjects. Notable English arts and crafts designers, such as C R Ashbee, either visited Chicago[4] or were published in local journals. English architect M H Baillie Scott's article 'On the choice of simple furniture'[5] gave expression to a number of issues that were to become central to the Prairie School philosophy and that the Griffins were to hold dear throughout their lives:

> the architect … must try to express in bricks and mortar the spirit of the countryside; he must then, having built the right kind of house to harmonize with a particular site … [furnish it] with the right kind of furniture.

> For it is not enough that furniture should possess intrinsic beauty, unless it also possesses this further quality of exquisite appropriateness to its position and its use. It should appear almost to be a piece of the room in which it is placed and in absolute harmony with its surroundings.

To this concept of 'total architecture', the interweaving of all aspects of a project into a unified entity, Walter was to advocate the use of an underlying modular structure as an aid to the creation of a harmonious whole:

> The aesthetic function of the furniture and furnishings is not now to attract attention to itself or to its individual specimens, but to carry out and express a larger creature of the imagination; a home as unique in general conception as in all its parts. Such a scheme in the first place should rest upon a given measure of rhythm or module, the necessary condition of harmony, supplying the scale of all the appurtenances as well as the envelopment and the structure itself.[6]

The proposition that interior design elements should express an intrinsic unity as well as mirror the aesthetic of the architectural whole was not, of course, original to Baillie Scott or Griffin or Mahony. Its exact genesis is difficult to determine, but by the turn of the nineteenth century it was becoming a common theme among progressive architects in Europe and America. Charles Rennie Mackintosh in Scotland, Josef Hoffmann in Vienna and Frank Lloyd Wright in Chicago were notable early advocates and gifted interior designers as well as architects.

Regardless of debate over the extent and nature of Frank Lloyd Wright's role as design mentor to both Marion and Walter, their employment in the Oak Park studio (Walter 1901–1906, Marion 1895–1909) during what is often regarded as Wright's most creative period, was unarguably of considerable consequence in the formation and consolidation of many of their architectural ideas. Wright's unique interior design vocabulary grew out of the arts and crafts philosophy, but gave to it a new aesthetic dimension that borrowed variously from the precedent of Louis Sullivan,

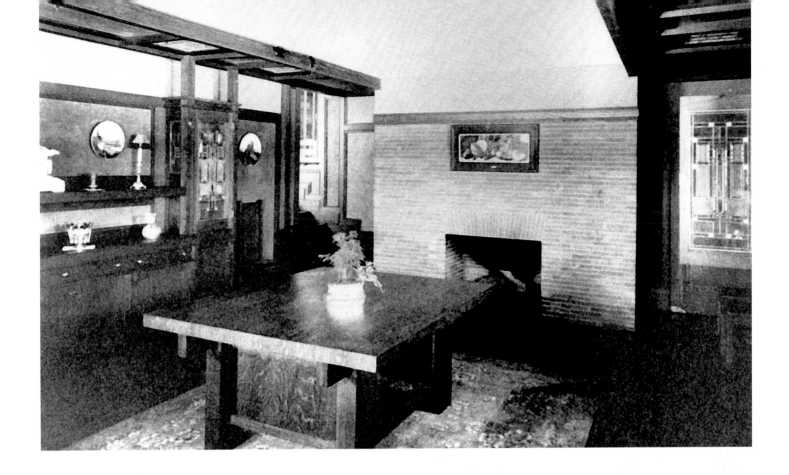

Japanese design principles and contemporary European and British design directions, and was inspired by the midwest landscape.

However, neither Marion nor Walter would have been drawn to, or employed by, Wright unless their own design ideas and interests were already sympathetic to his. That is, rather than deriving their inspiration from Wright, they shared common inspirational sources with him. Working in the highly creative environment of the Oak Park studio no doubt provided a unique opportunity to learn from Wright and to contribute ideas, as well as to develop their own aesthetic vocabulary and philosophy.

Certainly Walter and Marion's first major commissions, produced independently of Wright but while employed in his office, substantiate the maturity and confidence of their own architectural practice. These two 1903 projects — Marion's Unitarian Church of All Souls, Evanston, Illinois, and Walter's house for William Emery, Elmhurst, Illinois — also involved substantial interior design detailing, including light fittings, built-in and free-standing furniture, and leaded glass panels.

Obliged to revise her original, highly inventive design for the Unitarian Church of All Souls (*see pp 23, 59 and 60*) to conform with the 'gothic' theme demanded by the client, Marion managed to design a number of elements — in particular the leaded glass skylights and suspended, pyramidal leaded glass light fittings — which, in their secular, 'Wrightian' references,[7] dramatically lifted the interior beyond the ecclesiastically conventional. The inverted pyramid form of these light shades was to reappear

Above: Walter Burley Griffin designed dining room, William Emery house, Elmhurst, Illinois, 1903 reproduced in the *Architectural Record*, vol 23, 1908, p 499. The furniture reflects an arts and crafts influence as well as Griffin's concern for integrating interior elements.
Courtesy Nicholls collection, Sydney.

Previous page: Walter Burley Griffin in a Newman College 'couch chair' in the Roy Lippincott house, Melbourne, about 1921. A fold-down footrest is concealed beneath the seat.
Photo courtesy National Library of Australia, Canberra.

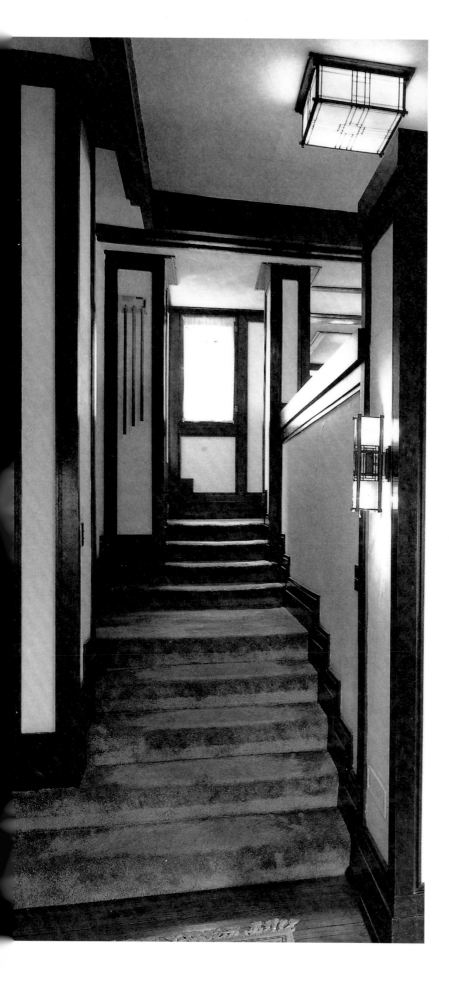

in several light fittings designed for projects in Australia, and the green and amber of their coloured glass was used recurrently in the Griffins' later interior design work. Examples of the light fittings survived the demolition of All Souls in the 1960s.

Walter's assured Emery house, (*see p 22*) with its interpenetrating interior spaces at once defined and unified by a dramatic interplay of horizontal and vertical elements, also featured built-in furniture and light fixtures that reflect his early confidence in detailing interior spaces. The dining room's built-in buffet, with its solid construction relieved by linear mouldings and abstract leaded glass panels flanking cupboard doors, is a simple complement to the interior scheme and has much in common with a similarly configured buffet in Frank Lloyd Wright's B Harley Bradley house dining room of about 1900. On the basis of the Emery house buffet's design, it is likely the solidly practical dining table featured in a 1908 photograph of the house[8] was also designed by Walter to complement the surrounding interior.

Perhaps the most telling indication of Walter's ability to focus on fine detail as well as the architectural whole is demonstrated in his design for the rectangular glass and brass bracket wall lights that survive today in the Emery house. Paul Kruty notes in his book *Walter Burley Griffin in America* that the light 'so pleased Wright that he subsequently used it on many of his own houses including the Dana and Little houses, and the George Barton and W H Heath houses in Buffalo, New York. (Of course, it is often removed and auctioned today as a Wright design.)'[9] The simple rectilinearity of these Japanese-inspired lights sits perfectly against the vertically defined rectangular wall elements within the house.

While Walter, having left Wright's office in 1906, was busy expanding his independent practice, Marion's architectural career was taking on new life. Frank Lloyd Wright's departure for Europe in September 1909 left a number of unfinished or barely begun projects. Wright employed Hermann Von Holst, a Chicago architect previously unassociated with the Prairie School, to complete the projects, and he in turn hired Marion to assist him. Of these houses, the David Amberg house in Grand Rapids, Michigan (1910) and the Edward P Irving and Robert and Adolph Mueller houses in Millikin Place, Decatur, Illinois (1910–1911) were the most substantial commissions. Marion designed the entire Amberg residence, completed the Irving house and designed the Mueller houses. Walter supplied a landscape plan for the Millikin Place site and Marion's bold, geometric streetlights complemented its architectural aesthetic.

But if the nature of Marion's contribution to the exterior architecture of these impressive Prairie style structures has been disentangled in recent years, the identification of the designers responsible for the equally impressive interiors and furniture of the houses is far less adequately resolved. Attributed variously in the past to Frank Lloyd Wright, Von Holst, Marion and the Milwaukee 'interior architect' George M Niedecken, it is relevant here to analyse documentation identifying Marion as the original interior designer.

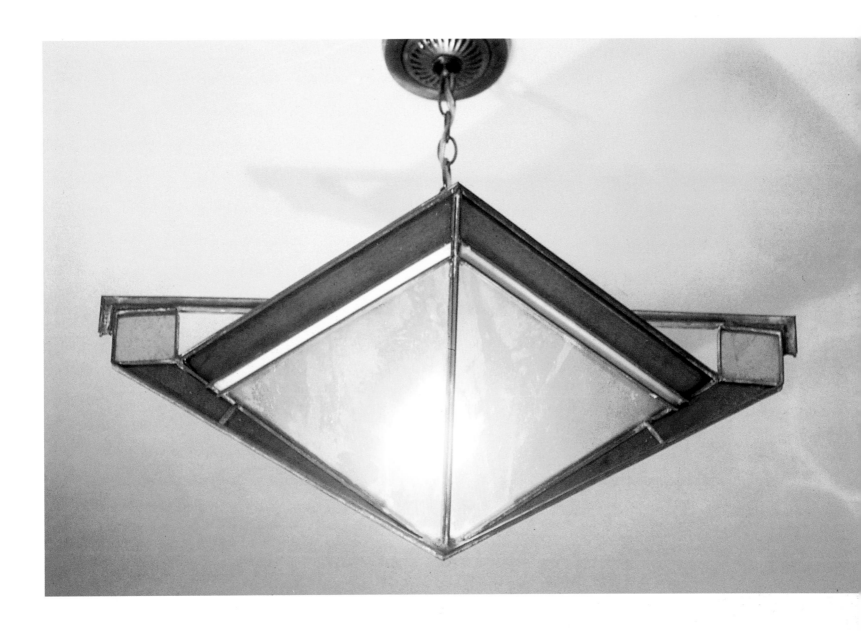

Above: Marion Mahony, ceiling light for the Unitarian Church of All Souls, Evanston, Illinois, about 1903 (now demolished), coloured glass and metal. The inverted pyramid design has much in common with the lights used in Frank Lloyd Wright's Susan Lawrence Dana house (Springfield, Illinois, 1903).
Courtesy Georgia Lloyd. Photograph courtesy Mati Maldre, Chicago.

Left: Walter Burley Griffin, glass and brass bracket wall light in an internal stairway of the Emery house, Elmhurst, Illinois, 1903. This recent photo shows how effectively the design of the light repeats and reinforces the vertical rectilinearity of the internal wall elements. The light is often mistakenly attributed to Frank Lloyd Wright and was used by him in several projects.
Photograph courtesy Mati Maldre, Chicago, 1989.

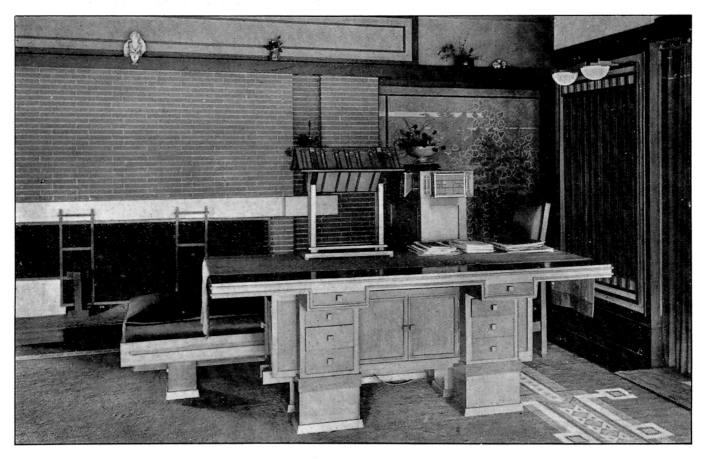

Portion of living room furniture, comprising library table, couch, reading lamp, book-case and desk with desk lamp.
Architect: MARION M. GRIFFIN.

In 1913 extensive articles on the Irving and Amberg houses were published in the *Western Architect*.[10] Each carried several photographs of the completed and furnished interiors, while the Irving house article also featured elevation drawings for some of its striking furniture. Images in the Amberg house article were captioned 'H.V. von Holst, Architect, Chicago. Marion M. Griffin Associate', while the Irving images carried the caption 'Frank Lloyd Wright, Architect — H.V. Von Holst, Associated'.

Although Marion's name is omitted entirely from the Irving house article and only 'in association' in relation to the Amberg house, she makes consistent claims in 'The magic of America' and elsewhere to having 'complete control of the design'.[11] This assertion is reiterated later in 'Magic' when Marion, adopting the pseudonym Xantippe, reminisces along similar lines.[12]

Elsewhere in 'Magic', captions in Marion's handwriting to several photographs of the Irving, Amberg and Robert Mueller house interiors assert her responsibility for interior fittings and furnishings. Accompanying two

photographs of the Amberg interiors is the caption, 'Amberg dwelling & furniture. MM & von H' (we can safely assume Marion is here acknowledging Von Holst because of his employer status rather than any direct design involvement), and the superb Irving living room is captioned, 'Furniture, carpets, draperies, radiator screens and glass, MMG & von H / Mural by Niedecken'.[13] Lest it be construed that such self attribution was the product of an elderly eccentric's meanderings, the same Irving house photograph accompanied an article by Walter, 'Standards for furnishing', published in the *Australian Home Builder* in 1923 and clearly credited responsibility for its contents to 'Marion M Griffin'. Photographs of all these interiors survive today in the Nicholls collection, an important archive of photographs, documents, drawings and ephemera passed on by Marion to the Griffins' architectural partner, Eric Nicholls in the late 1930s.

The bold and accomplished Prairie style combination desk and couch in the Irving house photograph is now in the collection of the Milwaukee Art Museum where, on the basis of archival documentation relating to George Niedecken's business activities, it is attributed to Niedecken:

> Dear Mr Von Holst:
> We are just barely able to complete the drawings for the Irving furniture. Mr Niedecken is not at all satisfied with them, but lack of time prevents our finishing them as we would like to.
>
> We hope that you can secure this contract for us and will appreciate anything that you can do to close it with Mr Irving. Our prices include making the details of the furniture and art glass ...[14]

Many of Niedecken's beautiful Japanese-inspired presentation drawings for the Irving and Amberg house projects survive in the Milwaukee collection, but do these and archival documentation prove Niedecken was actually the designer of these interior elements? Marion was certainly not in the habit of claiming undue credit; on the contrary, like most of her female contemporaries, she endured a lifetime of under-acknowledgment, with Wright, Von Holst, even Walter, among others, commonly being given sole credit. In view of her obvious architectural leadership of these projects, is it not inconceivable that Marion's professional relationship with Niedecken was the reverse of that which had existed between Wright and herself? That is, is it possible that Marion, this time assuming responsibility for overseeing the complete project, produced the initial design concepts that were then worked up into presentation drawings for clients by Niedecken, just as she had worked from initial sketches produced by Wright in earlier projects?[15] And what are we to make of her remark to Walter, reproduced in 'The magic of America': 'Mr Von Holtz sent me a copy of the letter he wrote Mr Felton concerning the publication of the Amberg dwelling [presumably the article in the *Western Architect*, October 1913]. N certainly has colossal nerve'?[16]

While constraints of space do not allow for a detailed analysis of this vexed question of authorship, it is worth bearing in mind not only Marion's own repeated claims over several decades to responsibility for these interiors, but also the breadth of experience she must already have developed working with Frank Lloyd Wright on the design of furniture, lighting and decorative glass.

The structural geometry of the furniture designed for these Decatur and Grand Rapids houses reiterated and reinforced their architectural features. Five years later and on another continent, Marion's reaction to the demands of an entirely different architectural space — as well as those of its users — engendered a very different furniture response. The tables and chairs designed for the Cafe Australia in Melbourne in 1916 are unique in the Griffins' work and underline the versatility and sensitivity of their approach to individual projects. Described in detail by Marion in 'Magic',[17] the Cafe Australia project involved the entire redesign of the entrance and interior spaces for the cafe's owner, A J J Lucas. These bold and lofty interiors, with their 'Sullivanesque' openwork plaster decoration, massive ribbed

Left: Photo of the Irving house living-room furniture which accompanied Walter's article 'Standards for furnishing', *Australian Home Builder*, August 1923, pp 34–35, 45. Note the clear attribution to Marion. The combination couch and desk is now in the collection of the Milwaukee Art Museum where it is attributed to George M Niedecken, despite Marion's claims in 'The magic of America' that she was responsible for the design of these pieces and other furniture in the house.
Photograph courtesy State Library of Victoria.

Below: Marion Mahony, streetlights, Millikin Place, Decatur, Illinois. In the background is the E P Irving house for which Marion was involved in designing interior furniture and fittings, about 1910. The design of the lights echoes the strong interplay of horizontal and vertical elements in the Irving house. Walter provided a landscape plan for the Millikin Place projects 1911–1912.
Photograph courtesy Mati Maldre, Chicago, 1991.

Following pages: Banquet Hall, Cafe Australia, 1916. The joinery of the blackwood chairs and tables and their combination of repeating circular and triangular motifs was unusually complex for the Griffins. The furniture was made by the H Goldman Manufacturing Company, Melbourne.
Courtesy Nicholls collection, Sydney.

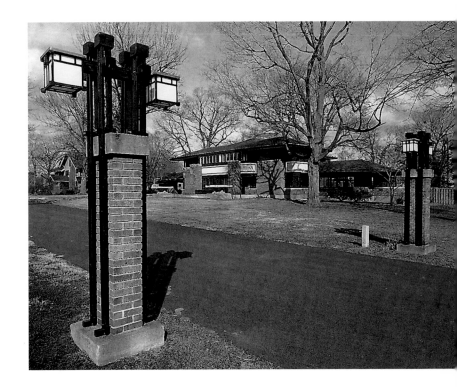

piers and exuberant sculptural decoration were the last word in elegant Melbourne dining:

> Of the Cafe Australia one could perhaps say it is the most beautiful cafe in the world ... It occupied the ground floor of a down town building under the light well ... and consisted of five rooms separated not by walls but by great piers which carried the structure of the building above.

> It is lighted in part by the open vaulted grill under the light well and partly by stained glass ceiling panels screening electric lamps. The tiles used were real gold Delft tiles brought from Holland. The sculpture was done by Miss Baskerville of Melbourne and the mural decoration by Miss Merfield of Melbourne.[18]

The cafe comprised several dining areas furnished with either cane chairs or the Griffins' leather-upholstered, high-backed dining chairs, and with circular-topped tables, suitable for a setting of four, or, as in the 'banquet hall', rectangular tables with the same elegant supporting structure. The latter tables could be joined together for multiple sittings as required.

The location of surviving examples of the cafe furniture had defied the best efforts of the most determined furniture aficionados until the recent discovery in Melbourne of one of the rectangular tables and an incomplete chair. Analysis of this purpose-designed furniture reveals it to be unusual for the Griffins in a number of ways. First, it is made of Australian blackwood, dark stained, rather than the preferred oak. Secondly, its design and construction is unusually complex. And, thirdly, its use of a repeating rhythm of curved elements is unprecedented.

A stamp on the underside of the chair seat indicates the furniture was made by the H Goldman Manufacturing Company, a Melbourne firm which specialised in custom-made, high quality furniture and won several gold medals at international exhibitions in the first quarter of the century.[19] Goldman's familiarity with the indigenous blackwood may well have influenced the decision to use this particular timber, but the company's long experience as makers of fine furniture would have been essential in resolving the chair and table's challenging joinery complexities.

Intricately constructed, the Cafe Australia furniture was a highly distinctive solution to the demands of a complex interior. Its integration within this interior was achieved through the repetition of shapes and motifs — the circularity of the tables and chair seats, the opposing curves of the chair back rails and table supports, the triangular thrust of the chair backs and table bases — and their articulation in the surrounding interior detailing. Reference in 'The magic of America'[20] to the cafe's use of the triangle and the circle as the chief unifying architectural motifs connects with Marion's later belief in the cosmic significance of these shapes (light for the triangle, warmth for the circle) and suggests the possibility of their deliberate symbolism within the cafe interiors. Instead of solid, arts and crafts style furniture the Griffins turned to the more curvilinear European art nouveau and Viennese secessionist design for inspiration. It is both puzzling and unfortunate that no

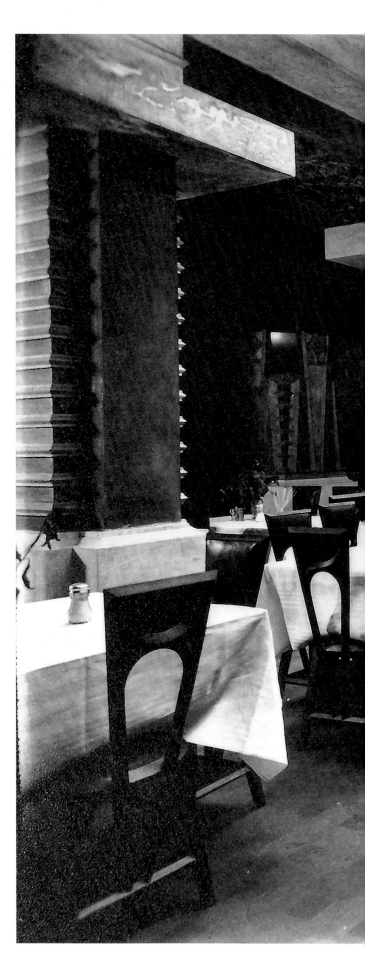

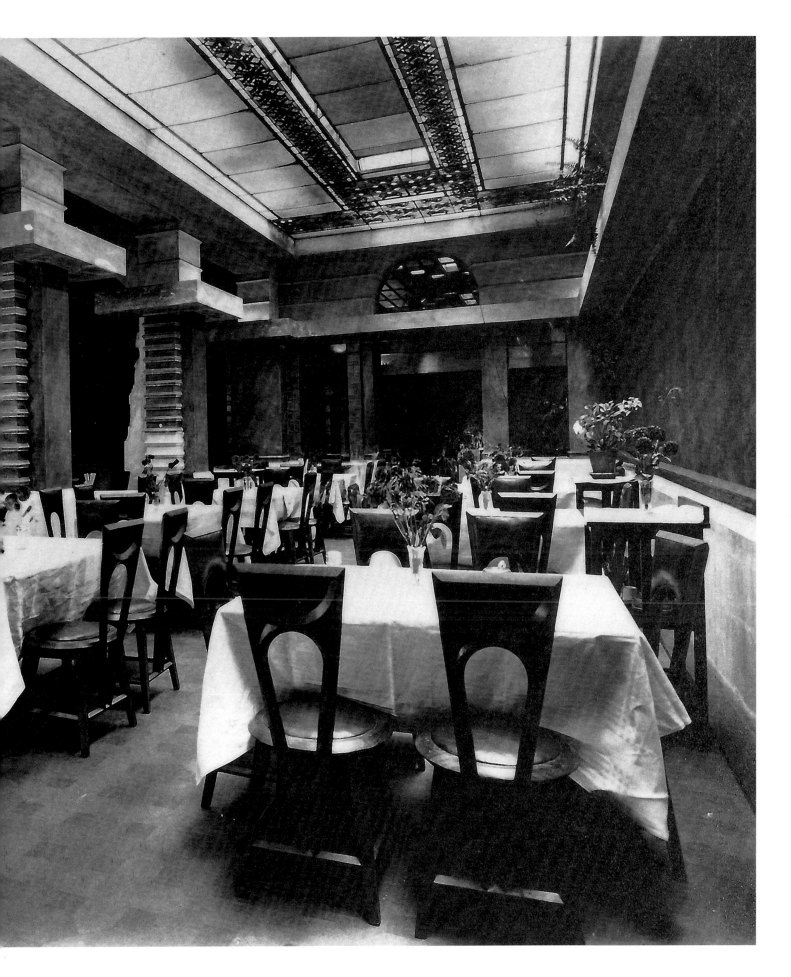

drawings, apart from a small sketch[21] of the cafe furniture remain and that not one of the cafe chairs or circular tables appear to have survived intact.

By contrast, the furniture designed by the Griffins for Newman College at the University of Melbourne in 1917, is relatively well-documented and well-represented through surviving examples. 'The Newman College project', wrote Jane Carolan in *The collegiate furniture of Walter Burley Griffin*, 'was to give Griffin an opportunity to realise a complete integration of architecture and interior design on a scale and in a completeness which he was unable to achieve elsewhere'.[22] This 'completeness' included the design of all the furniture for each of the two-roomed students' quarters — study table, swivel chair, table lamp, bed, chiffonier, bookcase and side chair — as well as a generously proportioned 'couch chair' for the library, lecture chairs and dining furniture. All were executed in Japanese oak (*Quercus acuta*) and, in contrast to the deliberate stylishness of the Cafe Australia furniture, returned to the solid arts and crafts values of the American years.

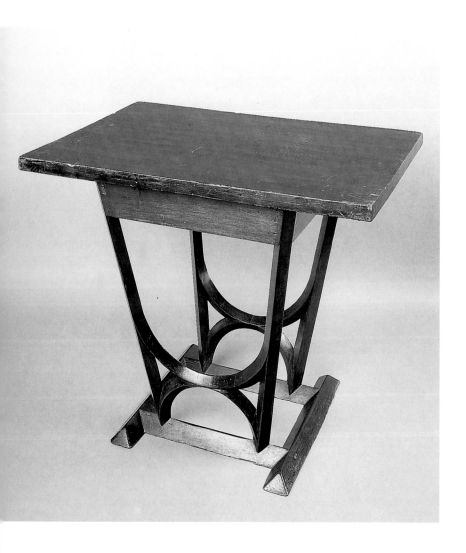

Almost abstract in conception, totally functional and capable of a high level of machine production, the Newman College furniture was a culmination of ideas absorbed to date and the physical expression of theories delivered in numerous lectures and writings. Perceiving no conflict between the use of machinery and the retention of natural surfaces, Walter wrote in 1925: 'There is an inherent beauty in all natural materials that can be brought out by mechanical working in a higher degree than any other way … For simple lines and plain surfaces the beauty is in the greatest degree provided by the material itself; Nature's contribution beyond all effective imitation'.[23]

Documentation drawings for various examples of the Newman College furniture show how completely the Griffins had grasped principles of economy, both in a design sense and in construction methods. The furniture has no curves or ornamentation and is designed to be relatively easily produced using standard cabinetmaking construction methods and hardware. Wherever possible Japanese oak is veneered onto a hardwood or lightweight wood carcase, thus considerably reducing the cost of materials and the weight of the finished pieces. Several examples of the Newman College furniture bear the label of James Moore & Sons, City Road, Melbourne.

The Capitol Theatre, Melbourne (1921–1924), presented the Griffins with a similar opportunity to pursue the ideal of integrated architecture on a large scale. Yet two more different projects could not be imagined: the one for an ecclesiastical client, conventional and uncompromising, the other providing a spectacular environment for no other purpose than the enhancement of the then novel movie-going experience. It is to the Griffins' great credit that they had the flexibility and imagination to approach each project on its own terms and that they delivered results entirely appropriate to the individuality of each project.

Unlike Newman College, however, the Griffins' brief for the Capitol Theatre did not, as far as can be determined, extend to the design of furniture. Given their adventurous 'modernist' approach throughout the interiors, one can only speculate what alternative they might have provided to the 'period trash' [24] — for example, Jacobean and Louis XIV style furniture — that was eventually scattered throughout the interiors, no doubt much to their consternation.[25]

The Griffins were responsible, however, for much of the Capitol's lighting, both fixtures and free-standing. Indeed, it was the theatre's astonishing lighting effects that thrilled audiences in the 1920s and that helped justify its preservation when threatened with demolition in recent times. Given the theatre's present sorry condition (it has been partially converted into a shopping arcade) one can now only imagine the effect on patrons of its startling prismatic plaster ceiling pulsating with coloured lights as the auditorium resonated to the booming chords of the Wurlitzer organ on stage.

As a complement to the prismatic effect of the main ceiling the Griffins also designed a series of imposing star-shaped lights that were affixed to the lowered ceilings around the perimeter of the stalls. These extraordinary,

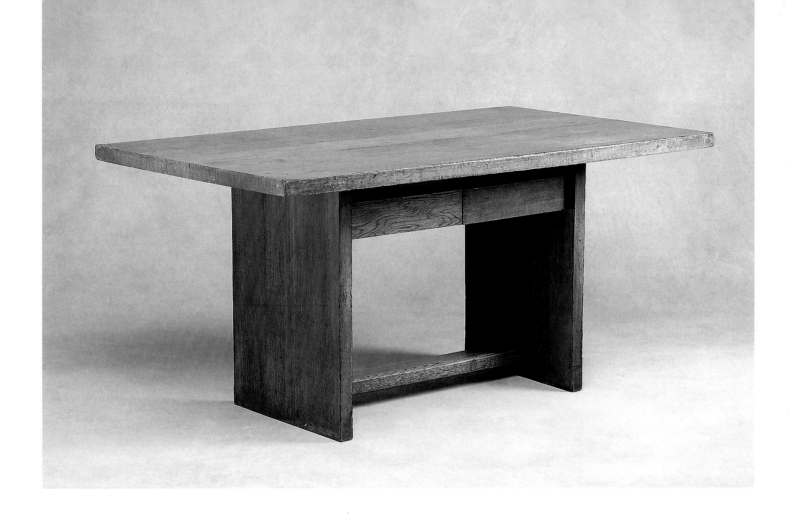

precociously 'art deco' style light fixtures, several of which have been removed and preserved, were composed of triangular panels of coloured and leaded glass held within a complex geometric, ribbed wood and plaster framework. Their glowing presence in the darkened theatre must have been truly awe-inspiring.

As a prelude to the breathtaking experience of the main auditorium the Griffins also paid detailed attention to the design of the series of foyers and stairways leading to it. Lighting again performed an important role. Positioned throughout the main foyer and adjoining lounge were a number of stylish light standards with the inverted pyramidal shades of which the Griffins were so fond. While no examples of these free-standing lights appear to have survived, they can be seen in several early photographs of the Capitol interiors. A design drawing for the light in the Art Institute of Chicago indicates that its clustered rod standard was made of cast iron and the shade of plaster and glass. Drawings also survive for several of the many smaller wall light fixtures the Griffins designed for the Capitol, including the strange, faceted spherical lights clustered on the foyer stairway columns that Griffin author, James Birrell, described in 1964 as 'reminiscent of Salvador Dali'.[26]

The opportunity that major projects such as the Capitol Theatre, Newman College and the Cafe Australia presented to design complete interiors was not to continue. On the contrary, with their energies during the 1920s and early '30s focused on the development of the Sydney suburb of

Above: Study table designed by the Griffins for the students' quarters at Newman College, University of Melbourne, about 1917, 69.5 × 152.5 × 42.5 cm. The simple design in Japanese oak was modern and functional and integrated with other college furniture.
Powerhouse Museum collection, 93/366/1. Photo by Scott Donkin, Powerhouse Museum.

Left: Blackwood table, Cafe Australia, Melbourne, 1916, the only known surviving example. Rectangular tables are visible in contemporary photographs of the cafe's 'banquet hall' and could be joined together for multiple settings.
Private collection, Melbourne. Photo by Andrew Simpson.

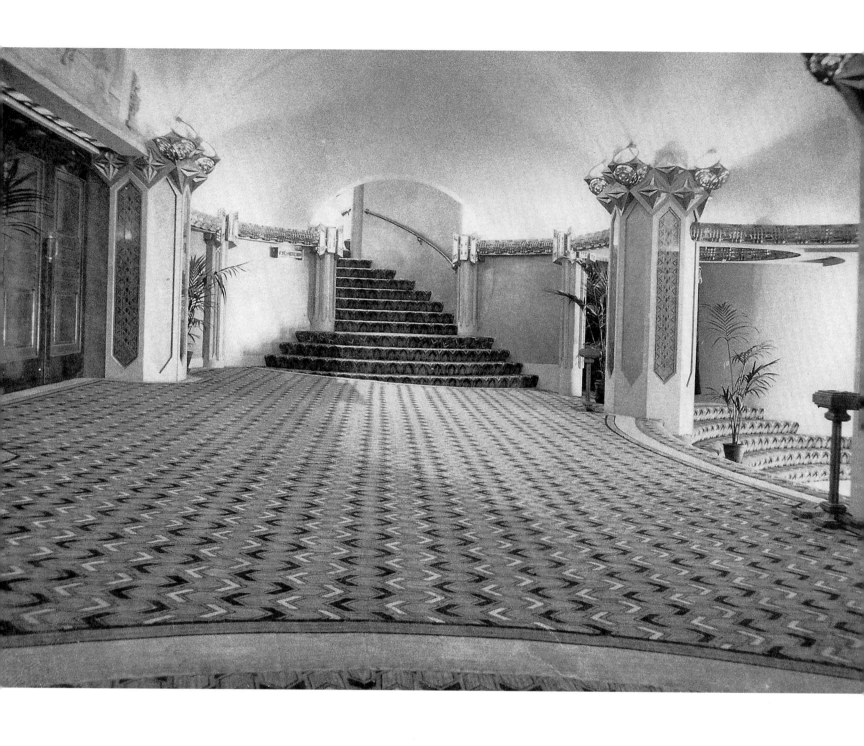

Castlecrag, Marion and Walter were to devote their attention to the very different problems of designing small houses with functional and flexible interior spaces. Such houses could accommodate only the most essential of free-standing furniture and relied on built-in cupboards, wardrobes, sideboards and shelving for their success as effective spaces:

> It is gradually becoming recognised now that the less furniture a house contains, consistent with its needs, the better. This is a phase of aesthetics which has been most evident among the people of the Orient. Australia is an Oriental country, and if our civilization embraces adaptation to environment, climatic influences may eventually bring about a corresponding reaction on the part of the people.[27]

The sale in 1997 of the Griffin-designed Cheong Cheok Hong house[28] in Castlecrag drew attention to its 1920s Bauhaus furniture, surviving from the time the house was owned by Jewish refugees Manfred and Friedel Souhami in 1941. Brought with them from Nazi Germany such starkly modern furniture was unavailable in Australia at the time, but well suited the house's equally minimal interiors.[29] One can only speculate if, given the availability of this furniture locally, it would have been preferred by Castlecrag residents over the light-weight cane or seagrass furniture that featured commonly in Castlecrag interiors in the 1920s and '30s. Certainly Walter's obvious preference for the very avant-garde French steel furniture seen in a number of the outdoor Castlecrag photographs signals his readiness to embrace the very latest in industrial technology.[30]

As well as informal cane furniture a number of the Castlecrag houses also featured what journalist Nora Cooper described in 1927 as the 'peculiarly shaped lamps'.[31] 'Peculiar' they may have generally appeared to Australians in the 1920s, but these handsome hanging lights, with their inverted pyramidal wooden shades and elegant horizontal mouldings, were a direct descendant of lights used by the Griffins twenty years earlier in the United States. The same inverted pyramid form also provided the inspiration for the imposing standard floor lights designed for the Guy house, Castlecrag, in the 1920s and for the hanging plaster shades used in several Melbourne residential projects. The importance that Marion and Walter attached to indirect incandescent illumination, either through cove lighting (which they pioneered in Chicago) or purpose-designed light fittings, is reinforced on several occasions by Marion in 'The magic of America':

> In the illumination of the home, the architect and illuminating engineer comes closer in contact with his client than in any other branch of his work. He is given a chance to work up many original and decorative ideas embodying special features which will harmonise with the general decorative schemes of the various rooms. Correct practice dictates that some way be devised to conceal the bare lamp from view. It is also believed that well diffused illumination very largely minimises the effect of glare and deep shadows making for a soft, efficient light.[32]

The extent of the Griffins' designs for furniture and lighting during their brief period in India (Walter from October 1935 to his death on 11 February 1937; Marion from May 1936 to

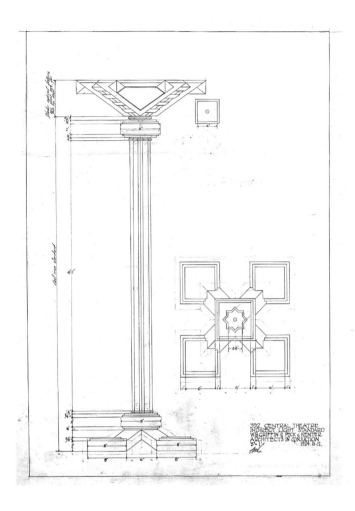

Above: Elevation and plan for an 'indirect light standard' for the Capitol Theatre, Melbourne, dated 3 November 1924 and initialled 'EMN' (Eric Milton Nicholls), ink on linen, 67 × 43 cm. Examples of this imposing standard light, specified to be made in cast iron and plaster, can be seen in early photos of the theatre's foyers.
Courtesy Art Institute of Chicago, gift of Marion Mahony Griffin through Eric Nicholls (KK/2#25–392).

Left: Stairwell leading from entrance foyer, Capitol Theatre, Melbourne, about 1924. The photograph shows various wall lights designed by the Griffins and underlines the importance they placed in the use of lighting to enhance the theatre's dramatic interior effects. The green, black and burnt orange carpet was also designed by the Griffins.
Photograph courtesy of Dorothea Irving, daughter of A J J Lucas, Melbourne.

Right: Ceiling light, Capitol Theatre, Melbourne, about 1924, coloured glass, wood, plaster, lead, 33 × 132 × 132 cm. Examples of this ceiling light were affixed to the lowered perimeter ceiling of the theatre's stalls. The light's sophisticated and complex art deco style indicates the Griffins' awareness of the latest European design development, well before the style's popularity in Australia in the early 1930s.

Powerhouse Museum collection, 97/308/1. Photo by Penelope Clay, Powerhouse Museum, Sydney.

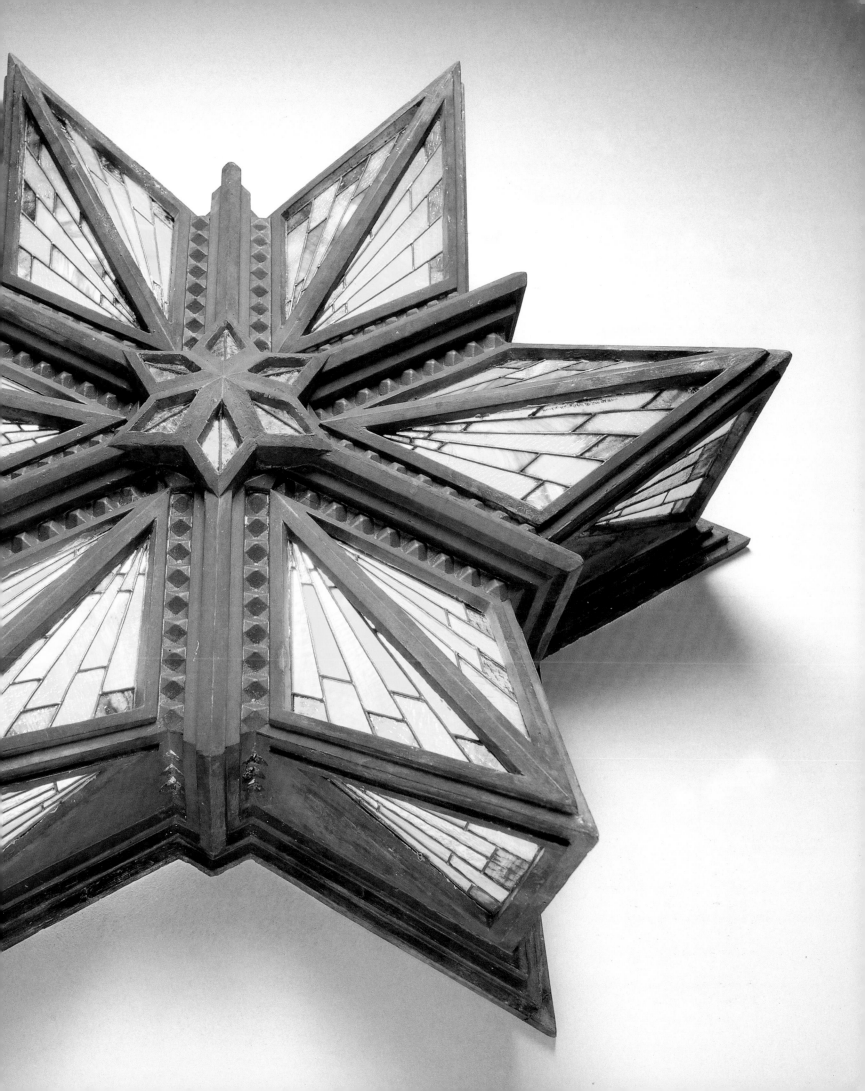

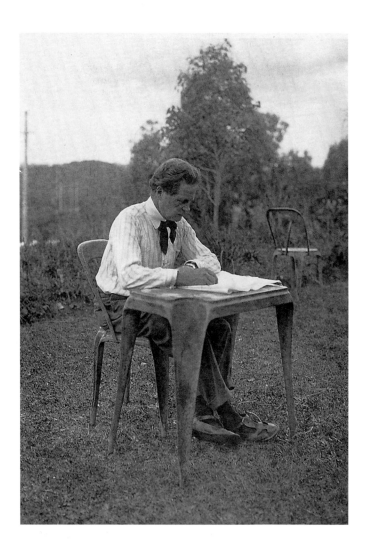

about April 1937) is difficult to determine. No known examples of their designs for interior elements appear to have survived — not surprising given that so few of their many remarkable Indian architectural projects were realised — but several references to the making of furniture occur in the extensive Indian correspondence from both Marion and Walter. Writing from Lucknow, India, to Marion in Sydney on 19 February 1936, Walter rather cryptically exclaims: 'At present I am checking and winding up as far as possible the Library [Lucknow University Library] details including the furniture lacking any item of which the Librarian says he will not bring the matter to a finality'.[33]

Three weeks later and exasperated with the slowness of progress he again complained to Marion: 'The Librarian has been a perfect pest with his procrastination and unwillingness to shoulder responsibility for action. A specimen chair is now being made in my bathroom!'[34]

The library was unfortunately never built to Walter's splendid design and we can only presume the furniture to which he refers suffered the same fate. In the absence of documentary evidence it is tempting to speculate that Walter's sensitive adaptation of traditional Eastern elements in the design of the library itself may also have extended to the library's furniture.

In addition to the furniture and lighting created for specific projects, the Griffins also designed furniture for their own needs. Several examples used in the Griffin office — desks, drafting tables and bookcases — survive today and have much in common with the solid and functional Newman College furniture of 1917. That the Griffins were in the habit of designing practical objects, in particular furniture, to meet their everyday needs is clearly, though poignantly, revealed in a letter written by Marion soon after Walter's death in India in February 1937:

> Genie darling … Under operation Walter died Wednesday night. Ruptured gall bladder, the consequence of his fall some three years ago … We thought at the end of three days that the danger point was passed. When I went over Wednesday morning, he gave me a thumb nail drawing of a bookrack to have the carpenter, who has been making furniture for us for some weeks, make it so that he could read in bed.[35]

The furniture and lighting designed by the Griffins over the 30 or so years they practised in America and Australia are significant not only for a more complete understanding of their design ethic, but also because they provide an important link between their architecture and those who inhabited it. The Griffins' humanist philosophy, coupled with their creativity and sense of 'fitness for purpose', ensured that their designs for interior elements served both the architectural context and human needs. In doing so they created a unique body of work that has made an important contribution to twentieth-century design.

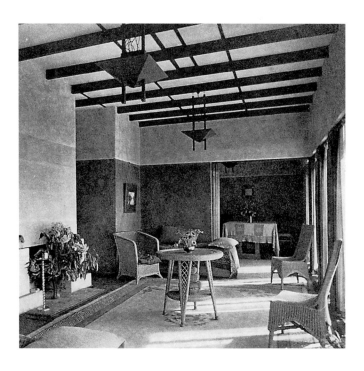

Notes

1. Stickley's highly successful 'Craftsman Furniture' business, based in Syracuse, New York, produced quality arts and crafts furniture, usually in oak, throughout the first fifteen years of the century. Stickley's furniture was marketed through his magazine *The Craftsman* and catalogues produced regularly from 1901 to 1913.

2. These include the Mary Bovee (1907), Ralph Griffin (1909), Comstock (1911) and Arthur Rule (1912) house interiors, all published in the *Western Architect* (vol 19, no 8, August 1913, pp 66–80), an issue devoted entirely to the Griffins' work.

3. Marion Griffin, 'The bungalow indoors' in Rogers & Manson, *100 turn-of-the-century brick bungalows*, Dover, New York, 1912, p 116. Interestingly, a typescript of an almost identical article is reproduced in 'The magic of America' (vol 4, 'The individual battle', pp 332–35, New York Historical Society typescript) where it is titled 'Underlying principles' and credited to 'WBG'.

4. Ashbee visited Chicago in 1896, 1900–1901 and 1908–1909. The interaction between progressive European, English and American architects at the turn of the century is dealt with in David A Hanks and Jennifer Toher, 'The decorative designs of Frank Lloyd Wright and his European contemporaries: 1895–1915' in *Frank Lloyd Wright: architectural drawings and decorative art*, Fischer Fine Art, London, 1985.

5. *House Beautiful*, vol 10, no 6, November 1901, pp 372–77.

6. Walter Burley Griffin, 'Standards for furnishing', *The Australian Home Builder*, August 1923, p 34.

7. Wright's Susan Lawrence Dana house (Springfield, Illinois, 1903) made similar use of arched leaded glass skylights and 'pyramidal' hanging lights. It is not inconceivable that Marion was involved in the design of these elements as well.

8. *The Architectural Record*, vol 23, June 1908, p 499. The photograph is notable for the absent clutter of dining chairs.

9. Paul Kruty and Mati Maldre, *Walter Burley Griffin in America*, University of Illinois Press, Urbana & Chicago, 1996, p 20. Documentation substantiating the attribution of the design of this light fixture to Griffin can be found in N K M Smith, ed, 'Letters, 1903–1906, by Charles E White, Jr. from the studio of Frank Lloyd Wright', *Journal of Architectural Education*, vol 25, Fall 1971, p 106 as cited in Kruty, ibid, p 34.

10. 'Residence for E P Irving, Decatur, Illinois', *Western Architect*, April 1913, p 38; 'Residence for D M Amberg, Grand Rapids, Mich.', *Western Architect*, October 1913, p 88.

11. 'The magic of America', vol 3, 'The municipal battle', p 172.

12. Ibid, vol 4, 'The individual battle', p 275.

13. Ibid, reverse of p 260.

14. John S Walbridge (Niedecken's partner) to Hermann Von Holst, 29 December 1910, cited in *The domestic scene (1897–1927): George M Niedecken, interior architect*, Milwaukee Art Museum, 1981, pp 70–71.

15. It is worth noting here that furniture designed by Niedecken independently of either Wright or Marion was much more subject to the influence of period styles and lacked the severity and purity of Prairie School design. See ibid.

16. 'The magic of America', vol 4, p 387.

17. Ibid, vol 2, 'The federal battle', pp 80–92.

18. Ibid, p 86.

19. Established by 1900 and active through to the 1930s, the company was located at 394 LaTrobe Street, Central Melbourne from 1913 until 1927, the year in which it moved to South Yarra. The Griffins also employed the Goldman company to make the splendid blackwood ceremonial casket and mallet, commissioned by the Australian Government for presentation to the Prince of Wales on the occasion of the laying of the foundation stone for the Capitol, Canberra in 1920 (National Archives of Australia: CRS A199, item 21/759). See Anne Watson, 'Walter Burley Griffin's "other" Canberra legacy', *Australiana*, vol 19, no 4, Nov 1997, pp 99–102, 110.

20. 'The magic of America', vol 2, p 84.

21. A small sketch of a chair similar to the cafe chairs occurs in the lower margin of a pencil elevation drawing for the cafe's 'Bower' room (Art Institute, Chicago, 1990.57.1–2). The drawing also includes sketches for cutlery.

22. University of Melbourne, 1993.

23. WBG, 'Standards for furnishing', op cit, p 34.

24. Walter's term for 'the monotonous procession of machine-made imitations of period furniture', ibid.

25. A set of now privately owned, wooden slatted armchairs, with circular upholstered seats and backs, salvaged from the Capitol Theatre in the 1960s may well be by Griffin, but no documentation has yet been discovered to confirm this attribution. A similar chair can be seen in Marion's presentation drawing for Walter's Ralph Griffin house (about 1909, Mary and Leigh Block Museum of Art, Northwestern University, Illinois).

26. James Birrell, *Walter Burley Griffin*, University of Queensland Press, Brisbane, 1964, p 167.

27. WBG, 'Standards for furnishing', op cit, p 34.

28. Built in 1922 this sandstone house was financed by the Rev Cheong Cheok Hong, a leader of the Chinese community in Australia.

29. For an account of the history of this furniture see H Greenwood, 'Design as politics', *The Sydney Morning Herald*, 29 March 1997, p 7s.

30. First manufactured in the mid 1920s by the Société industrielle des meubles multiples, Lyon, these stackable chairs and tables were the forerunners of today's moulded plastic furniture.

31. 'What constitutes the perfect small house', *Australian Home Beautiful*, 1 October 1926, p 31.

32. 'The magic of America', vol 4, p 219.

33. Ibid, vol 1, p 77a.

34. 6 April 1936, ibid, vol I, p 95a.

35. Marion to Genevieve Lippincott, 13 February 1937. Cited in Anna Rubbo, 'Marion Mahony Griffin: a portrait', in J Duncan and M Gates, eds, *Walter Burley Griffin: a re-view*, Monash University Gallery, Melbourne, 1988, p 19.

Above left: Walter Burley Griffin in the garden at Castlecrag, 1930. The chair and table feature in a number of the Castlecrag outdoor photos and were obviously favoured by residents including the Griffins. Of pressed steel, the furniture was first designed in the mid 1920s by a French company based in Lyon and is the forerunner of today's moulded plastic furniture.
Courtesy National Library of Australia, Canberra. Photo by Dr Jorma Pohjanpalo.

Below left: Living room of the Grant house, Castlecrag, about 1925 showing the wooden hanging lights used in several of the Castlecrag houses. 'Oriental' rugs and woven seagrass furniture complete the simple and informal setting.
Courtesy Nicholls collection, Sydney.

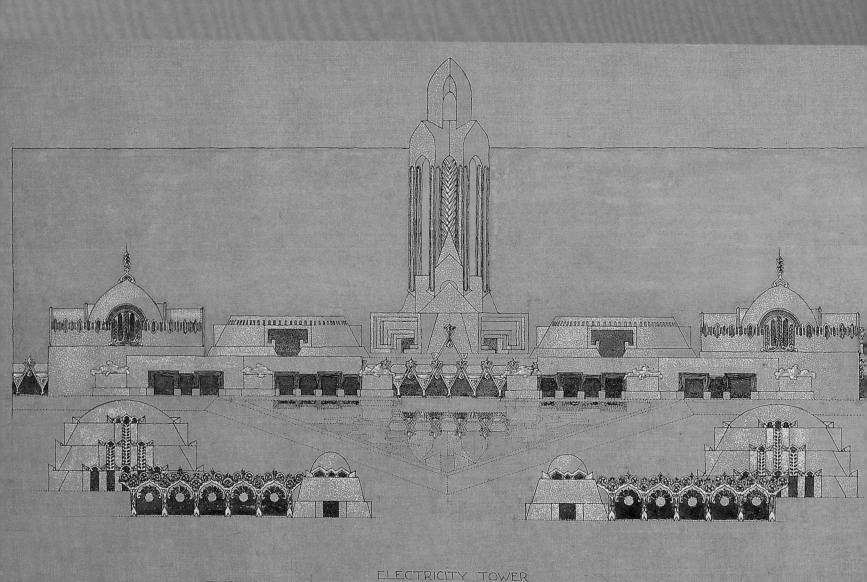

ELECTRICITY TOWER

ENGINEERING BATTERY   BATTERY

ROTUNDA   ROTUNDA
        THEATRE   JEWEL ESPLANADE   CABARET
                             FOUNTAIN PAVILION
HORTICULTURE STUPA   AGRICULTURAL   PYLONS   FLORAL ARCADE   STUPA
                    INDUSTRIAL AXIS

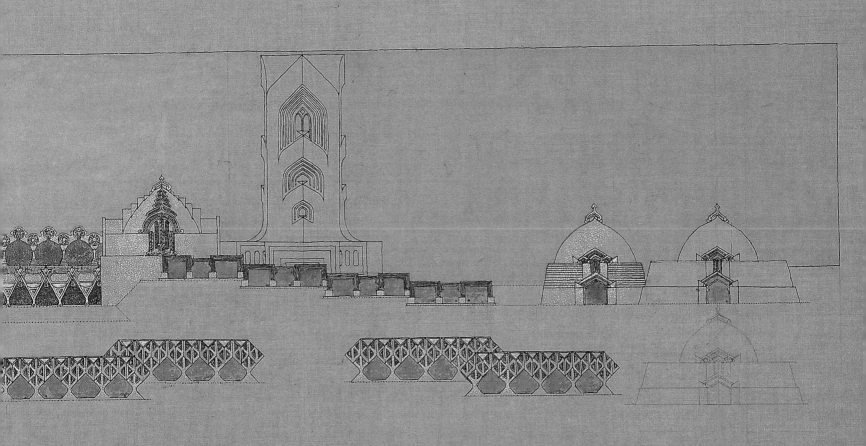

FORESTRY   ESCHELON STEPS   WOOD WORK

Walter Burley Griffin was almost 59 years old in October 1935 when, temporarily leaving Marion Mahony Griffin, then 64, and his friends and colleagues in Sydney, he travelled to the northern Indian city of Lucknow by way of Colombo, Bombay, Agra, and Delhi.[1] If Griffin felt that much of his life had been a preparation for this journey, in many ways the experience affected him more profoundly than he could have imagined. Griffin's Indian adventure produced a creative outpouring that, because of his untimely death fifteen months later in February 1937, was also his final testament. Here I propose to sketch the outline of the story, to introduce the major designs, and to analyse several of them in terms of Griffin's avowed aim to create a modern, Indian architecture.[2]

Griffin's immediate connection with India began through his close friend and supporter, Ula Maddocks, and her friend Ronald Craig, an Australian journalist who was living in India. By mid 1935 Maddocks' and Craig's 'conspiracy' to arrange for new commissions had resulted in Griffin's advising Alagappan Mudalir, a contractor in Benares (Varanasi), about the foundations of a Buddhist temple about to be constructed. Through Alagappan, Griffin was invited to submit a proposal for a new university library in nearby Lucknow. When his design was favourably received, Marion and his Australian partner, Eric Nicholls, urged him to accept the university's invitation to travel to Lucknow for further discussions. Nicholls and a competent staff would manage his Australian practice, while at home the circle of friends at Castlecrag would similarly be guided by Mahony, as they had been for more than a decade. The plan was set: Griffin was to direct construction of the library and return to Sydney within three months.[3]

With these assurances and hopeful about the prospects of constructing a major building, Griffin left Sydney on 8 October 1935 aboard the SS *Mongolia*, which departed Fremantle in Western Australia four days later, and arrived at Colombo, Ceylon (Sri Lanka), a week later. After an excursion to the ancient city of Kandy, Griffin continued to Bombay, where he was met by Ronald Craig. The pair visited the sixth-century Hindu caves on the island of Elephanta. Arriving a few days later at Agra and the very image of India itself to westerners — the Taj Mahal — Griffin found it 'no less breath-taking than to any devotee who has ever sung its praises, and quite independent of the fact that, architecturally, I could see many things that should have been altogether different'.[4] Still, they lingered for a full day. Griffin's rapid immersion in India's historic architecture concluded with visits to several more monuments to Islamic rule in northern India at Agra and at Fatehpur Sikri. Exploring the latter by moonlight, Griffin said, 'How altogether pusillanimous, puny was the effort of the civilization of Australia toward a Continental Capital compared with this, perfectly conceived and as perfectly completed monumentally, and then replaced by another in a fraction of the time consumed by merely talking about Canberra'.[5] A few days later, Griffin recorded his impressions of New Delhi, designed by Herbert Baker and Edwin Lutyens

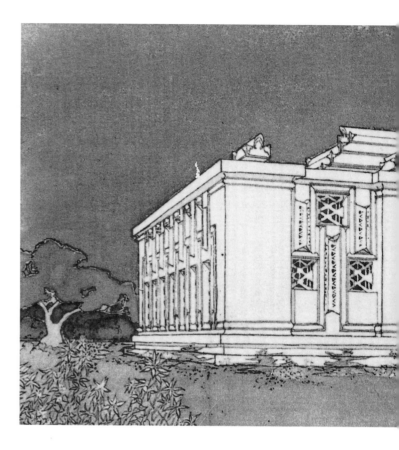

shortly after his own Canberra, and much more developed in 1935 than the Australian capital, noting 'the governmental terrace with vast stone buildings and several domes and extensive colonnades effectively massed is essentially Roman, even to the togas of the statues of the Viceroys despite the efforts to supply local color in all of the details'.[6]

Griffin arrived in Lucknow on 11 November 1935. The city, set on a level plain on the south bank of the Gumti River, was to Griffin 'a vast garden, with roads shaded by magnificent trees in many ways reminding one of the Mississippi valley' of his native Illinois.[7] The urban fabric, however, was unlike any western city. The densely packed ancient district of narrow lanes — the *chauk* — contrasted with open areas of vast palaces and gardens, colonial civic buildings, Islamic imambaras and mosques, and 'suburban' neighbourhoods for British officials and Anglicised Indians. The Lucknow of the 1930s was a rich mix of diverse cultures, religions and political groups. Hindus spoke Hindi, Muslims spoke Urdu, and almost no one outside of the government, the university, and the Indian ruling classes spoke English. Although Muslims were distinctly in the minority, they continued to control the major political and many of the cultural institutions, and their architecture was highly visible. As Griffin wrote to Mahony, 'graceful bulbous domes are everywhere ... in fact, domes and minarets play the same part in the landscape around here that "eggs and darts" play in Renaissance buildings'.[8]

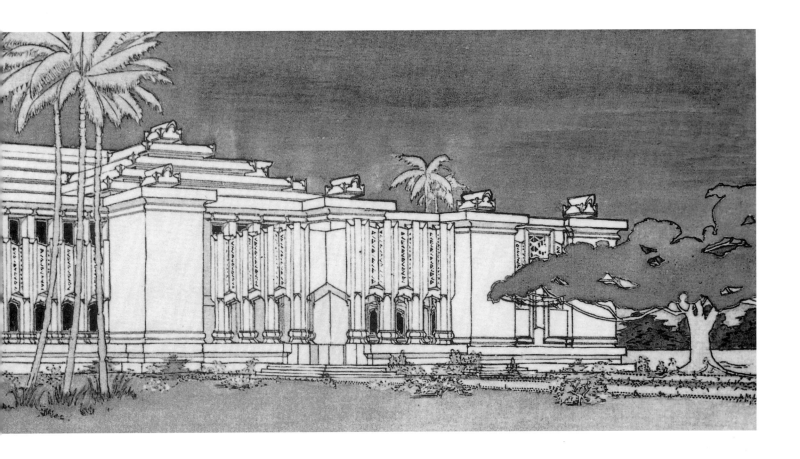

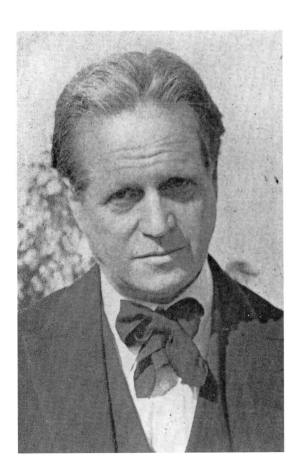

Above: Griffin designed the first version of the Lucknow University Library in mid 1935 while still in Sydney. This rendered perspective, now lost, was drawn by Eric and Molly Nicholls in the style of Marion Mahony Griffin. Photograph courtesy Nicholls collection, Sydney.

Left: The last known photograph of the architect, this portrait was published by Griffin's client, the Raja of Mahmudabad, in *Indian Wild Life*, vol 1, no 5, 1936, opp p 181.

Previous page: Mahony prepared this unusual elevation drawing of the United Provinces Industrial and Agricultural Exhibition in July 1936 to convince the fair's organisers of the power and beauty of Griffin's buildings. It shows both the Electricity Tower (left) and the Postal Tower (right), looking south along the Industrial Axis from the amusement area. Ink and watercolour on linen, 51 × 148.4 cm. Courtesy Avery Architectural and Fine Arts Library, Columbia University, New York, (1000.015.00094).

Following pages: Jwala Bank, Jhansi, India, 1936, Marion Mahony Griffin, delineator. Ink and watercolour on paper, 52.8 × 77.8 cm. Courtesy Avery Architectural and Fine Arts Library, Columbia University, New York (1000.015.00064).

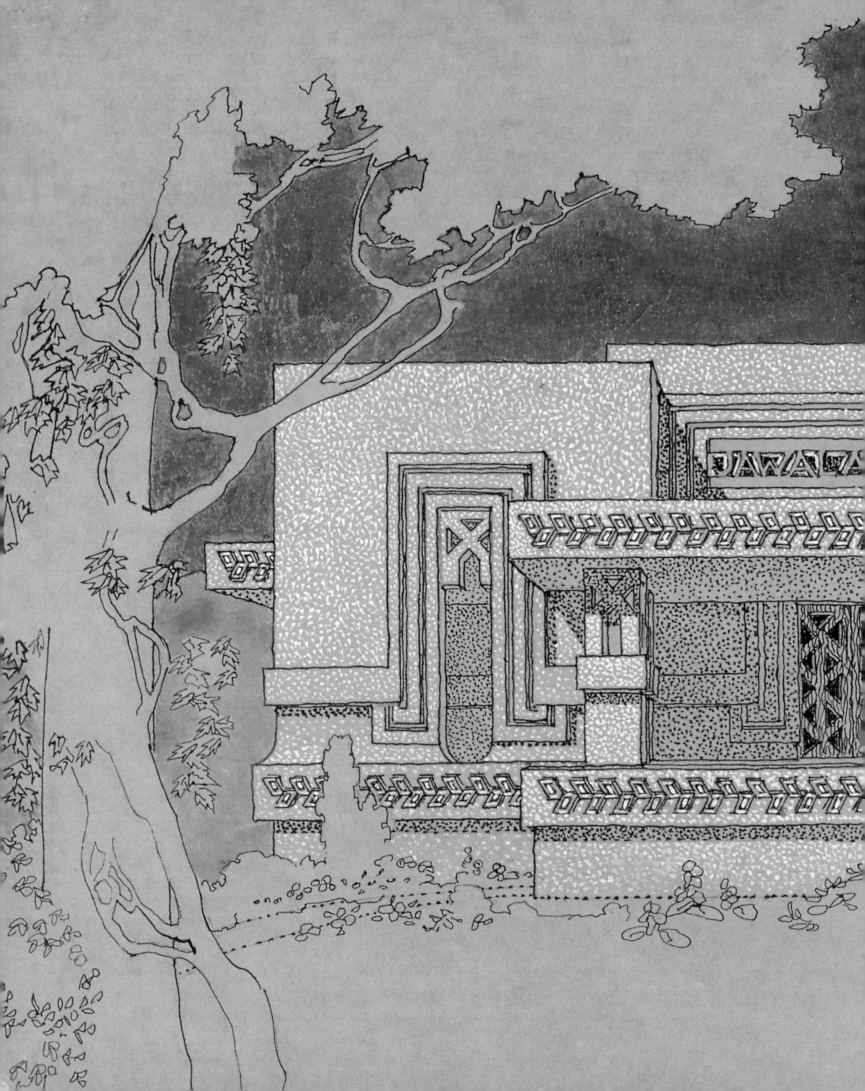

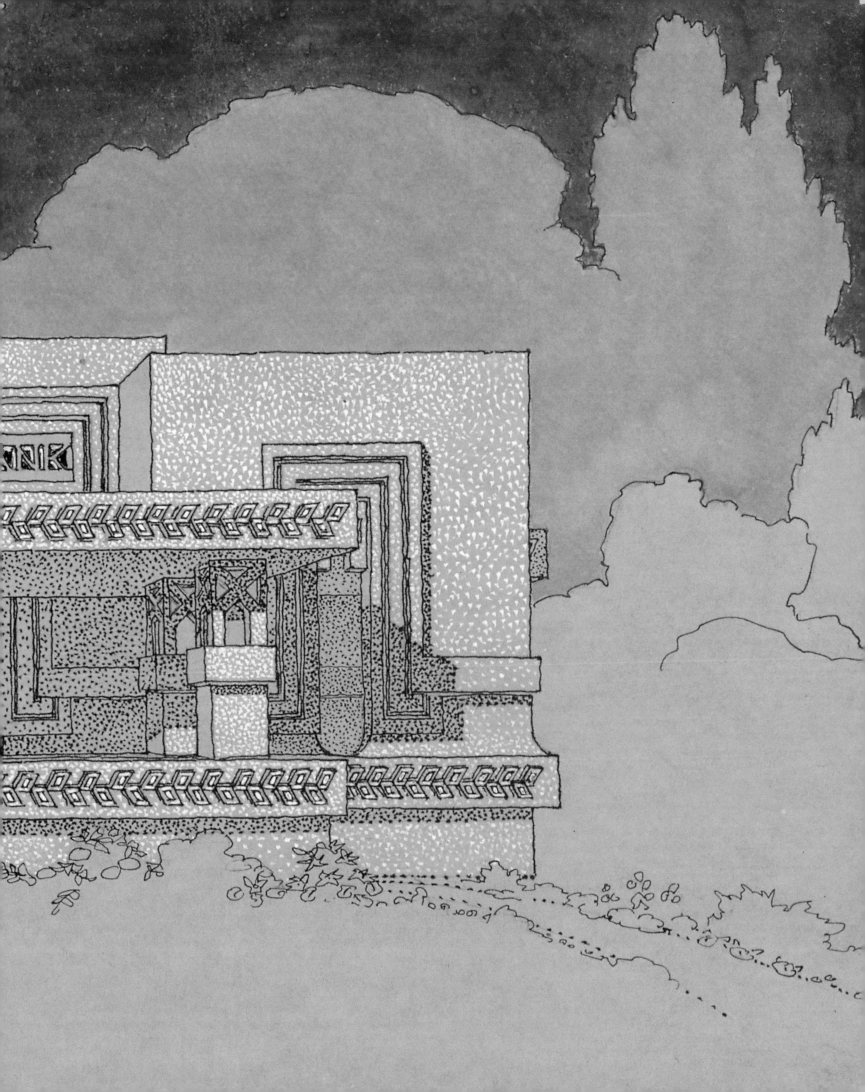

Much of this diversity was not immediately obvious, even to a visitor open to every new stimulus and sensation. For example, Griffin persisted in using a dome for a bank for a Hindu client, despite resistance from his contractor, Alagappan, until the latter told him, 'Hindus do not use domes, which are the prerogative of the Mohammedans'.[9] Yet Muslim and Hindu cultures could be unexpectedly mixed in Lucknow. The house for Griffin's client, Pirthi Nath Bhargava, a Hindu of the Brahman class, was to include a *zenana*, the quarters where elite women spent their lives in *purda*. Traditionally associated with Islamic practice, *purda* was part of Indian culture for both Muslim and Hindu families. Religious life was similarly subject to fine distinctions, not immediately apparent to a western outsider. Griffin's two clients who were Muslim leaders came from different Islamic sects: the Raja of Mahmudabad was a Shiite, while the Raja of Jahangirabad was a Sunni. These complicated affairs, however, were not troubling to Griffin; he seems to have enjoyed attempting to understand them. By the end of December, he was ready to tell his father, 'I am comfortable here and find endless source of interest in the environment of an ancient civilization'.[10] Indeed, Griffin the anthroposophist felt so at home in Lucknow that he had already decided that he belonged by right in India, that he may have spent a previous life there and certainly wished to return in a future life. 'As to my next incarnation, I cannot think of anything better in this poor old world than the job I am now on, though I fear the fixed star of my entelechy did not indicate that. My physical appearance does not suggest much of the Indian, but I have a hunch that much of my architectural predilections must have come from Indian experience.'[11]

Practising architecture there, however, was a different matter. Given a room in the Physics buildings of Lucknow University to use as an office, Griffin discovered to his dismay that officials had changed the proposed library site and wanted him to redesign the building. He encountered the first of what became an endless series of bureaucratic delays. As he worked to convince the building committee and its truculent chair of his point of view — even creating a new campus development plan — he was introduced to prominent academics, administrators and trustees associated with the university, all of whom began to seek his advice about their various building projects, real or imagined. Professors, rajas, contractors, Muslims and Hindus, young and old, all fell under his spell. He confessed to Ula Maddocks, 'It is a great relief to feel that there is a demand for such abilities as I have, which are of a kind foreign to Australia's requirements as the generality of them see things'.[12] Without hesitation — alone, and with neither a staff, nor a network of builders and suppliers — he set aside the three-month deadline and went to work.

Griffin's first building designed wholly in India — the addition of a *zenana* to the palace of the Raja of Jahangirabad — was in every way outside of his personal experience. The client, the building type, the way decisions were made and work undertaken — all were very new to

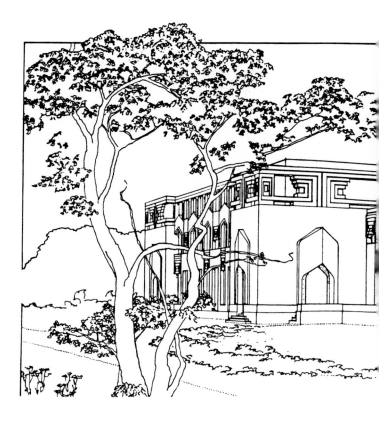

him. Timing itself became an issue: 'I am rushing the drawings because the Raja finds on consulting his almanac that Saturday of this week, the last of the lunar month, will be the most auspicious day for a long while to start my work'.[13] During that Saturday, he also discovered that there were 'unlucky' numbers among his room dimensions that had to be 'corrected'. Yet by late morning his revised design was approved by the raja. Returning after lunch, Griffin found 'all the trenches for every room accurately set out with lime lines checked with diagonal measurements to the nearest half inch awaiting our approval! Then 50 men were set to incising all these lines and inbedding brickwork corner- and bench-marks, and soon after all the trenches were under full blast, with another 50 on-lookers, when the coconut sweets were distributed to all, as is the custom in starting works'.[14] Griffin was astonished to report further that the raja 'came around here again Monday afternoon for the ground story plan, as already, during Sunday, the trenching had been completed and the concreting started!' This experience led Griffin — this great democrat and 'Single-Taxer' — to a startling conclusion: 'Aristocracy has much to commend it, not the least of which is the will and the power to make decisions. How different from the fear of

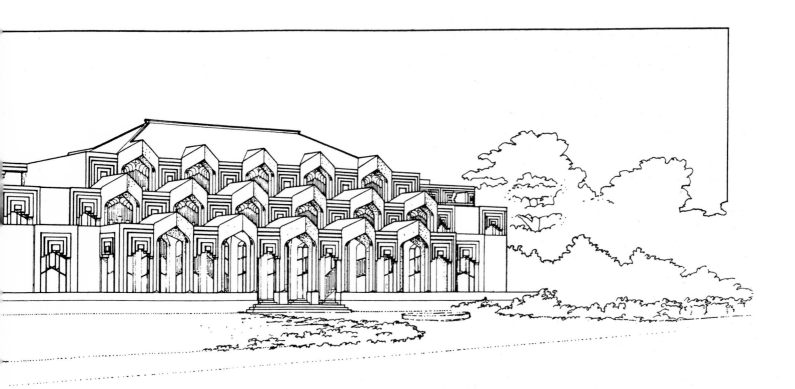

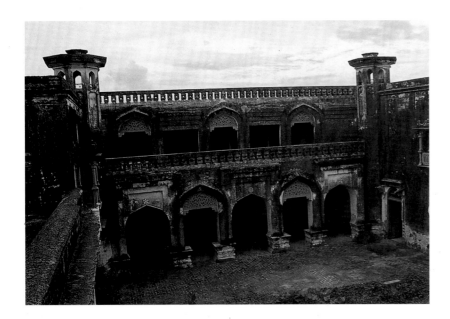

Above: Griffin and his contractor, Alagappan Mudalir, submitted this proposal for an addition to the municipal offices in Ahmadabad in January 1936. The public hall on the second level was entered directly from the main entrance through an elaborate divided stairway that was open to the outside but screened by the projecting porch on the ground floor. Because no perspective drawing of the complicated facade was prepared by Mahony, this sketch was created by Chicago architect Nathalie Belanger in 1997.

Left: In January 1936 Griffin designed a *zenana* addition to the rural palace of the Raja of Jahangirabad, which the delighted raja decided to build immediately, much to the architect's amazement. In 1974 James Weirick took this photograph of the abandoned building in a ruinous state. Courtesy Weirick collection, Sydney.

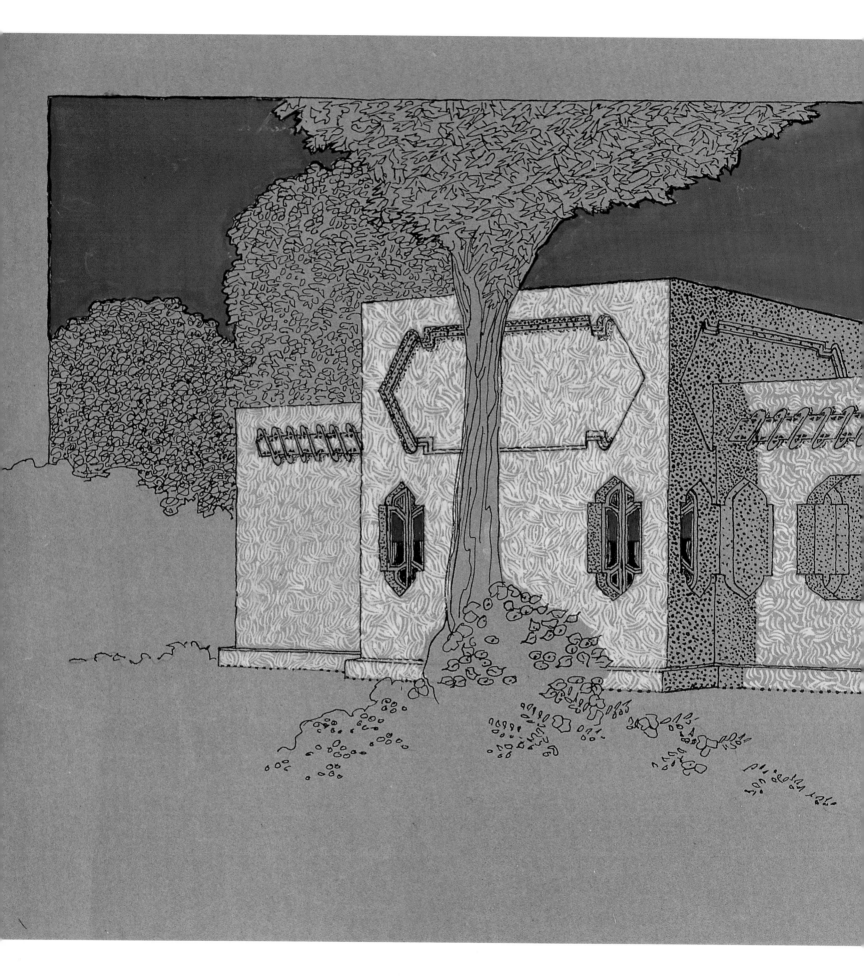

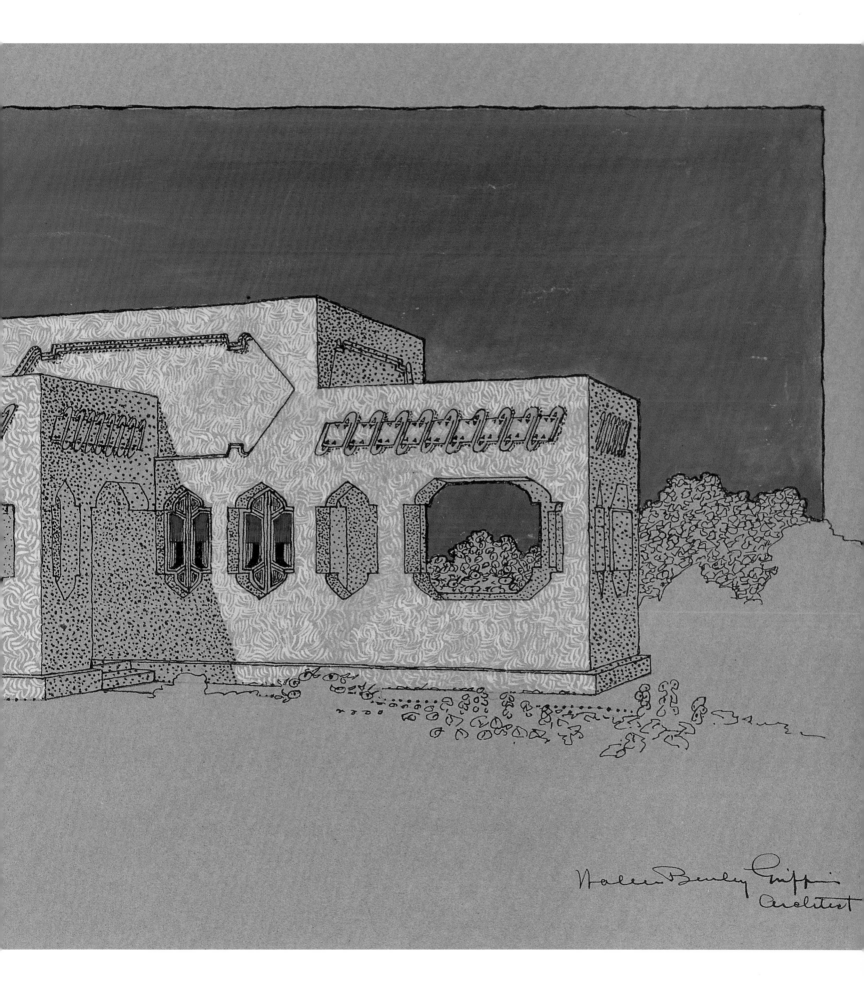

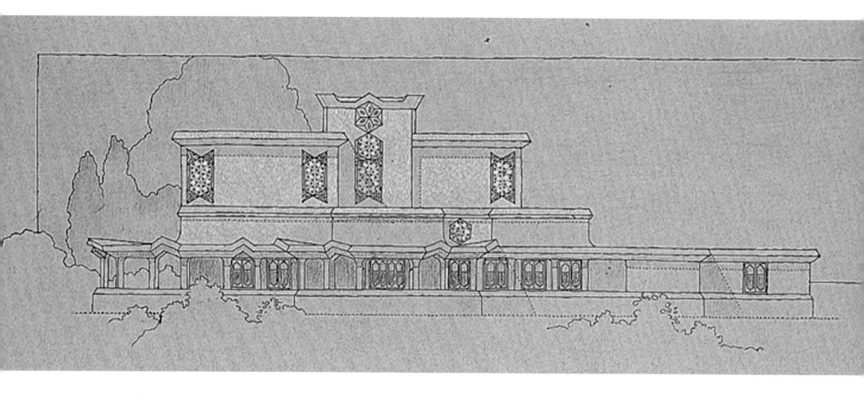

Above: In April 1936 Griffin reported to Mahony that Dr Birbal Sahni, a prominent figure at Lucknow University, was pleased with his new plans and elevations, but was too busy to authorise completion of the specifications. Although Sahni did not build the house, Mahony drew this elevation the following year. Griffin's design provided for a continuous verandah wrapped around its generous 432 square metres (4800 square feet). While the hexagonal window decorations reveal Griffin experimenting with new ornamental figures, the raised projections on the verandah harken back to the last designs of his American years. Detail, ink, gouache and coloured pencil on paper. Courtesy Avery Architectural and Fine Arts Library, Columbia University, New York (1000.018.00032).

Previous page: This small speculative house of staggered interlocking cubes of two different sizes was designed for Narain Singh in November 1936 and built in Benares. In Mahony's rendering it stands before a startling red sky. Ink and gouache on paper, 55.9 x 72 cm. Courtesy Avery Architectural and Fine Arts Library, Columbia University, New York, (1000.015.00033).

criticism, the subservience, the rationalization and inhibitions and paralysis that characterizes the sordid modern world'.

With the *zenana* for the Raja of Jahangirabad, Griffin's Indian career had begun in earnest, even with the university library job completely stalled. Griffin prepared plans for an addition to the municipal offices of the west Indian city of Ahmadabad, and for a new student union at Lucknow University. Unfortunately, neither project was built. But Griffin had better luck with faculty members. By April he could report, 'I am engaged with the third Professor's house sketches and have inspected the site for a fourth'.[15] Among the academics who came to him for help, four commissioned houses from Griffin that survive as fully conceived designs, two of which were built. Dr Birbal Sahni, for whom Griffin designed a house in April, was a noted botanist and palaeontologist. Dr Bir Bhan Bhatia's fields were pharmacology and medicine; as a physician he also maintained a private practice in the house Griffin built for him. Griffin built a verandah at Dr Sahni's house, and provided Dr Bhatia with a large *chabutra*, a kind of paved patio that was usually raised. The house for Dr Mathur, who taught physics, also sported covered verandahs around an open *chabutra*. Later in the year, Griffin designed a dwelling for a fourth faculty member, the mathematician Narain Singh. The small house bearing Singh's name, was built in Benares as an investment.

Despite the promise of these domestic commissions, the turning point in Griffin's decision to stay in India came in mid March 1936 when he was invited to prepare a scheme for a major trade fair in Lucknow that was planned for the autumn: the United Provinces Industrial and Agricultural Exhibition, to be built in Victoria Park between the *chauk* and the Gumti River. The project was to involve dozens of pavilions and scores of display booths, an amusement district, restaurants, and two large towers. His imagination ablaze, Griffin prepared a site plan for the exhibition that organised the rambling park into two powerful axes and a central circle and part of an oval.[16] The United Provinces exhibition was Griffin's last venture in town planning. Although meant to be a temporary fair, the project elicited a design of great significance to Griffin, for which he prepared an analytical program nearly as detailed as he had for Canberra almost 25 years earlier. And he created dozens of new buildings for the plan.[17]

Marion Mahony Griffin arrived in India on 30 May 1936, and helped Griffin to complete this vast enterprise on time. Although Walter had been hinting for Marion to join him since February, in April he had put enormous pressure on her until she agreed to help with the drafting. Marion had not participated in the design of the Indian buildings before her arrival, by which time almost half of the Indian saga was over, and the evidence suggests that the remaining Indian designs were also substantially Walter's. However, her appearance marked a sea-change in the workings of the Lucknow office. Forcing Marion out of her virtual retirement from architecture, Griffin also inspired her to new heights of visual expression in the renderings she created to show his new work.[18]

Among the residential and institutional buildings created by Griffin in India is a single civic monument: a memorial to King George V, who had died in 1936. It is also the design most obviously linked to British imperialism. Griffin's one British client, Desmond Young, was the conduit for several of his most important commissions, including the United Provinces exhibition. Young, who was publisher of the *Pioneer*, the largest English language newspaper in northern India, had come to India five years before to revive the moribund newspaper, founded in 1865 and famous for such past luminaries on its staff as Rudyard Kipling. By April 1936 Griffin and Young were talking about a new building. As Young recalled, 'It was both a pleasure and an education to discuss the plans' with Griffin.[19] By the following November, Griffin had conceived of the building in three sections: two office towers flanking the central printing plant. Unlike so many of Griffin's other clients, Young did Griffin the honour and courtesy of constructing the building in general accordance with the architect's plans. The city of Lucknow was less understanding when it permitted Griffin's most completely realised Indian design to be demolished in 1991.

In Lucknow Griffin befriended two influential rajas. Both were landholders with country estates in addition to their Lucknow palaces. The Raja of Jahangirabad, who had commissioned Griffin's first Indian building, arranged for Griffin to meet the young Raja of Mahmudabad to discuss the design of a library and museum for the raja's collection of rare Islamic books and manuscripts. In the Raja of Mahmudabad, almost 40 years his junior, Griffin found a true friend and the raja found a westerner he could honestly admire.

Perhaps the strongest bond between architect and raja was a mutual interest in the preservation of wildlife and its habitat. In July 1936, the raja launched a new magazine, *Indian Wild Life*.[20] As the magazine's patron, the raja commissioned a special building for the United Provinces exhibition from Griffin. Unfortunately, the design was a casualty of the fair's misfortunes. Griffin's most important commission from the raja was the library and museum for his book collection. In September 1936, Griffin visited the estate at Mahmudabad, where he was offered three possible building sites and selected the one 'just outside the moat and overlooking a long reach of it', as he recalled.[21] And so the library evocatively stands, captured in Mahony's perspective drawing. What the future would have held for this blossoming friendship between Walter and his most important Indian client cannot be answered, for the architect died four days after Marion presented the young raja with her breathtaking rendering, the only tangible evidence that survives of the design.

On Friday, 5 February 1937, Griffin complained of stomach cramps, of the kind he had first reported the previous October. On Saturday he was found to have a ruptured gall bladder, for which he was operated at King George Hospital in the medical complex overlooking the exhibition grounds.[22] Marion sat by Walter's bed through the night and was there when he awoke from the operation at five o'clock on Sunday morning. She visited her husband daily during the week and by Wednesday was expecting a full recovery — 'everything seemed to be going so well', as she later recalled.[23] In fact, peritonitis had set in; in a few short hours the infection overwhelmed Walter's weakened body. Marion recounted the final day, 11 February, to Ula Maddocks:

> As the end drew near, I talked to him, telling him what a wonderful life I had with him, how he was beloved by everybody; and suddenly he turned, as if with a great effort, and looked straight in my eyes, his own wide, startled, as if it had never occurred to him that he could die. His eyes never left mine till he drew his last breath and I closed them … He didn't want to go. Things were pouring in on him and he was happy.[24]

A plot was quickly found in one of the Christian cemeteries and Griffin's body was buried in an unmarked grave.[25]

'Walter B. Griffin is no more!' lamented the Raja of Mahmudabad in *Indian Wild Life*.[26] 'Blessed with noble vision, lofty ideals, unassuming personality and simple habits — he was a saint.' Desmond Young eulogised his architect, 'With great charm of character, and fund of humour and good spirits, he was so entirely and so obviously selfless that there was something almost saintly about him'.[27] Thus were the perceptions of a Muslim raja and a British colonial united in their appraisal of the Australian architect, landscape architect and town planner from Chicago.

Marion, numbed with grief, but also in turn bitterly disappointed by Walter's death and quietly accepting of it as anthroposophically inevitable, stayed in Lucknow for perhaps two more months to complete what was essential.

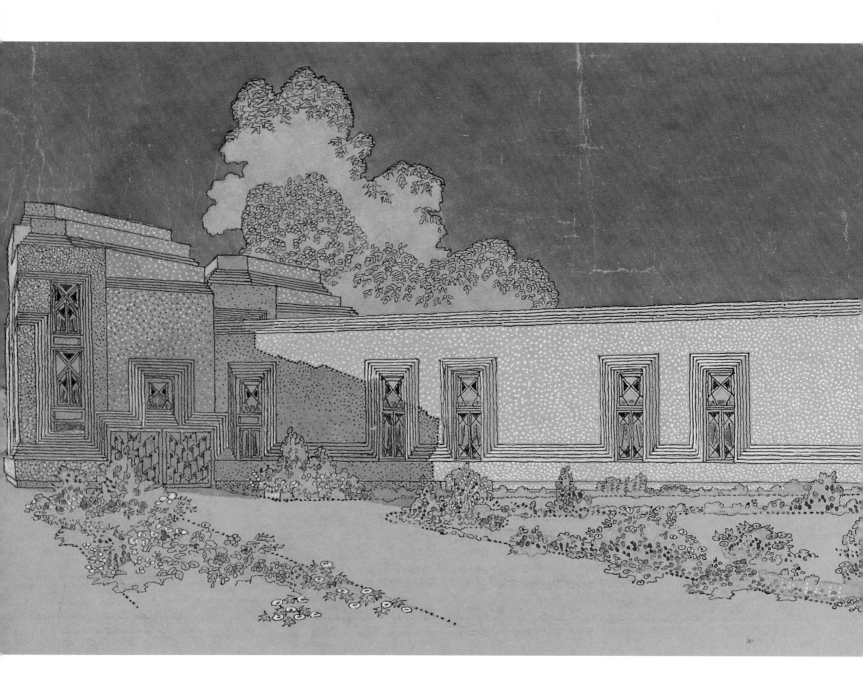

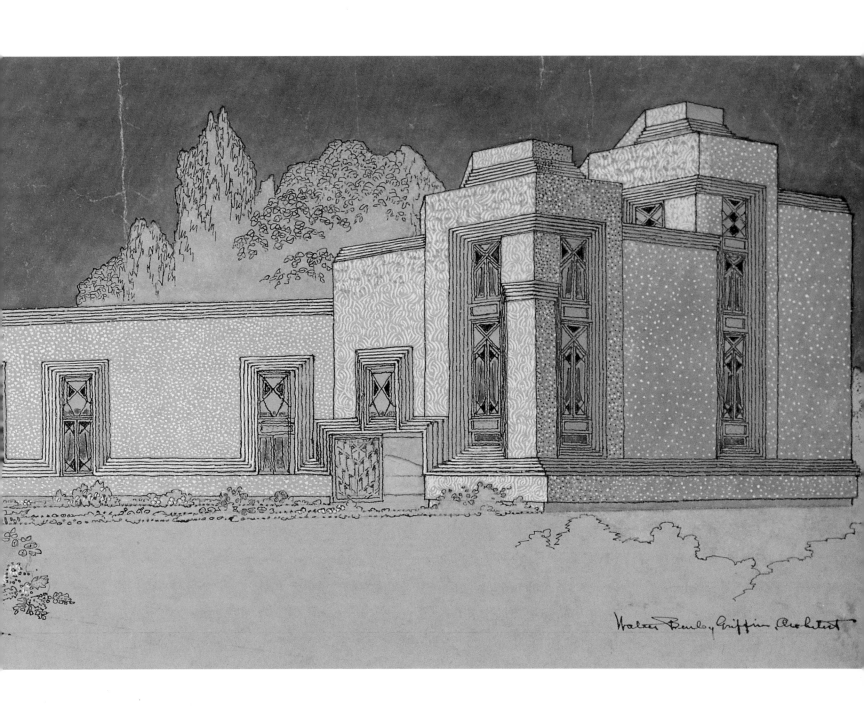

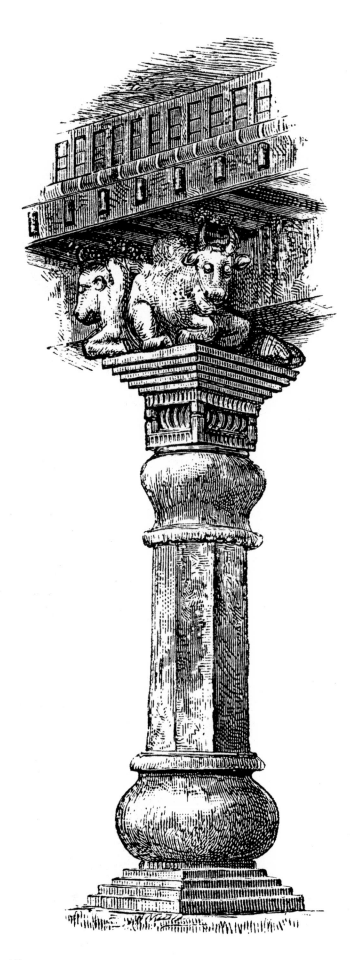

When it was clear that no one from the Australian office would join her in India, she returned to Castlecrag. Within a year, she had moved to Chicago where she valiantly if futilely fought for the next twenty years to keep the memory alive of the blazing Indian sunset to the careers of these two remarkable American architects.

The moving story of the Griffins' Indian episode leaves unanswered the questions of just why the buildings look the way they do and how we are meant to respond to them. The contexts for this work are at once Griffin's approach to a universal modernism and his response to a specific environment. The creative challenge posed for him was to produce designs that were a synthesis of the two positions. Griffin's first response to India was to unite them. A month after his arrival, he stated categorically, 'In the buildings of all sorts, I recognize most of the "motifs" I have used or even thought of in my lifetime of [the] practice of architecture'.[28] To his evident pleasure, Griffin found in India a vernacular landscape that 'is certainly for me the earthly paradise of flat roofs and not those factory-like "modernist" introductions but rich and imaginative ones, where the masses are composed and the wall finished with modeled and per-forated copings and balustrades'.[29] He could be describing his own William F Tempel house of 1911 (see p 29), or the house he would design later in the year for Narain Singh.

Secondly, he imagined the possibility of applying native solutions to a modern but localised architecture. These included attempts to adapt vernacular construction techniques, such as bent bamboo with plaster infill, to the buildings for the United Provinces exhibition. They also included less tangible responses. Early in his travels, Griffin declared to Ronald Craig that the caves at Elephanta near Bombay were not aesthetically complete but rather were 'something that contained many of the rudiments of good architecture'.[30] Clearly such 'rudiments' could become the foundations of a Griffinesque form of modern Indian architecture, if wedded to his established practices.

Griffin discussed the problem of creating a modern Indian architecture in an essay, 'Architecture in India', published the month before he died.[31] Here he cited two unfortunate developments: 'a loss of feeling for design' among native builders; and 'a hankering after stark, logical, European modernism'. Griffin called for architects to reject the International style and to produce modern buildings that satisfied the real needs of the age. He cautioned that this new architecture should not be too localised: 'the spirit of the times rather than of the localities finds consciousness in these days of world-wide contacts'. Yet he argued that architects must strike a balance between universal modernity and the particular context: 'the stamp of the place is an essential element of each architectural problem and any building … that is unsympathetic with its natural, human-natural and artificial environment is neutralised and vitiated thereby'. Griffin was asking for a great deal: creating an architecture that fulfilled the charges to reflect the 'spirit of the times' and yet reveal the 'stamp of the place' would

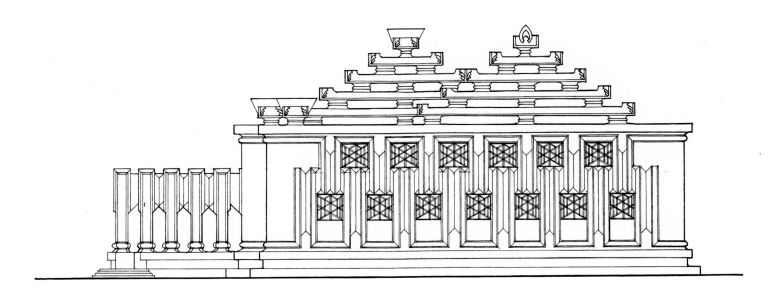

require an extraordinary imagination coupled with enormous energy.

Griffin had grappled with the issue of an appropriate Indian style in the Lucknow University Library — his first building designed for India, but created before he left Australia. Marion reported to her sister that Walter's design 'looks and feels quite Indian and yet is the last word in modernism'.[32] But of what exactly do the two elements — 'Indian' and 'modern' — consist? The library is dominated by six massive pier-like pilasters, a Griffinesque feature that appears on such American buildings as the F P Marshall house (1910) (*see p 30*). However, the bases of the columns of the projecting porch, set on a series of three rectilinear base courses, are moulded in a most unusual manner for Griffin. Before 1935 Griffin rarely used curving forms of any kind in his architecture; but here the column begins with an upward curve, then bulges out to form a flattened sphere before rising. In fact, this detail apparently is based on an ancient Buddhist column-type dating from the first century.[33] Yet Griffin does not literally 'quote' the column in a historical sense. It becomes a building block for the design of the exterior walls. He uses the form as a moulding to articulate the base of the entire building, mirrored at the top of the pylons as a cornice moulding, and used to frame the large, off-set windows lighting all sides of the building in a complex alternating rhythm. This single example of the application of historical precedent suggests the ways in which Mahony — and Griffin — could claim that the first version of the Lucknow University Library was both Indian and 'modern', that is, a part of Griffin's personal style.

Taken as a whole, Griffin's Indian designs share one or more general characteristics. Most striking, perhaps, is the complex surface treatment. Sometimes this takes the form of an exuberant ornament, while the surfaces of other designs

Above: East elevation of the first version of the Lucknow University Library, redrawn by Nathalie Belanger, Chicago, from the original working drawings.

Left: A column from a Buddhist rock cave at Nasik, northeast of Bombay, probably dating from the first century AD. From James Fergusson, *A history of Indian and Eastern architecture* (John Murray, London, 1891, p 150), a work known to Griffin since his student days at the University of Illinois and specifically mentioned in his Indian letters.

Previous pages: Griffin's design for the printing plant and offices of Lucknow's *Pioneer* newspaper, which was the only major building erected in India to his plans. Because the rectangular lot was set back from the main thoroughfare and was approached by a narrow access road, Griffin placed the building diagonally on the site with the two end towers aligned with the entrance drive, and provided circulation for delivery trucks through the building. In December 1936 the Viceroy of India set the building's cornerstone, and the newspaper published Mahony's perspective. Ink, crayon and watercolour on paper, 53.6 x 77.9 cm.
Courtesy Avery Architectural and Fine Arts Library, Columbia University, New York, (1000.015.00087).

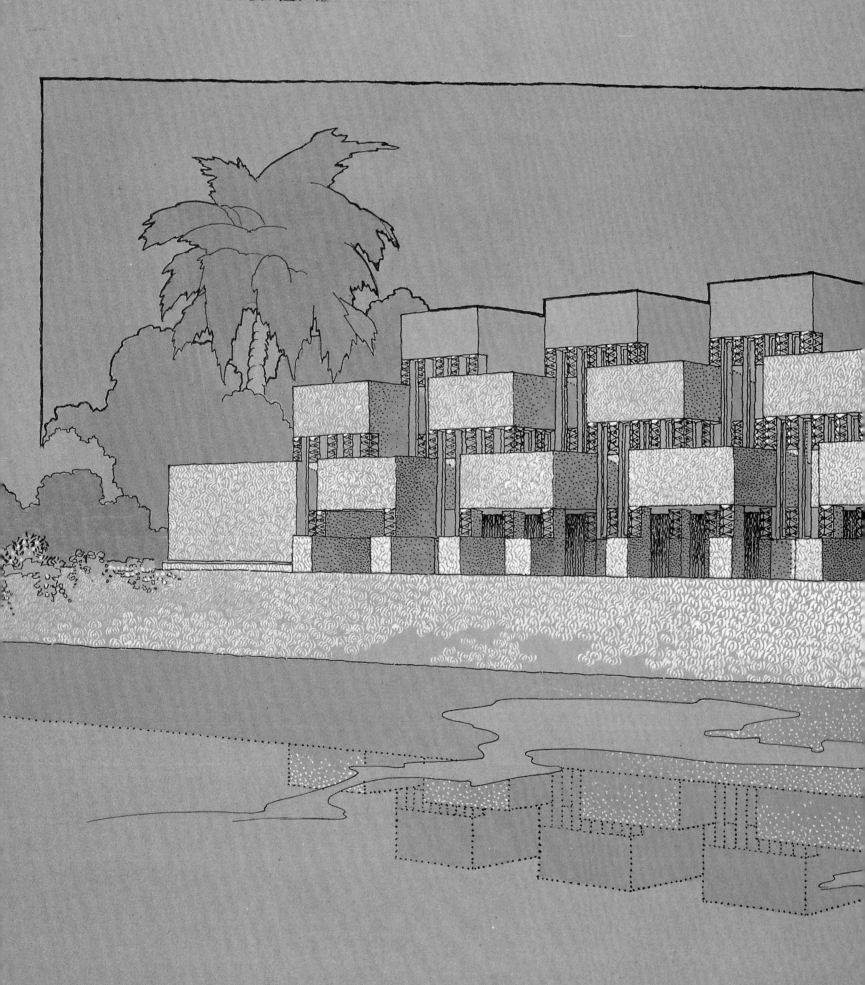

LIBRARY and MUSEUM
RAJA MAHMUDABAD

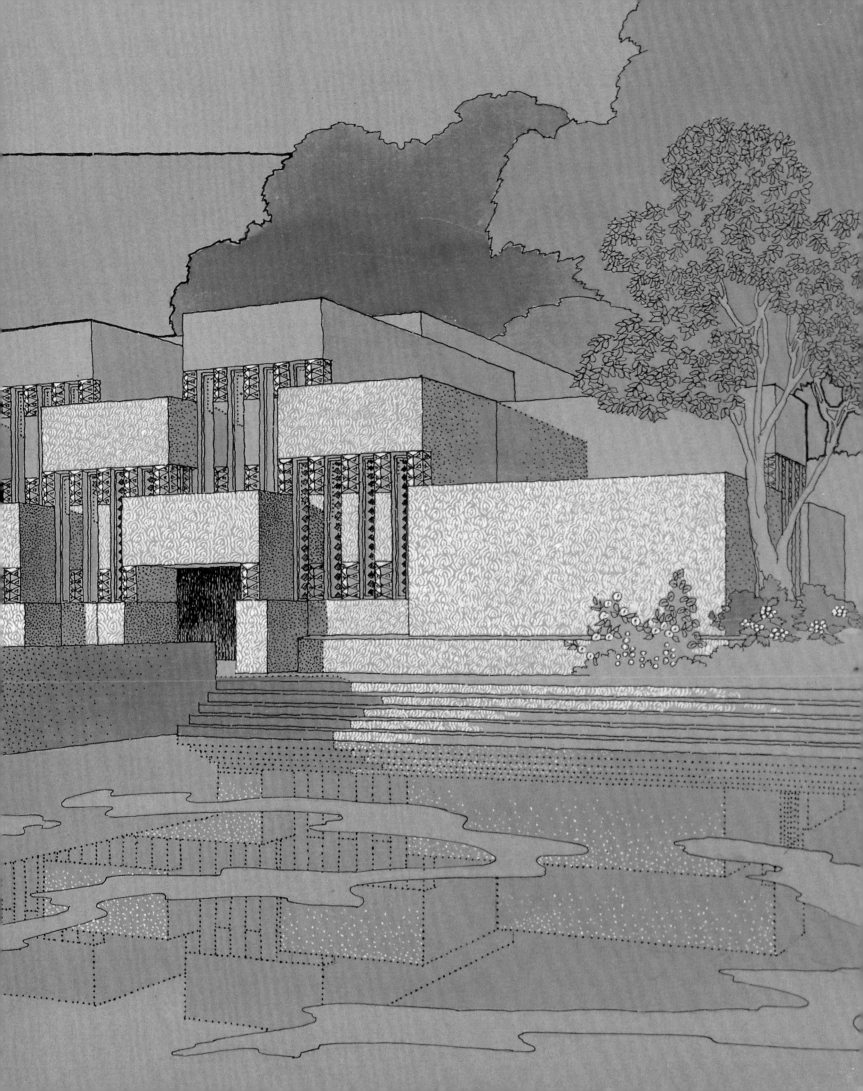

are covered by receding bands, found on the Pioneer Press building. The composition of several works — including the King George V memorial — is conceived, not as simple shapes detailed with clearly defined ornament, but as groups of repeated geometric solids that coalesce to form a complete structure. These characteristics — the generous use of ornament and the sculptural conception of a building — may strike us as essentially 'Indian'; yet neither is new in Griffin's work, and their expression in India, whatever it reveals about Griffin's intentions, reflects tendencies that were developing in his designs over the previous two decades.

Many of the Indian buildings, including the King George V memorial, have centralised plans. Perhaps this is a local response. Such plans are rare in Griffin's earlier work, the few examples including the Clark Memorial Fountain at Grinnell, Iowa, and the proposed garden plan for the Joshua Melson house in Mason City, Iowa. However, they are common in historic Indian architecture, even appearing in the interior temple of the great cave at Elephanta visited by Griffin.

Finally, the single most common feature found in Griffin's Indian designs that is new in his work is the pointed arch with flat haunches rising from curved springers — the so-called Mughal arch. Absent from western architecture, it is a ubiquitous motif of north Indian architecture. And it is everywhere in Griffin's first Indian designs, dominating the facade of the Ahmadabad municipal offices and many of the pavilions of the United Provinces exhibition. It is even employed as slightly projecting gables of the three levels of the exhibition's Postal Tower.

We can seek to understand Griffin's Indian buildings by dividing them into three chronological phases: designs conceived in winter and spring 1936; those created in the summer and autumn destined for the United Provinces exhibition; and the final buildings designed in autumn 1936 and winter 1937. In Griffin's first buildings designed wholly in India — the *zenana* and the Ahmadabad municipal offices — he experimented with stylistic elements found locally and attempted to incorporate them into his own style. The project for Ahmadabad presented him with the opportunity to review his thoughts about an appropriate language of Indian modernism — to design a major public building that 'looks and feels quite Indian and yet is the last word in modernism', to repeat Mahony's words. Consciously seeking a design to be 'worthy of the architectural traditions of boldness, taste and skill that constitute the basis of this town',[34] Griffin created a complex composition of balconies, covered verandahs, uncovered *chabutras*, and screened walkways. The walls are articulated with receding and projecting bands. Here is a modern edifice that feels strongly related to India's past of decorated, arched public buildings.

Yet the particular vocabulary is not really Indian. The bands, apart from the complex, repeating surface pattern they produce over the facade, are not actually Indian. If anything, the effect more nearly suggests designs of the Austrian secessionists Otto Wagner and Josef Hoffmann than the Taj Mahal or mosques in Lucknow. In fact, they are closest to Griffin's own previous work, from the entrance to the Cafe

Australia, built in Melbourne in 1916, to his submission to the Chicago Tribune Tower competition of 1921.

Similarly, the projecting gable hoods that dominate the composition at Ahmadabad, which seem to come directly from Mughal architecture, signal this as 'Indian modern' as does no other single feature. Actual Mughal arches, however, are almost always heavily ornamented with incised patterns; Griffin's are without applied ornament. Most importantly, Mughal arches are never developed as plastic forms in three dimensions. The expression of the arch as a gable is purely an invention of Griffin's. As with the banding, we can find expressive projecting gables in Griffin's earlier work, such as Newman College in Melbourne (1915–1918). Finally, the decorated, sculptural massing of the whole building has nothing particularly to do with Indian architecture, but prototypes can be found in Griffin's work before his arrival in India, dating as far back as his own house for Trier Center of 1912. Yet the relationships at the municipal offices between solid and void, wall and ornament, angle and curve, are strikingly new in Griffin's work.

An approach to design has emerged. At the Ahmadabad municipal offices, Griffin used the general tendency in Indian architecture, whether Hindu or Muslim, to break up surfaces with elaborate decoration, and he employed a common historical motif, the Mughal arch, to create an 'original' modern form that is also consistent with his own earlier buildings.

Following these first designs, Griffin provided a public expression of his aspirations for a readable Indian modernism for the United Provinces exhibition. The designs show a remarkable diversity of form and decoration at the same time that they are subordinated to the master plan. Some of them, including the numerous rotundas, draw their inspiration from Muslim domes or Buddhist stupas. Others consist of purely geometric creations; for example, the photography pavilion is hexagonal, while the administrative office is simply a cube whose layered surfaces recede in bands. The Postal and Electricity towers, as signposts without practical functions, perhaps reveal Griffin's additive approach — universal Indian references integrated with a personal vocabulary of form — most clearly of all. The contrasting compositions are both based on the Mughal arch, easily recognised and prominently displayed. In the Postal Tower it is expressed as a projecting gable, while it appears in the Electricity Tower, in an original and unorthodox way, as the termination of the tower itself. The shapes of the two towers, in contrast, are anything but clear and comprehensible. Each has a centralised plan that generates complex forms in three dimensions by rotated squares and squares-in-circles as it rises through the many levels. Although these complex plans suggest a new esoteric, perhaps theosophical, symbolism, they are a private, not a public, response to India.

The buildings designed after the United Provinces exhibition between October 1936 and February 1937 form the aesthetic culmination of the Indian venture. The group includes three public designs — the Pioneer Press, the library for the Raja of Mahmudabad, and the King George V memorial — and a handful of houses[35] that constitute a new phase in Griffin's Indian work, and present us with what must be termed his mature Indian style. None is overtly 'Indian' in the manner of the exhibition's pavilions and booths. For example, none of them is domed or has the Griffinesque Mughal arch. All are rectilinear. Gone are the great swathes of vibrant ornament that are characteristic of the Indian work until now. For example, the alternating projecting gables of the early Ahmadabad municipal building nine months later have become the stately, planar reading spaces at the raja's library. In these sculptural compositions mass and decoration are one and the same. All are variations on the theme of the fragmented wall, produced by projecting and receding masses or similarly stepped bands that dissolve individual forms. Griffin integrated the banding most perfectly in the conception of the wall of the Pioneer Press building, where they articulate the corners, mark the towers and define the entrances.

These last buildings show a tendency toward the most elemental building blocks of architecture, on the one hand, and a cutting away of that simplicity, on the other, to create layering of form, which culminates in the interlocked geometry of the King George V memorial. At the Singh house, these alternating forms become large and small cubes. The six cubes are arranged as two sets of three, each set a large cube flanked by smaller ones. The two sets are placed side by side, but shifted by one cube, to make a six-room house of great versatility, a house type that can easily be imagined as a prototype for a large-scale development. The simple scheme provides both roof terrace and verandah. The result is at once modern, Griffinesque, and Indian — adapted to local conditions and responding to local traditions.

By Griffin's own measure, he had created a modern Indian architecture whose forms were consistent with his life's work yet were characteristic of their cultural settings. He had experimented with new construction techniques and responded to new sources of visual inspiration. After their initial appearance, these had become less explicit and more integrated into his established style. Griffin's architectural language was so rich that, with the support of Marion Mahony Griffin coupled with his faith in the anthroposophical rightness of his Indian endeavour, he was able to expand his aesthetic vocabulary to create an exuberant, expressive architecture reflecting both the 'stamp of the place' and the 'spirit of the times'.

Previous pages: The culmination of the Griffins' work in India, the library and museum for the Raja of Mahmudabad, were designed by Walter in the first week of February 1937 and drawn by Marion the following week as Walter lay dying. 'The staggered and set back cubes', in Paul Sprague's words, 'provide a powerful image of scholarly detachment and quietude in a subdued yet monumental composition, a place where readers, withdrawn from the world and protected from it by both a moat and elegant ornamental screens, can reflect upon the inner truths provided by the books and artifacts housed within'. Ink and watercolour on paper, 55.8 x 79 cm. Courtesy Avery Architectural and Fine Arts Library, Columbia University, New York, (1000.015.00088).

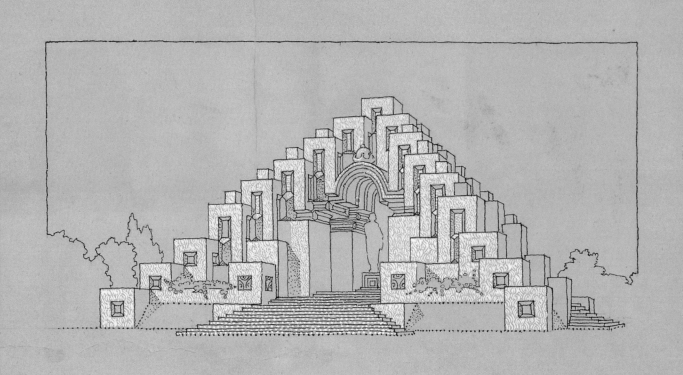

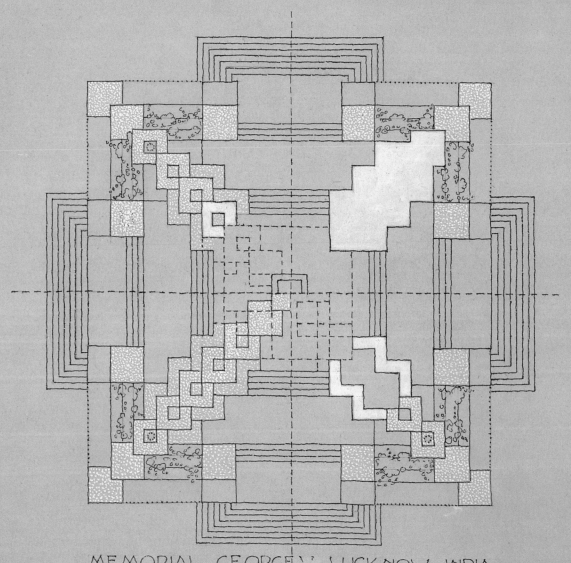

MEMORIAL GEORGE V LUCKNOW INDIA
MR CHOWDHRAY SCULPTOR
WALTER BURLEY GRIFFIN ARCHITECT

Notes

1. For a more thorough examination of the issues raised here, see Paul Kruty and Paul E Sprague, *Two American architects in India, Walter B. Griffin and Marion M. Griffin, 1935–1937*, University of Illinois, School of Architecture, Champaign, Illinois, 1997. The present essay is adapted from my three chapters in this book.

2. The major source of information about the Griffins in India is preserved in the first book of 'The magic of America'. Subtitled 'An American architect's year in India', this is primarily an exchange of letters between Walter and Marion, with additional letters to Ula Maddocks, Eric Nicholls, George W Griffin (Walter's father), Georgene M Smith (Marion's sister), and several explanatory passages written by Marion. References to particular letters will take the following form: 'WBG to MMG, 6 February 1936, 'Magic', vol I, 75a', meaning: Walter to Marion, date on letter, 'The magic of America', volume 1, page 75a (as marked in the lower right-hand corner of the copy in the New York Historical Society Library). The principal collections of Indian drawings are preserved in the Avery Architectural and Fine Arts Library, Columbia University, New York, and the Art Institute of Chicago.

3. MMG to Georgene M Smith, 8 October 1935, 'Magic', vol 1, p 10a.

4. WBG to MMG, 8 November 1935, 'Magic', vol 1, p 31.

5. WBG to MMG, 8 November 1935, 'Magic', vol 1, p 31.

6. WBG to MMG, 12 November 1935, 'Magic', vol 1, p 34a.

7. WBG to George W Griffin, 26 December 1935, 'Magic', vol 1, pp 59–60.

8. WBG to MMG, 20 November 1935, 'Magic', pp 38a–39.

9. WBG to MMG, 12 March 1936, 'Magic', vol 1, p 83.

10. WBG to George W Griffin, 26 December 1935, 'Magic', vol 1, p 58.

11. WBG to MMG, 11 December 1935, 'Magic', vol 1, p 44.

12. WBG to Ula Maddocks, 20 February 1936, 'Magic', vol 1, pp 76–77.

13. WBG to MMG, 30 January 1936, 'Magic', vol 1, p 66.

14. WBG to MMG, 30 January 1936, 'Magic', vol 1, p 70. The subsequent quotations are from this same letter.

15. WBG to MMG, 20 April 1936, 'Magic', vol 1, p 102a. For the revised date of the Lucknow University Union building, see Kruty and Sprague, *Two American architects in India*, pp 22, 77–78.

16. For a full description of the fair buildings, as well as a detailed plan of the grounds, see Paul E Sprague, 'The United Provinces Industrial and Agricultural Exhibition', pp 49–64, in Kruty and Sprague, *Two American architects*.

17. Griffin's program for the fair, 'United Provinces of Agra and Oudh, All India Exposition, Lucknow, India, General Plan', may be found in 'Magic', vol 1, pp 102d–115a. A copy of the illustrated brochure, *The U. P. Industrial & Agricultural Exhibition, Lucknow: Album*, Pioneer Press, Lucknow, 1936, survives in the Mitchell Library, Sydney.

18. The United Provinces exhibition itself, however, did not fare so well. A fierce monsoon and a tight budget delayed construction and compromised the architecture; yet the plan did follow Griffin's ideas (perhaps more closely than Canberra does) and, as a national trade fair, it was a solid success.

19. 'A Home to be proud of', *The Pioneer 75th anniversary supplement*, 15 March 1940, p 25.

20. So impressed was he with Griffin's ideas about the human use of land compatible to nature that he reprinted Griffin's recent essay, 'Occupational Conservation' (originally published in *Australian Wildlife*, vol 1, October 1935, pp 24–25), in his magazine, *Indian Wild Life*, vol 1, no 5, 1936, pp 181–85.

21. WBG to Ula Maddocks, 20 September 1936, 'Magic', vol 1, p 161a.

22. MMG to George W Griffin, 11 February 1937, Peisch collection, Avery Architectural and Fine Arts Library.

23. MMG to Ula Maddocks, 11 February 1937, 'Magic', vol 1, p 199a.

24. Ibid, p 200.

25. For an account of the rediscovery of the grave, see Graeme D Westlake, 'Walter Burley Griffin's Final Days in India', *Inland Architect*, vol 33, January/February 1989, pp 64–67.

26. 'Editorial notes', *Indian Wild Life*, vol 2, no 1, 1937, p 247.

27. *Pioneer*, 13 February 1937, p 3.

28. WBG to Clamyra [Marion's niece], 24 December 1935, 'Magic', vol 1, p 57.

29. WBG to Stella Miles Franklin, 25 November 1935; Miles Franklin papers, Mitchell Library, Sydney.

30. Ronald Craig to Ula Maddocks, 8 November 1935, 'Magic', vol 1, p 26.

31. Walter Burley Griffin, 'Architecture in India', *Pioneer*, vol 17, no 19, 9 January 1937.

32. MMG to Georgene M Smith, 8 October 1935, 'Magic', vol 1, p 10a.

33. Our illustration is taken from James Fergusson's *History of Indian and Eastern architecture* (1891), a work known to Griffin since his student days at the University of Illinois, and specifically mentioned in his Indian letters.

34. WBG to MMG, 6 February 1936, 'Magic', vol 1, p 74.

35. These include the remodellings for Pandit P N Bhargava and Begam M Raza, the Singh house, and the mansion for the Prince of Nepal near Benares.

Left: King George V memorial. The 1937 design, based on a 6-foot module presumably related to the statue's height of twelve feet, called for a pyramidal canopy of stacked rectangular solids to rise from its square base to a height of 14 metres (46 feet). Ink, pencil and watercolour on coloured paper, 63.5 × 50.8 cm.
Courtesy Avery Architectural and Fine Arts Library, Columbia University, New York (1000.018.00061).

PYRMONT INCINERATOR

AND ITS PRECEDENTS

PETER Y NAVARETTI

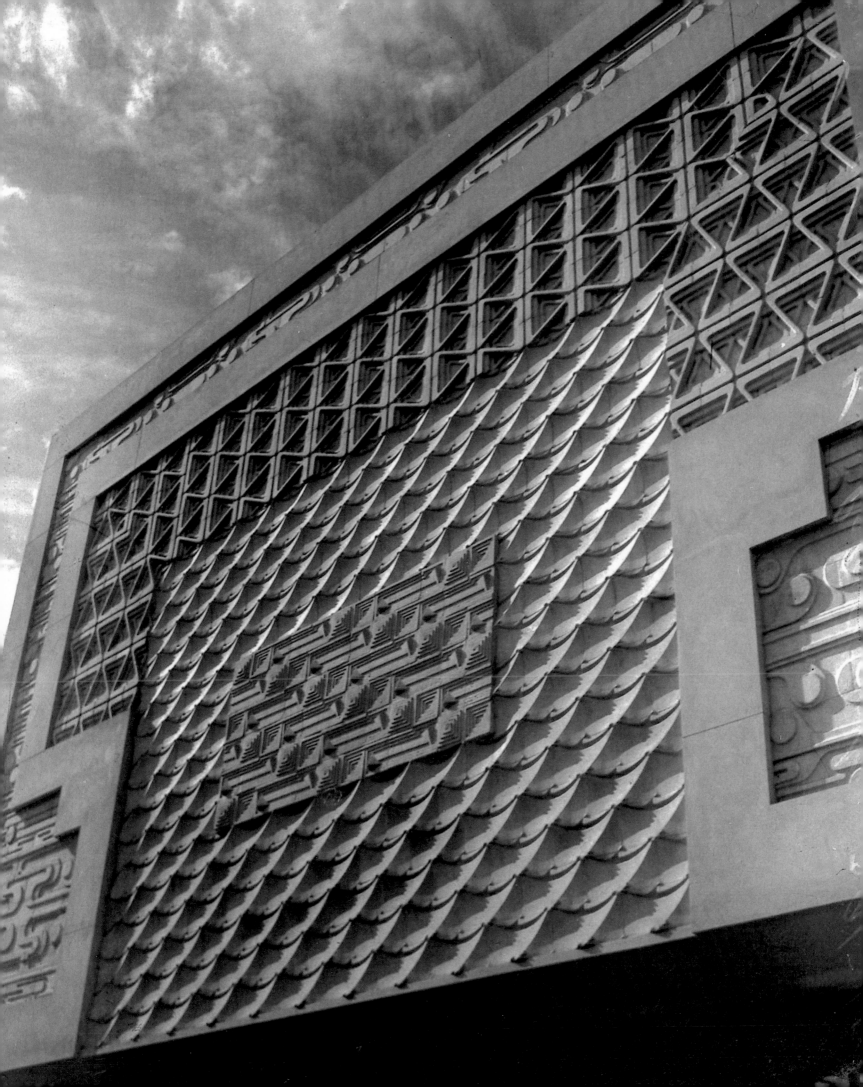

The Pyrmont incinerator in Sydney was Griffin's visible expression of the interlocking of town planning and architecture. 'One could not ask for a more telling monument to his [Griffin's] work in this ancient continent. In the basic arts of architecture and music, Australia is now ready to lead the world.'[1] These words by Marion Mahony Griffin, in her memoirs 'The magic of America', summarise the importance she saw in this magnificent architectural expression of the envelope for a basic functional process.

During the 1920s and early 1930s, municipal councils were gradually becoming aware of the value of incineration as a means of disposing of garbage. These authorities were concerned with both the shortage of suitable waste lands within their boundaries for the tipping of garbage and household refuse, and the growing public protest about the danger to health of council tips. The horrors of the two epidemics which swept through the Australian cities after the First World War were still fresh in the minds of the citizens.

At that time the most popular methods of garbage disposal were by dumping at sea or by burial to reclaim waste lands. From the point of view of hygiene these methods left much to be desired and councils, with the health of the people uppermost in their minds, decided to build incinerator plants.

One of the most successful incinerator companies in Australia was the Reverberatory Incinerator & Engineering Company (RIECo). Its advertisement in the *Australasian Engineer* of February 1930, describes the benefits and features of their product:

> At Last! An ideal Incinerator has ... such a high state of efficiency in the elimination of dust, smoke and noxious fumes, and the thorough destruction of municipal garbage, as to make this Incinerator a most valuable asset to any municipality.
>
> Amongst its outstanding features are: low cost of installation and upkeep, one attendant only required for each furnace, cost of burning lower than burying garbage. The gravitation feeding of furnaces and the ideal conditions for the stokers, must appeal to municipal officers. The furnaces are constructed of heavy steel plate and housed in handsome buildings which are an architectural feature in any district.

On 22 July 1926, John Boadle (1873–1963), an engineer from Moonee Ponds in Victoria, lodged his invention titled, 'Reverberatory Incinerator especially applicable for the destruction of refuse', at the Commonwealth Department of Patents.[2]

The first incinerator designed on the reverberatory principle was erected by John Boadle for the Sandringham Council in Victoria, in 1926. It proved so satisfactory that the plant was duplicated by the addition of another furnace. Plants were subsequently erected at Box Hill (1927) and Geelong (1928) in Victoria, and Bexley (1929) in New South Wales. Evidence from these plants convinced other municipalities to select this type of incinerator.

Not long after the incorporation of RIECo in August 1929,[3] the Essendon City Council in Victoria decided to construct an incinerator in Holmes Road, Moonee Ponds.

The site selected, situated as it was adjacent to parkland and in close proximity to residential areas, demanded a building that would, as far as possible, harmonise with its surroundings. The design of a suitable building was one of the requirements of the contract that was awarded to RIECo. The managing director of the company, Mr Nisson Leonard-Kanevsky, had commissioned Walter Burley Griffin in 1922[4] to design Leonard House at 46 Elizabeth Street, Melbourne, as his firm's head office. In addition, Griffin had his Melbourne drawing office in Leonard House from 1924.[5] It was therefore quite natural that Mr Kanevsky should ask Griffin to design a building of architectural merit, in keeping with the residential area, to house the incinerator plant. The inspiration for the design of the Essendon incinerator came from the Peters house in Chicago, which Griffin designed in 1906.

As Eric Nicholls was architect-in-charge of Griffin's Melbourne office in 1929 (Griffin had moved to Sydney in 1925), it was he who actually obtained the commission to design this building. When it was realised that there would be further commissions from RIECo for other incinerators, Griffin formed the partnership of Griffin and Nicholls, which continued after Griffin's death in 1937. The association between the Griffin and Nicholls partnership and RIECo concluded with the Canberra incinerator designed by Eric Nicholls in 1938,[6] a second unit for the Ipswich incinerator in Queensland in early 1940 and a couple of unsuccessful tenders also in 1940.[7]

So successful was the reverberatory type of incinerator that in 1940 RIECo proudly proclaimed that it had installed every municipal incinerator in the Commonwealth of Australia, with the exception of two, in the last ten years.[8] During that time eighteen incinerators had been constructed, and the thirteen designed by Griffin and Nicholls had each been individually designed to suit their site and the size of the incinerator plant required.

By February 1932, the New South Wales municipalities of Bexley, Kuring-Gai, Waratah and Randwick were all operating RIECo incinerators. Just prior to the Sydney City Council deciding to build an incinerator, John Boadle and Walter Burley Griffin went to the United States to investigate the latest methods of incineration and combustion. They were away several months at the expense of Nisson Leonard-Kanevsky.[9]

The garbage destructors built in the 1900s were not only unsightly structures but the method of garbage disposal was inefficient and unhygienic. These early destructors required much manual labour to operate and work was carried out in appalling conditions. The workers had to endure the intense heat from the open furnace while they stoked the furnaces with putrid rotting garbage, one shovel load at a time. When the ash and clinker residue built up in the bottom of the furnace it had to be scraped out into bins, so the air on the working level was filled with dust, making seeing and breathing impossible without injury and discomfort to the hot, sweating stokers. For some distance around the old destructors the air would be filled with smoke and ash would fall onto nearby homes and streets. These

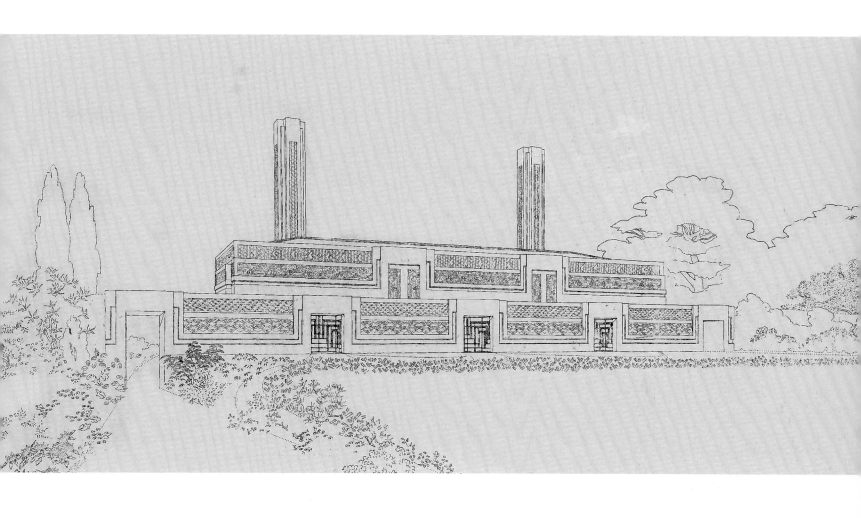

Above: Preliminary design for the unbuilt Moore Park incinerator, about 1932. Print of drawing on board, 63 x 129 cm, artist unknown.
Courtesy the Mary and Leigh Block Museum of Art, Northwestern University, Illinois (1985.1.82).

Previous page: Facade of Pyrmont incinerator showing the different concrete tile patterns representing the four 'ethers' — light, warmth, sound and life — defined by Dr Guenther Wachsmuth in his 1923 book *The etheric formative forces in Cosmos, Earth and Man.* Marion translated this book from German prior to 1932.
Courtesy Fairfax Photo Library, Sydney.

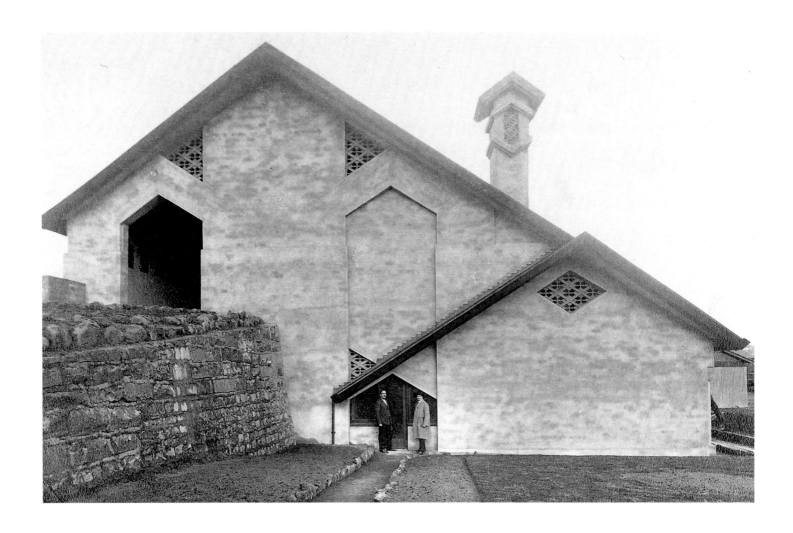

Above: Essendon municipal incinerator, Melbourne, in 1930 with Nisson Leonard-Kanevsky on the right at the entrance. It was the first of the Griffin/Nicholls RIECo incinerators and one of the few still standing.
Courtesy Nicholls collection, Sydney.

Right: Section rendering of Essendon incinerator, dated 28 October 1929 and signed 'E M Nicholls, architect'. Ink and watercolour on paper, 40 × 80 cm.
Courtesy City of Moonee Valley, Melbourne (C2272).

Following pages: Perspective rendering of the second design for Moore Park incinerator, Sydney, 1933. Ink on paper, 56 × 96 cm, artist unknown.
Courtesy the Mary and Leigh Block Museum of Art, Northwestern University, Illinois (1985.1.104).

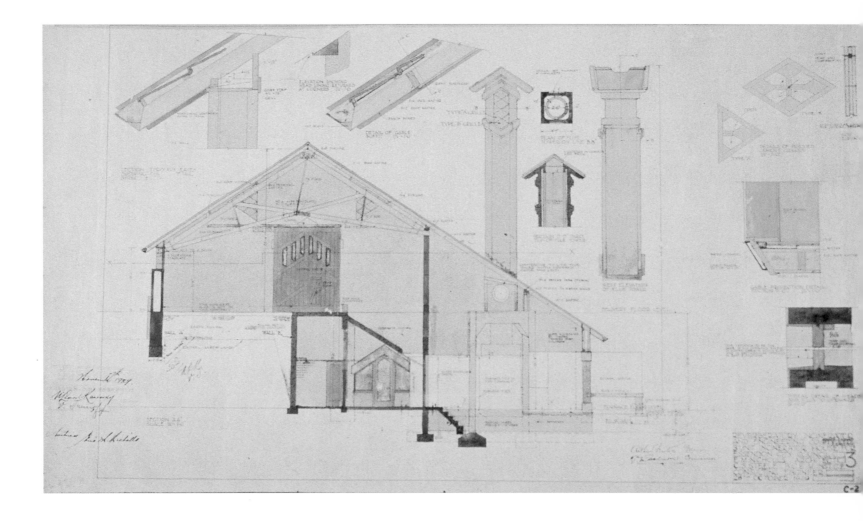

unhealthy aspects of garbage disposal were eliminated by the invention of the gravity-feed reverberatory process.

The Pyrmont incinerator was the largest ever built by RIECo and it incorporated the latest improvements in reverberatory incinerators. Because of the large quantity of garbage collected by the council lorries each morning, it was necessary to construct within the incinerator building a garbage trough which extended virtually the full width of the structure. Above the trough was a travelling gantry mechanical scoop which was able to pick up the garbage from the trough and drop it into one of the sloping hoppers that conveyed the garbage by gravity into the furnace. In this way the furnaces were kept fully charged all day.

The rotation of a wheel on the lower level opened a controllable door, allowing the required quantity of garbage to fall into a preliminary chamber, into which hot air was forced, thus drying up and eliminating the moisture of which there is a large amount in most household refuse. Being now much more easily burnt, the dried garbage was thrust down sliding slotted bars into the furnace. The temperature attained in the furnace varied between 1200 and 2000 degrees Fahrenheit, although 1500 degrees was sufficient for the destruction of the garbage. The extra

temperature ensured that the smoke and fumes, as well as the 'green gases' rising from the refuse on the drying hearth were thoroughly consumed and rid of their noxious qualities in the furnace prior to their discharge as a 'thin film of clear vapour from the flue tower'.[10]

This pollutant-free emission was achieved by deflecting or reverberating the hot gases of combustion over the material to be consumed and under the reverberatory arch which was at incandescent heat: thus complete combustion of the mixed gases took place during their passage into the second chamber. The employees worked at a lower level, separated from the garbage hoppers. They merely assisted the garbage combustion process by rodding through small port holes in the furnace walls.

The clinker pit was below the combustion chamber. The stoker, having pulled over sufficient clinker onto the chamber floor doors, then revolved a pair of horizontal cast-iron doors to the vertical hanging position and the clinker and ash fell through into a metal skip. The residue chamber was thus sealed to prevent a rush of cold air into the furnace. The clinker was then considerably cooled before its removal from the residue chamber. The clinker skip when full, was then wheeled on rails to the east end of the building where

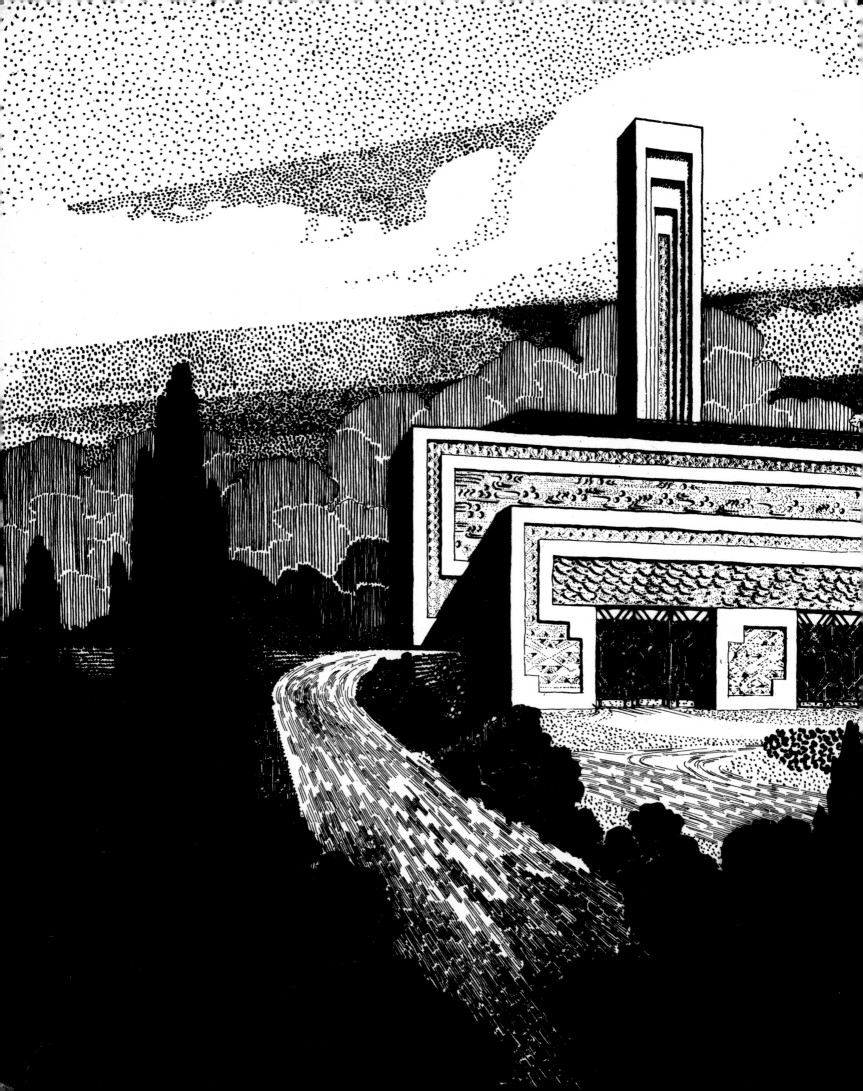

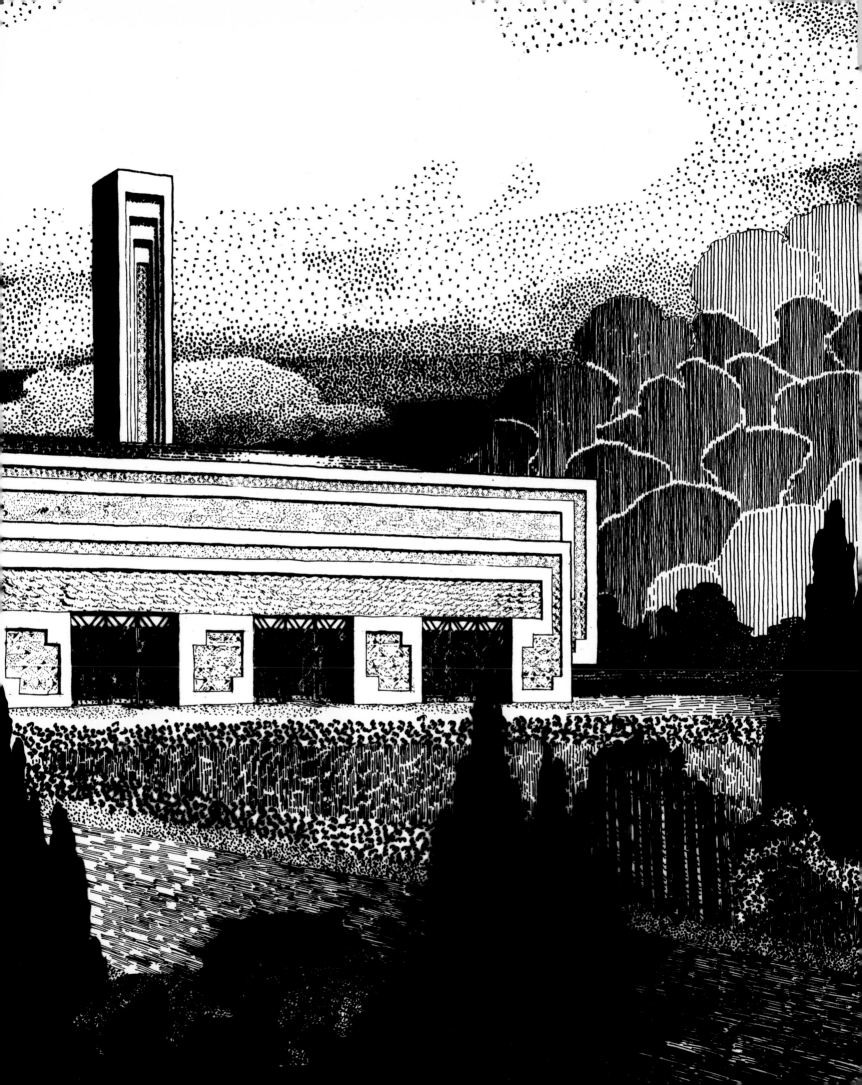

the same overhead gantry picked up the skip, raised it to the top level of the building and tipped its contents into the ash hopper above a waiting lorry that would take the clinker and ash away to be subsequently used as municipal road ballast or fertiliser for council parks and garden plantations.

Prior to 1932 the Sydney City Council had two English cell-type incinerators in operation, one at Pyrmont and one at Moore Park. Both had been in operation for many years, were no longer running efficiently, and were not able to cope with the increasing quantity of garbage being collected in central Sydney. The residue from the Pyrmont plant was carried out to sea in punts and sunk five miles from the Sydney Heads.

One Sydney City Council alderman, O'Dea, moved that a subcommittee of the Works Committee should be formed to investigate and report on the disposal of the city's refuse, particularly with regard to the question of incineration as against punting to sea.[11]

At the Works Committee meeting of 4 May 1932 it was approved in principle that Sydney's garbage would in future be disposed of by incineration. The recommendation to council was that a new incinerator be erected at Moore Park and the Pyrmont incinerator be remodelled. Initially tenders for the new incinerator would be called from Australian firms, but in the event of Australian tenders proving unsatisfactory, tendering would be extended to manufacturers from abroad. The site chosen to erect the new plant was at the south-western corner of Moore Park, about a quarter of a mile beyond the old destructor.

In *The Sydney Morning Herald* of 14 December 1932, it was announced that the City Council had agreed to spend £40,000 on the construction of a new incinerator at Moore Park, only half the original expenditure proposed. Eighteen tenders were received and that of RIECo Ltd, Sydney, amounting to £37,691 was accepted.

The newspaper reported that: 'provision will be made for the construction of the building to an aesthetic design'. RIECo in its tender offered to maintain the plant free of cost for four years and for a further six years for £100 a year.

Only one week later, however, the Minister for Local Government, Alderman Jackson, called a special meeting with the object of rescinding the decision of the council to erect an incinerator at Moore Park. He had twice previously been out-voted to defer the decision on the tenders. In addition, representatives from an unsuccessful tenderer waited on the Lord Mayor, Alderman Wallace, stating that their incinerator tender was £5000 less than the one accepted by the council. On 20 December 1932, the City Council declined to rescind the decision to award the contract to RIECo. It was revealed at this special meeting that the City Engineer favoured another tenderer and there were weaknesses in the specifications of the RIECo tender which it was proposed to overcome by special guarantees. The Lord Mayor admitted that the building to be erected by RIECo was a better one than that of the unsuccessful tenderer, but the City Council should think of the utility of the plant rather than the appearance of the building.

Right: Perspective of the Griffin–Nicholls alternative design for Brunswick incinerator, Melbourne, 1934 (incinerator project no 5). Pen and watercolour on paper, 48.2 × 78 cm. Courtesy National Library of Australia, Canberra (R4116).

BEYOND ARCHITECTURE

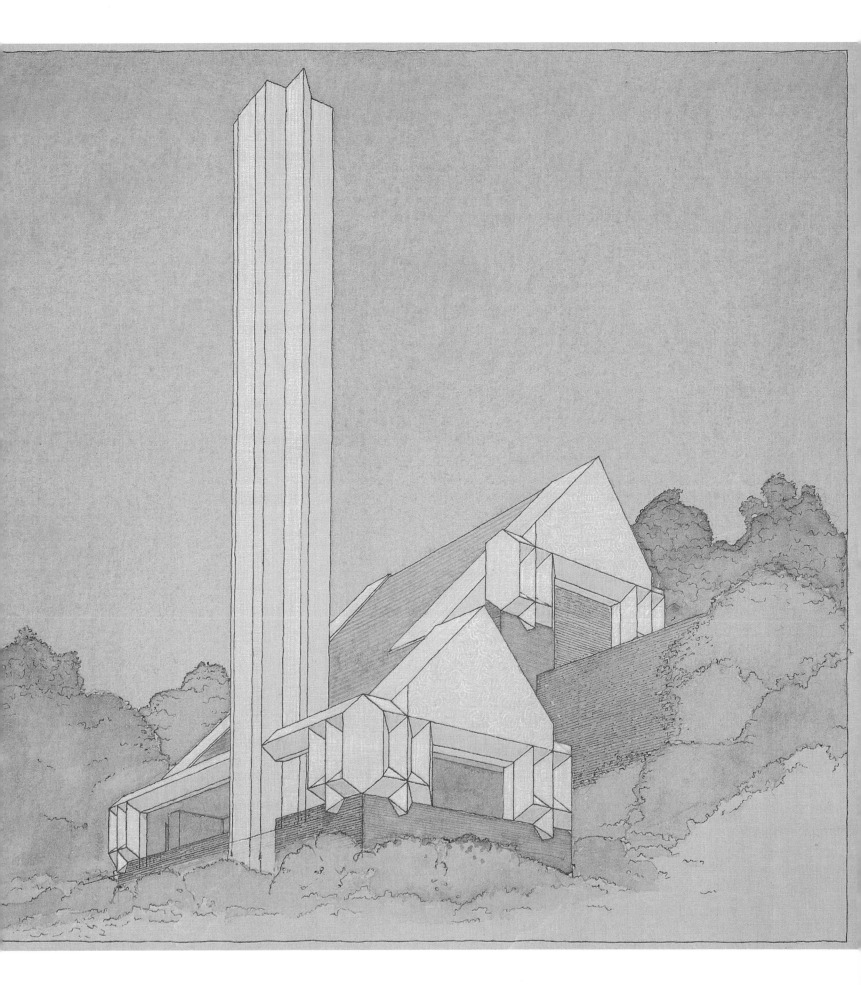

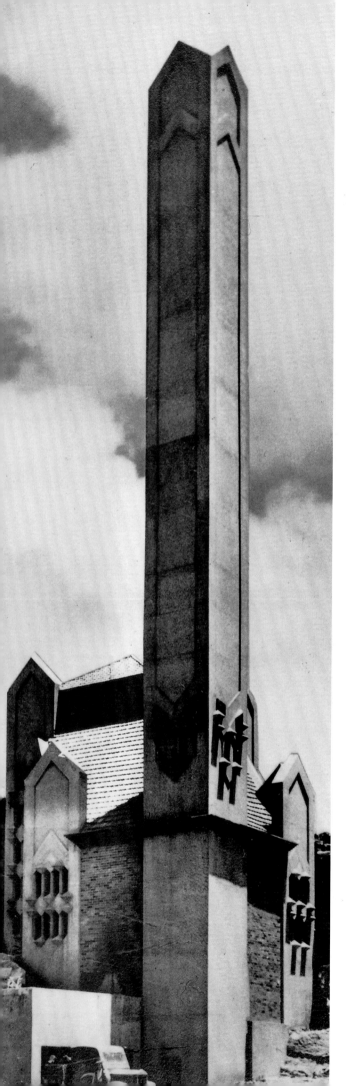

Alderman Garden said that:

> the accepted tender was not the lowest submitted by the
> successful firm. They had [submitted] another tender as low
> as £16,250, but the committee of experts, as well as the City
> Engineer, recommended the higher tender as being the most
> efficient to meet the special requirements of the City Council
> and the class of garbage that it would have to deal with.[12]

The contract between the City Council and RIECo to build the incinerator at Moore Park was signed on 27 January 1933. It was reported in *The Sydney Morning Herald*, for the first time, that the building was 'designed by W. Burley Griffin [*sic*] and E. M. Nicholls, architects' on 28 January 1933.

At the City Council meeting of 7 February 1933, a letter was received from the Property Owners' Association suggesting that the council should review the proposed expenditure of £37,000 on the erection of a garbage incinerator at Moore Park. 'We will be forced to take extreme action if the matter is not reconsidered', the association said. It suggested that a committee should be appointed to inquire fully into the project. The council did not act on the association's demands.

Then followed an objection to the site of the proposed incinerator, from the British-Australasian Tobacco Co Ltd. The objection claimed that fumes and smells from the proposed incinerator would have 'a deleterious effect on tobacco products in manufacture, and would be detrimental to the health of employees'.

On 18 May 1933, the council's intention to build an incinerator at Moore Park took a turn for the worse. The Property Owners' Association, whose request for an inquiry into the erection of an incinerator at Moore Park had been denied by the City Council, then made representations to the Minister for Lands, who immediately instituted a Land Board Inquiry to commence on 30 May 1933. This effectively took the choice of the site for the incinerator out of the control of the City Council.

The Metropolitan Land Board, on 10 July 1933, announced that it would recommend to the Minister for Lands that the City Council should be refused permission to build an incinerator on a site in Moore Park. The chairman, Mr Connolly, stated that there were objections in the public interest, both to the continuance of the present destructor and the dedication of another area in the park for garbage destruction. The Board found, however, that a modern incinerator of the type proposed, if carefully and efficiently operated, would not be a source of danger to the health of residents or employees in the immediate vicinity, nor would it be likely to create any serious nuisance to manufacturers conducting businesses in the neighbourhood. With this finding the Land Board had inadvertently boosted the reputation of the RIECo type reverberatory incinerator, an endorsement that must have encouraged other municipalities to seriously consider installing RIECo incinerators.

The Board pointed out that the public had been deprived of the use of a considerable area of the park by different buildings, which had been erected there, including

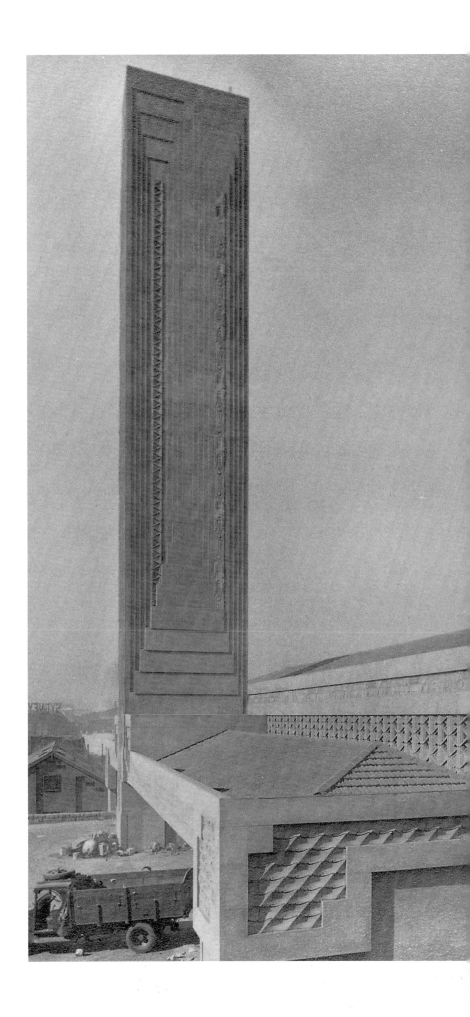

Left: Leichhardt municipal incinerator, Sydney, built in 1936, now demolished. Its soaring triangularity expressed Griffin's belief in the aesthetic possibilities of industrial buildings.
Courtesy Nicholls collection, Sydney.

Right: View of Pyrmont incinerator showing the 'art deco' chimney, whose height and commanding position made it one of Sydney's landmarks.
Courtesy Nicholls collection, Sydney.

Following page: An early photograph of Pyrmont incinerator clearly showing the decorative complexity of the juxtaposed tile patterns.
Courtesy Nicholls collection, Sydney.

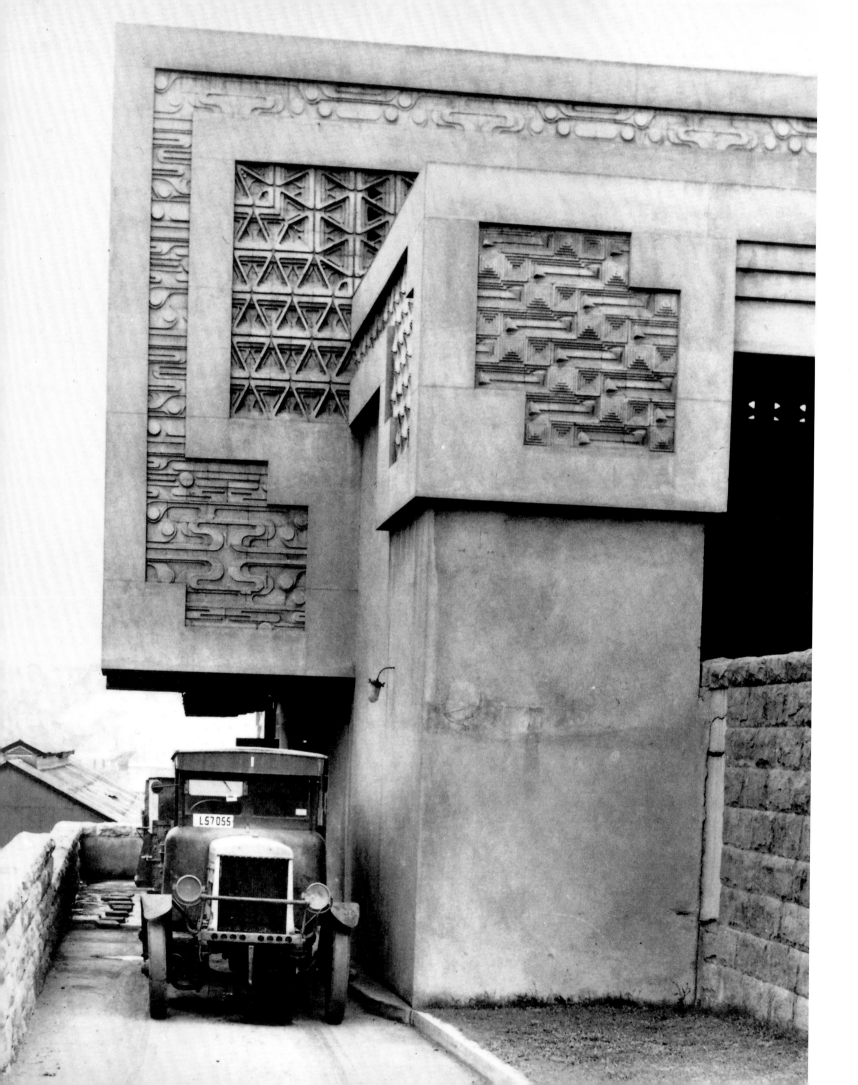

the existing destructor. The evidence tended to show that the park was already overcrowded, as far as the playing areas were concerned. The natural growth of population and the ever-increasing demand for suitable areas for outdoor recreation rendered it necessary for the retention of the proposed site as a recreational area, and for the same reason the present site of the destructor should be restored to the park.

The Board suggested several other sites that would be suitable for the proposed incinerator, but if the site of the existing destructor at Pyrmont were used the capital cost in the acquisition of a new site would be avoided. On 18 August 1933, the State Cabinet disapproved of the proposal to build the incinerator at Moore Park, saying that it was opposed to areas dedicated for parks being used for other purposes.

At a special meeting on Monday 30 October 1933, the City Council 'rejected a proposal to dispose of the city's refuse by punting [it] to sea, and decided to proceed with the construction of an incinerator on a site adjoining the existing garbage destructor at Pyrmont'. The amendment motion to construct the incinerator at Pyrmont was moved by Alderman Sir Samuel Walder. The voting was nine votes to three in favour of incineration at Pyrmont.

It was reported in *The Sydney Morning Herald* on 10 January 1935, that the Pyrmont incinerator would be in operation by the end of the year. It would be large enough to dispose of the amount of refuse previously burnt by the old destructors at Moore Park and Pyrmont. The incinerator was expected to cost £37,000, but roads and other necessary work would bring the total expenditure to about £45,000.

The site chosen was extraordinarily steep, requiring two levels of sandstone retaining wall to support the three-storey reinforced concrete incinerator building. Consequently, the only vehicular access to it was from Saunders Street, Pyrmont. A new design with only one chimney stack was selected by the Sydney City Council. The building form accurately follows the functions that took place within it. Through this design Griffin expressed the philosophy of his mentor, Louis Sullivan, which is, that form follows function.

Externally, the design by Griffin and Nicholls was strongly influenced by the Pre-Columbian architecture of the Zapotek people of Mitla in Mexico. The building's proportion and method of inserting tile decorations between plain geometric bands on the facade is strikingly similar to the temple ruins at Mitla. At Pyrmont, however, Griffin created a version of this ancient form in reinforced concrete and precast concrete tiles, with cantilevered end bays and wide-span openings for the garbage trucks to pass under. His design was thus at the forefront of building technology in 1934.

The Pyrmont incinerator was one of Sydney's most prominent buildings of the 1930s. Its art deco flue tower, which actually contained two cylindrical stacks, was one of Sydney's landmarks and could be seen from many parts of the metropolis.

The building contained the largest incinerator plant in the Commonwealth, costing approximately £50,000, and it served the whole of the city of Sydney. No less than 100 truck loads of miscellaneous refuse, some containing as much as 15 cubic yards (11.45 cubic metres) each, were delivered to the plant each day, and the whole was reduced to an innocuous residue within sixteen hours daily.[13]

Marion's account in 'The magic of America' indicates that she, Walter and possibly Eric Nicholls treated the design of the Pyrmont incinerator with the spiritual zeal and enthusiasm usually associated with ancient religious monuments. Marion states that by the reverberatory 'method of incineration, matter is practically reduced to primeval elements — heat, light, sound and magnetism'. She described the Pyrmont incinerator as the 'Alpha–Omega', 'the final expression and dissolution of Matter'.[14]

As in the motifs of ancient architectural decoration, the motifs of the decoration of the Pyrmont incinerator are not conventionalised physical forms but are rich expressions of the basic forces and states of all nature.

> The four formative forces which have already manifested in nature express themselves in four basic forms: the Circular, the Triangular, the Wave [or Crescent] and the Rectangular. Within this building, [which is] a powerful expression of substantiality, matter reverses its steps moving from solid to liquid to light to heat and disappears. It would be absurd to say that something has been destroyed (other than form or appearance). So here we find architecture expressing these spiritual facts, not through feeling, as in the past, but by emotion controlled and directed by the trained intellect which, through discipline, can move on to conscious imagination and inspiration.[15]

> The Sydney Incinerator erected on the high rock promontory of Piermont [*sic*] will stand we think as an historical record of 20th Century architecture. It is as beautiful, as majestic as unique as any of the historical records of the past. Historically it records the basic fact of the 19th Century civilization later emphasised by the smashing of the atom.[16]

The Pyrmont incinerator is believed to have been the only building by Griffin in which the design and ornamentation were influenced by his interest in anthroposophy.

> The ornament is the record of what remains when matter is destroyed — warmth which manifests in the material world in the spherical form: the only form of matter when the solar system came into material existence, the Saturn period; the triangle, when the gaseous condition came in the Sun; the crescent or wave form of the Moon period when there was the liquid condition of matter; and the rectangle, the controlling form of the solid condition as seen in the human being's blood crystals …

> … warmth … is the basic factor in incineration which takes all of the refuse of the great city and reduces it to elements. Because of this method [of reverberation], an incinerator can be placed anywhere, in a park or wherever a monumental building will emphasize a beautiful landscape. It can be right in the center of things for there is no unpleasantness in the process. Municipality after municipality realized this and adopted the method. The cost of the building was always included in the bid. Griffin was the architect of the company so every municipality had to accept the architect with the method, and the company so invariably won that the other competitors gave up bidding.[17]

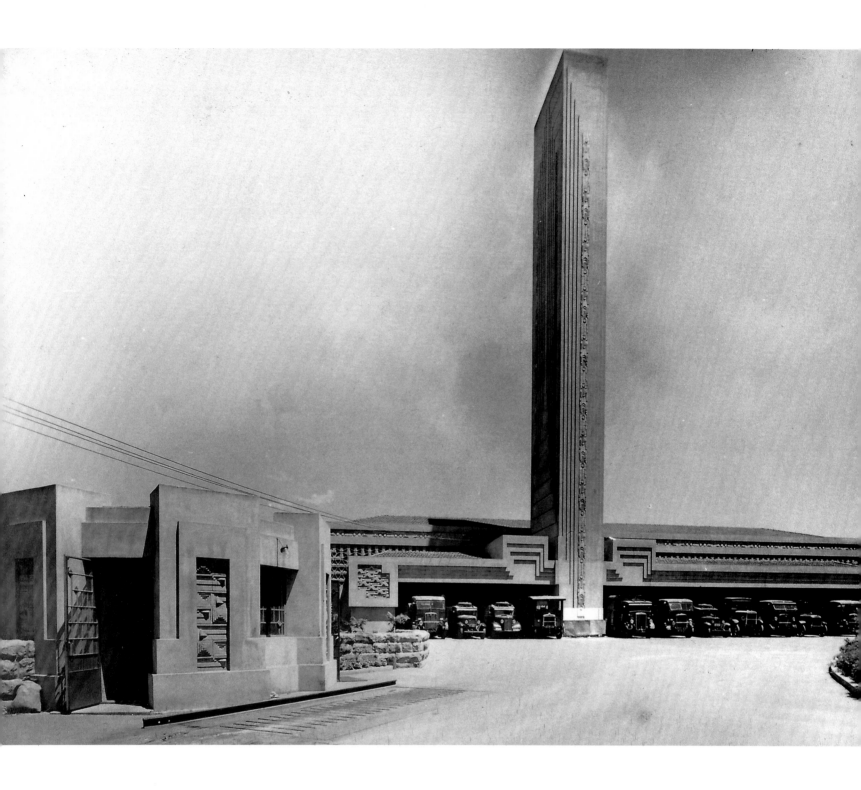

Above: View of Pyrmont incinerator, Sydney, showing
council trucks lined up at the refuse unloading bays.
Courtesy Dianne Betts, grand-daughter of Nisson Leonard-Kanevsky,
Melbourne.

The Pyrmont incinerator became a clear statement and proof of Griffin's design philosophy which he used in all his works: a beautiful design was less expensive than an ugly one. By this Griffin meant that if a building was well designed for its function then the savings in economic use would outweigh any additional capital expense to make it beautiful.

It is believed that there was always at least one furnace burning at the Pyrmont incinerator from 1936 until its closure in 1971. No alternative use was found for the building and its condition deteriorated to the point where the flue stack was declared structurally unsafe. The enormous chimney was demolished in stages at great cost in 1986.

In time however, it was the destructive forces of heat from within the furnaces and flues, and the rain from without, that ultimately tore the concrete building apart. An engineering report stated that the building had deteriorated too far to be restored. In the end the City Council sold the incinerator and site to a property developer. The council issued a demolition permit on 6 May 1992, and the incinerator was demolished in the following days. The Pyrmont incinerator is lost, except for a number of the ornamental facade tiles that were collected by Griffin enthusiasts, prior to its demolition and subsequently acquired by the Powerhouse Museum.

RIECo incinerators designed by Griffin and Nicholls

1930	Essendon, Victoria
1930	Kuring-Gai, New South Wales
1931	Waratah, New South Wales
1932	Randwick, New South Wales
1933	Glebe, New South Wales
1934	Willoughby, New South Wales
1935	Pyrmont [Sydney City Council], New South Wales
1936	Leichhardt, New South Wales
1936	Hindmarsh, South Australia
1936	Brunswick, Victoria
1936	Ipswich, Queensland
1937	Thebarton, South Australia
1938	Canberra, Australian Capital Territory

Notes

1. Marion Mahony Griffin, 'The magic of America', New York Historical Society, vol 3, p 422.
2. Commonwealth of Australia Patent no 2912/26. Dated 22 July 1926.
3. Victorian Companies Office, company file no C 0014832 M: doc.1.
4. Melbourne City Council archives. Building Permit Application is dated 8 November 1922.
5. Sands & McDougall, *Victorian directory*, 1926. Griffin's office was on the fifth floor, Leonard House.
6. *Shire and Municipal Record*, November 1938, p 335. 'Work has commenced on Canberra Incinerator'.
7. *Shire and Municipal Record*, February 1940, p 484. RIECo advertisement.
8. Ibid.
9. Interview with Marshall R Fordham, 1971. (Member of Griffin's staff from 1930; manager from 1932.)
10. *Essendon Gazette*, 9 January 1930.
11. *The Sydney Morning Herald*, 17 February 1932, p 12.
12. *The Sydney Morning Herald*, 21 December 1932, p 15.
13. *Australasian Engineer*, December 1938, pp 188–89.
14. Marion Mahony Griffin, 'The magic of America', New York Historical Society, vol 3, p 421.
15. Ibid, vol 3, p 422.
16. Ibid, vol 3, p 424.
17. Ibid, vol 3, pp 424 and 425.

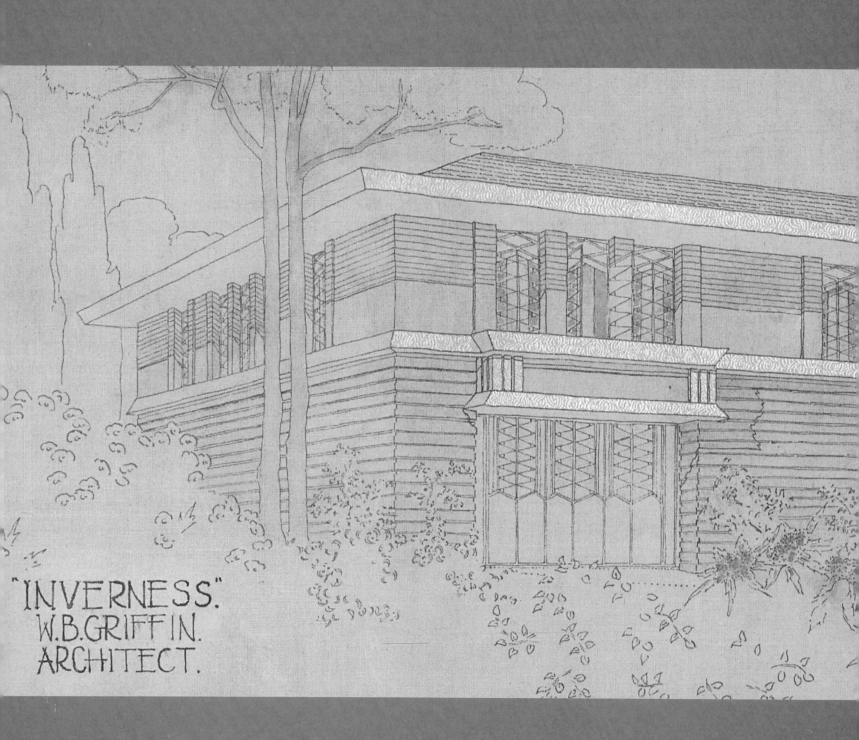

"INVERNESS."
W.B. GRIFFIN.
ARCHITECT.

GRIFFINS   DAVID DOLAN

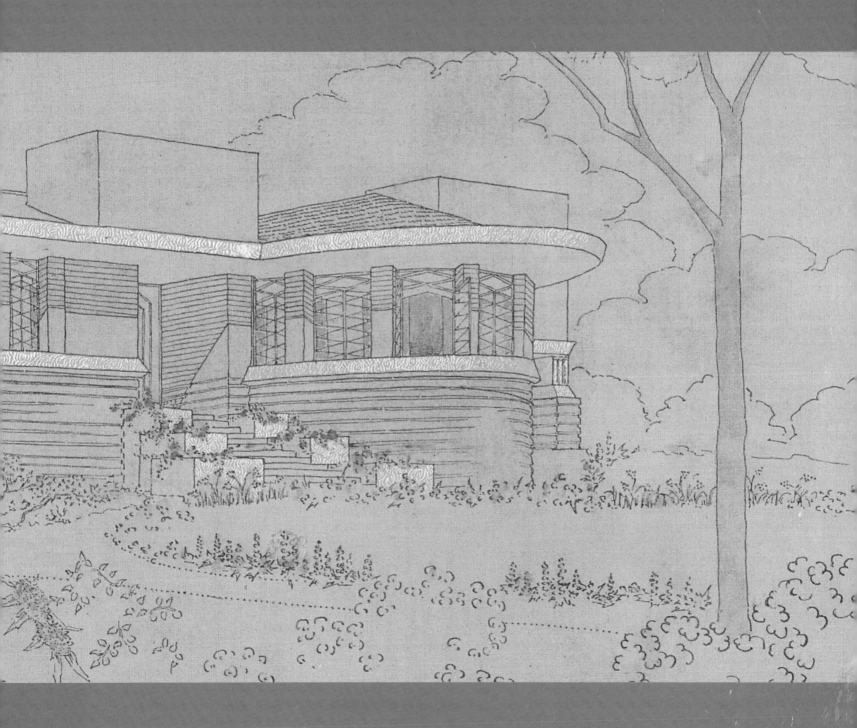

It has always been difficult to assess the scope of the life and work of Walter Burley Griffin and Marion Mahony Griffin, both in Australian and in international terms. Despite their importance in Australian history particularly, and the fact that over 80 years have passed since the Canberra competition, there have been no comprehensive biographies about the Griffins, although there have been many articles and several books about aspects of their architecture, planning and landscape design. The late Peter Harrison, author of *Walter Burley Griffin landscape architect*, believed that 'the complete story of Griffin is never likely to be tracked down'.[1]

Was Walter Burley Griffin a major talent in the history of American architecture who was half-forgotten and under-rated because he left the USA at age 36? Were Walter Burley Griffin and Marion Mahony true internationalists whose partnership was the most important and original architectural and planning venture ever seen in Australia? Or were they followers of Frank Lloyd Wright: minor provincial figures who briefly captured international attention with their beautifully presented competition-winning plan for Canberra, but whose careers were otherwise undistinguished? Over the years, particularly in Australia, these questions have been discussed and debated but rarely before addressed systematically.

This book provides evidence for the claim that they were highly significant figures whose activities spanned three continents and cultures, who drew knowledgeably upon diverse and powerful intellectual and conceptual sources, tackled some of the biggest architectural jobs then available, and produced distinctive designs and structures which often seem ahead of their time. Yet from another perspective theirs can seem a story of frustration, marginalisation, bad luck, bad timing, and even failure.

Direct comparison with Frank Lloyd Wright, often implied but seldom expounded, is sometimes used to relegate the Griffins to the status of minor talents. Contrary to popular perception, they were not dependent on Wright for their style, career start, or original prominence. The architectural historian Roxanne Kuter Williamson rates both Griffins highly in *American architects and the mechanics of fame*, but does not see the Wright–Griffins connection as a strong example of her theme of the transference of 'design strength' between architects at critical points in their careers. Williamson notes that Walter contributed to the development of some of Wright's designs;[2] and while admitting that 'to an unpractised eye, Griffin's houses are indistinguishable from Wright's own work' adds that 'it is undeniable that Wright's very best designs surpassed the Prairie style houses done by Griffin'.[3] This is generally agreed, but overlooks the fact that comparing their North American houses is a comparison between the work of architects at different ages and stages of maturity.

Wright spent almost all his working life in the USA, with more and richer clients, and at a time of US cultural and media dominance of the modern world. He had the advantage of living longer than Griffin by some 30 years, which enabled him to produce his best late work, and also to

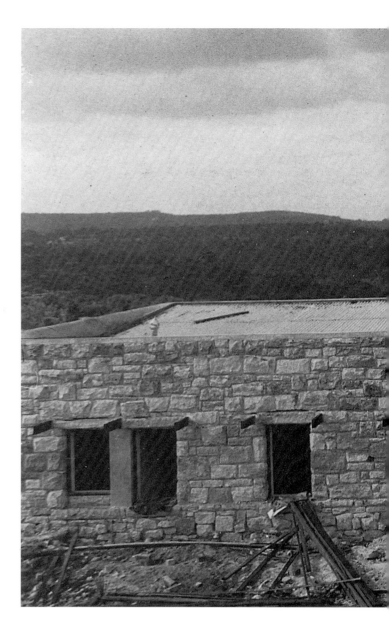

build his own legend. Unfortunately, in order to make a fair comparison we are reduced to speculation; but it is necessary to say that if Walter Burley Griffin had lived a few more years and been able to build some of his spectacular geometric colourful Indian designs, comparison with Wright would do him no harm, and the world history of modern architecture would be different. This is speculation, but it is not nonsensical fantasy: the designs exist and show Griffin moving into a new phase of unprecedented imaginative creativity. James Weirick has spoken of this and other examples of the Griffins' best work as pointing to a lost style: 'the great decorative modernism that might have been'.

Both Griffins were influenced by their association with Wright, but they had their own (joint and separate) mature styles. The importance of the Wright connection is probably over-emphasised in most accounts of their life and

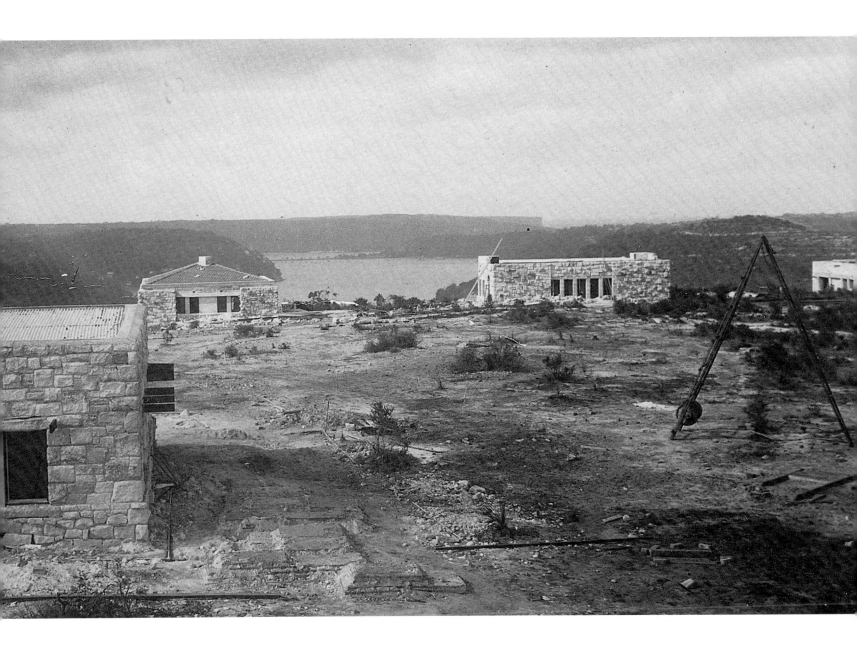

work because they first met in his Oak Park studio. Their marriage and work partnership was and is central to their life stories. In terms of how they have been (mis)understood by history, their brief involvement with Wright seems to have been exaggerated by the circumstance that they came together under his roof.

The impossibility of separating their professional and private lives is reinforced by the fact that their marriage occurred in the year that changed their lives in another respect as well: 1911 saw the announcement of the competition for a plan for the proposed but as-yet unnamed federal capital city of Australia. In hindsight, we may feel that life might have been easier for the Griffins if Walter had accepted the other job offered him that year and returned to the University of Illinois as professor. It is not surprising that he chose to go to Australia, however. Few architects in any

Above: This photograph of Castlecrag in 1922 is a reminder that the project involved re-establishing — not preserving — native vegetation in a suburban setting. The exposed harbourside hilltop land had been denuded and was suffering continuous soil erosion.
Courtesy Nicholls collection, Sydney.

Previous pages: Alan Cameron house, 'Inverness', Killara, Sydney, designed in 1933 by Walter Burley Griffin. Ink and watercolour on linen, drawn by unidentified artist from the Griffin office, 31.5 × 59.5 cm.
Powerhouse Museum, Sydney, gift of Ewen Cameron (93/342/1).
Photo by Sue Stafford, Powerhouse Museum.

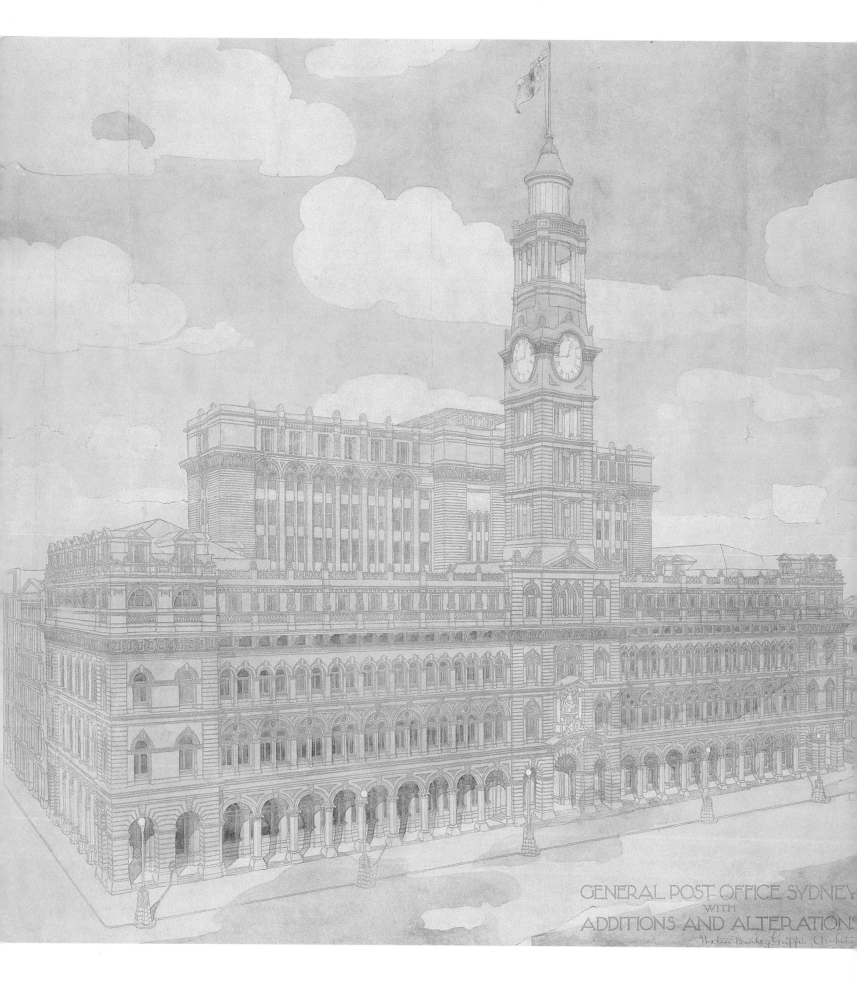

GENERAL POST OFFICE SYDNEY
WITH
ADDITIONS AND ALTERATIONS

era have the opportunity to plan and build a major city, let alone a federal capital for an emerging nation with apparently limitless future prospects.

Among the most persistent Griffin myths is the common belief, still occasionally stated in history texts, that the Griffins left Wright's employ to go to Australia. This is incorrect, as Wright had left Chicago to go to Europe in 1909, and Walter had successfully branched out on his own in 1906 at the age of 29. His career had been building well, but it really took off after he won a degree of international fame for the Canberra plan. This is an important point because it refutes the impression Wright later tried to give, that the Griffins were merely a couple of his junior assistants. Before leaving his studio both had held senior positions in his team, and both had reached professional maturity before 1911, and their formative experiences were well digested and transcended by then.

In recent years there has been a revisionist myth that Walter was just a front-man for Marion's ideas. Thanks to Anna Rubbo's and Paul Sprague's chapters, readers of this book will also be aware that this is a caricature.

Another confusing irony lies in the fact that in Australia, Walter Burley Griffin is best known as the designer of Canberra. Most visitors to Canberra think they are seeing his vision realised. There are important indicative echoes of the Griffin vision in elements of the layout and street patterns of old inner Canberra as it has been built, but the vision is grossly diluted and adulterated. In a vain effort to preserve the integrity of their plan, the Griffins fought a long losing battle with the federal authorities.

In hindsight, it seems that Canberra made and unmade Griffin. At the time of their marriage, the Griffins may have had personal as well as professional reasons for abandoning their American career and coming to Australia. Walter could have basked in his success and continued his American practice, or taken the university job. Instead, he and Marion showed their commitment to their ideals by deciding to try to implement the prize-winning concept. But the frustrations involved cost them dearly. In *The architecture of Walter Burley Griffin*, Donald Leslie Johnson blames 'the bitter years of Canberra' for the decline he sees in the quality of Griffin's domestic architectural designs, reluctantly suggesting 'the burden of the Canberra affairs must have taken a heavy toll on the sensitive man ...'[4] Writing about this crucial turning point in Walter's career, Peter Harrison suggested that the stubborn idealist in him meant that 'it is unlikely, even had it been possible to foresee the outcome, that he would have adopted any other course'.[5]

In previous chapters, Paul Kruty discussed the Griffins' Indian experience, their Melbourne practice is examined by Jeffrey Turnbull, Peter Navaretti outlined the remarkable story of their municipal engineering architecture, and Anne Watson examined their interior and furniture design. These essays show that the Griffins produced much outstanding and original architecture, and played an important part in the development of Australian culture in their time, embodying key trends as diverse as

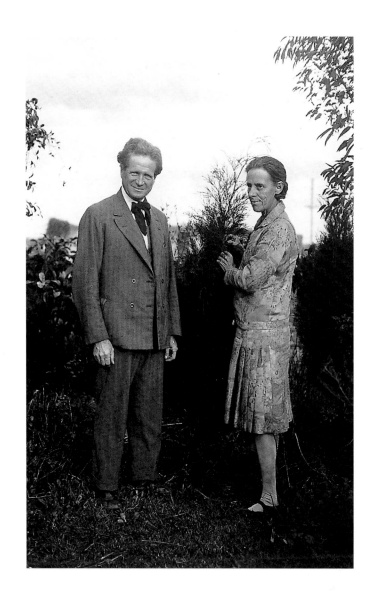

Above: Walter and Marion in Castlecrag, 27 July 1930. In early twentieth-century Australia they were a distinctive, almost exotic couple.
Courtesy National Library of Australia, Canberra (Pictorial collection). Photograph by Dr Jorma Pohjanpalo.

Left: Walter Burley Griffin, proposed additions to the General Post Office, Sydney, 1917. Hand-coloured dyeline print signed by Griffin's assistant Roy Lippincott, 40 × 50 cm.
Courtesy National Archives of Australia, New South Wales (400 1/2, item 11).

spreading American influence and increasing interest in growing Australian native plants. Yet there is also a strong sense of under-achievement. This is most obvious in the regrettable situation that neither Canberra nor Castlecrag developed as the Griffins had intended. They lived in difficult times, and the political and economic disasters of the First World War and then the Great Depression respectively placed insuperable obstacles in the path of these two major projects.

The sense of failure is not, however, limited to these grand schemes which fell short of expectations. All architects have designed some buildings which were never built, and some which were commenced but never completed, for a variety of reasons, usually financial problems on the part of the client. The research to quantify this would be impracticable, but the Griffins seem to have had a very high proportion of both non-starters and non-finishers in their career, especially in Australia and India. This situation is keenly felt in Perth, which has no Griffin works because neither of the two projects for that city — a campus landscape design for the University of Western Australia, and a headquarters for the Young Australia League — was carried out.

The coincidence of personal and professional landmarks continues to the end of the Griffins' partnership. Encouraged by a substantial commission for Lucknow University Library, Walter went to India in 1935, and it is easy to blame his death after just over a year in that country for the lack of realised projects. It seems another example of the Griffin jinx that the biggest job he actually completed in India, a set of stunningly inventive buildings for the United Provinces Exhibition at Lucknow in 1936–1937, was always meant to be temporary so was duly demolished. Several of his Indian projects were abandoned in his lifetime, and others on the drawing board at the time of his death could have proceeded had the clients or authorities wanted to see them built.

This sense of frustration or failure cannot be dismissed as just an example of the Australian tall-poppy-lopping syndrome, or a part of the Griffin legend mischievously and misleadingly developed since their lifetimes. Marion, in 'The magic of America', sees their lifework as an exhausting struggle against mediocrity and bureaucracy. On the basis of the evidence in this book, readers can form their own opinion as to whether this perception is justified, and whether the Griffins were just unlucky, or whether their individualistic originality put them out-of-step with their times, or whether there were other forces at work. James Weirick's account in this book, more detailed than any previously published, shows that the reasons for their frustration were complex, multiple, and more political than mysterious.

Discussion of these questions in Australia often brings forth the accusation, almost part of the Griffin legend, that they were too idealistic and impractical, personally eccentric or difficult to work with. Perhaps Marion's strong personality and unconventional views on some matters raised conservative hackles in an era when professional women were rarer than today and females were less often

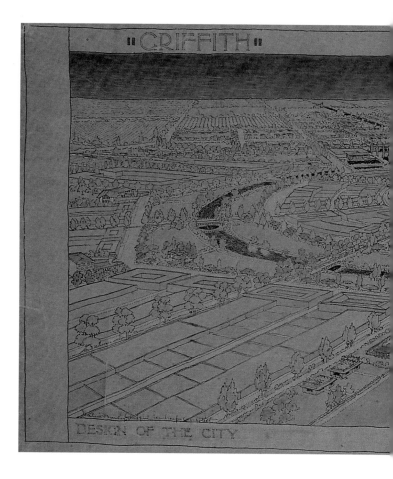

encouraged to be assertive. Similarly, their interest in theosophy and anthroposophy, far more common in educated circles in their time than now, can be misconstrued to suggest weirdness. In fact, Walter's career, particularly in the USA, provides plenty of counter-evidence that he was adaptable, diplomatic, practical, good at communicating with clients and often able to get his way.

Professional life was possibly made more difficult for the Griffins by the lack of precedents for the kind of professional practice they tried to operate for many years. Only the railways facilitated their efforts to commute between and across Canberra, Melbourne and Sydney at a time when most architectural practices in Australia were locally based. By spreading themselves across several Australian states and cities they compounded the effect of also moving between continents. Although they produced important work in many places, there was no one city where they really belonged and which adopted them, maintained their creations, preserved their documentation, and boosted their reputation in the crucial years: the first few decades after death or retirement when the work of artists and architects goes out of fashion before being rediscovered and 'revived'.

Today, the Griffins are recognised and respected by architectural historians and fortunate property owners in the USA, and celebrated in several parts of Australia —

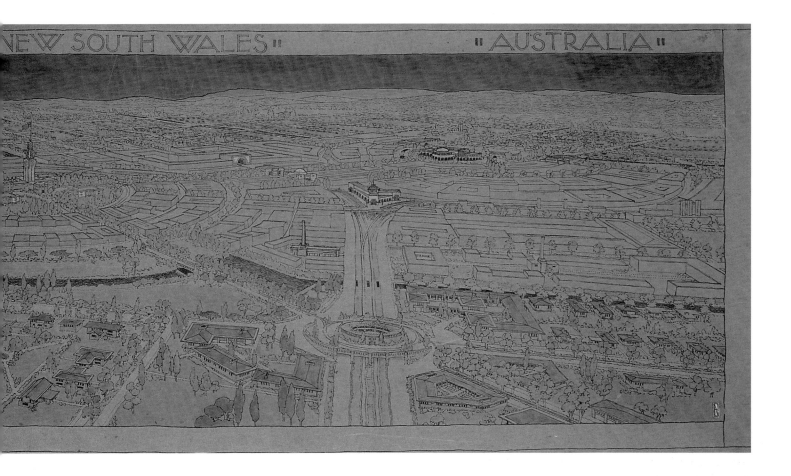

specifically Canberra and Castlecrag — though ironically in both the latter places their vision has been ruthlessly compromised. During the years while their vision was being debased by politicians and planners who should have known better, the swings of taste and fashion told against them. Two decades after it was built, the Fishwick house, one of Griffin's grander creations at Castlecrag, was marked down by a professional valuer because of its unconventional design.[6]

The Griffins attracted and inspired extensive press and magazine coverage, and wrote their share of articles and speeches, but less ephemeral, more extended study of their work was late in appearing. J Birrell's 1964 *Walter Burley Griffin* suffers from lack of information. An expatriate American resident in Australia, Donald Leslie Johnson, published *The architecture of Walter Burley Griffin* in 1977 followed by the first thorough Griffin bibliography in 1980. Peter Harrison's master's degree thesis on landscape architecture was written at the same time as Johnson's text, and was frequently revised by its author who died in 1990, but it did not appear in book form until 1995. By then, public and media interest in the Griffins was the highest it had been since their lifetime, and the publication trickle was looking like a regular flow, with two titles in 1994: Walker, Kabos and Weirick's *Building for nature: Walter Burley Griffin*

Above: Walter Burley Griffin, 'Design of the City', Griffith, New South Wales, 1915. Ink and watercolour on silk sateen aerial perspective by Roy Lippincott, 41 × 106 cm. Walter's design, which had much in common with Canberra, proved too ambitious for this town and never developed to the extent anticipated.
Courtesy Archives Authority of New South Wales, Sydney (AO doc 225).

Following pages: Elevation rendering of the second design for Lucknow University Library, 1936. Ink and watercolour on coloured paper, 45.7 × 60.8 cm.
Courtesy Avery Architectural and Fine Arts Library, Columbia University, New York (1000.015.00078).

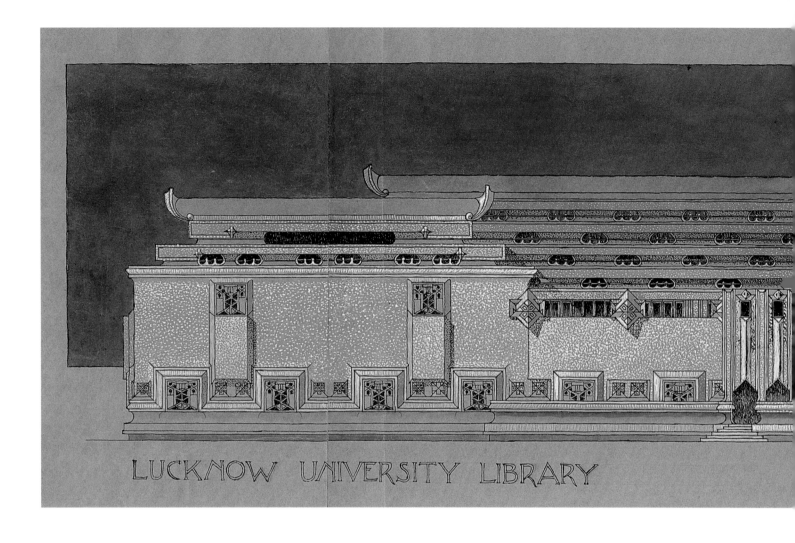

LUCKNOW UNIVERSITY LIBRARY

and *Castlecrag*, and Peter Proudfoot's provocative *The secret plan of Canberra*.

The lack of detailed biographical information about the Griffins not only inhibits our understanding but encourages speculation, particularly regarding the impact of their personalities and private life on their work and careers. The notion that the Griffins were cranky or difficult to work with was contradicted in a 1993 interview Anne Watson and David Dolan conducted with Mr David and Mrs Violet Pratten, then probably the Griffins' last surviving clients.[7] Mrs Pratten remembered going to deliver some documents to the Griffins' home in Castlecrag in 1934 and Marion telling her seriously (in the best theosophical tradition) that she had fairies at the bottom of her garden. Yet the Prattens were adamant that the Griffins were friendly, likeable, practical, easy to deal with, and able to compromise when appropriate.

The Griffins had no children together in 26 years of married life, which is hardly surprising considering that Marion was 40 when they wed. It is reasonable to suggest, however, that their childlessness has been a factor in their confused and ambiguous personal and professional reputation. Children often play a major role in collecting

and retaining information and objects relating to their parents, and in shaping their posthumous image.

In February 1937, when Walter died suddenly in India and was buried in an unmarked grave, Marion was 66. With no family to keep her in Australia, she returned to the USA. In her late writings, and her handling and disposition of the drawings, documents and few other items she retained from her partnership with Walter, she tried to record and preserve her version of their life and work, but it was not to good effect. Old, ill, lonely, poor and disillusioned, she lived in retirement with a niece until 1961 when she died aged 90. The death of this proud, creative, history-making professional woman, born in the apocalyptic year of the great Chicago fire, and whose drawings helped give Australia its national capital, went unremarked.

When Marion left Australia, the Griffins' junior partner Eric Nicholls worked on for many years, and Griffinesque echoes can be seen in some of his own designs. Eric and later his architect daughter Marie remained loyal to the Griffins' memory and conscientiously preserved many of their drawings, pieces of furniture and personal items including books. But no firm has survived bearing the Griffin

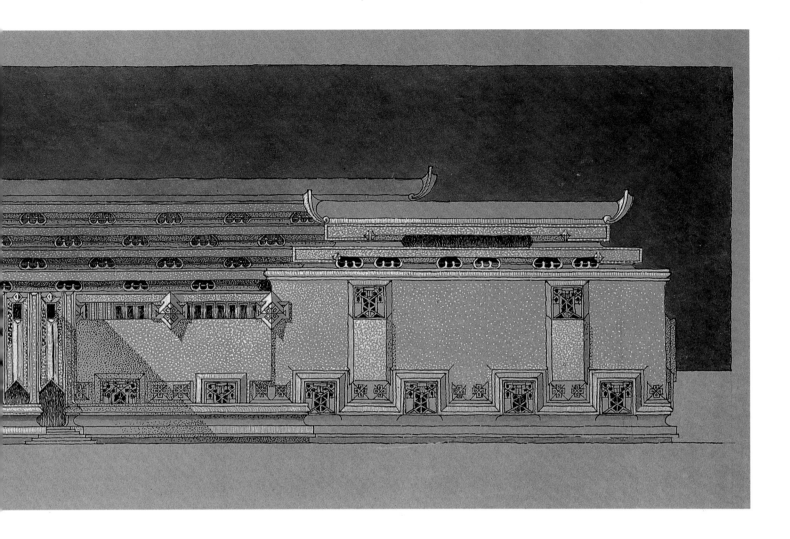

name, while in every city there are architectural firms proudly bearing the names of founders and forebears of varying levels of distinction. These offices often preserve drawings and records spanning several generations. As a result, it is far easier to reconstruct the careers of innumerable mediocre or competent practitioners than it is to document and understand the life work of two of the most talented, original and ambitious architect-planners of their day.

This leads to the question of whether professional artistic and architectural reputations were or are generally national, or can be truly international. At first glance it seems odd to suggest that movement between countries could prevent rather than facilitate international recognition. Yet this can happen, because so-called 'international' recognition is often really just an extension of recognition in a single powerful centre or nation which exerts cultural hegemony by presenting its own values and developments as universal. Overall, the evidence suggests that the Griffins' international relocations limited rather than enhanced their opportunities, achievements and recognition.

Walter Burley Griffin and Marion Mahony Griffin were important members of the Prairie School of Chicago,

and arguably the most important international architects ever to work in Australia. This book and the exhibition which inspired it should remove any whiff of failure from their reputations, but a certain frustrating sense that more might and should have been achieved will probably always, justifiably, remain.

Notes

1. Peter Harrison, *Walter Burley Griffin: landscape architect*, Robert Freestone, ed, National Library of Australia, 1995, p 2.

2. Roxanne Kuter Williamson, *American architects and the mechanics of fame*, University of Texas, Austin, 1991, p 46.

3. Ibid.

4. Donald Leslie Johnson, *The architecture of Walter Burley Griffin*, Macmillan, Melbourne, 1977, p 97.

5. Harrison, p 34

6. Documents in possession of the family of Vanessa Mack, Sydney.

7. Thanks to Alison Germaine McSweeney for arranging and facilitating this meeting.

SELECTED BIBLIOGRAPHY

References have been selected for their comprehensive coverage of the Griffins' work or their relevance to the chapters in this book. Much more has been written by or about the Griffins. For a bibliography of these references prior to 1976 consult Donald Leslie Johnson, *Canberra and Walter Burley Griffin: a bibliography of 1986 to 1976 and a guide to published sources*, Oxford University Press, Melbourne, 1980.

Anon. 'Residence for E P Irving Decatur, Illinois', *Western Architect*, April 1913, pp 38–39.

Anon, 'Walter Burley Griffin and community planning', *Western Architect*, vol 19, no 8, August 1913, pp 67–80.

Anon. 'Residence for D M Amberg, Grand Rapids, Michigan', *Western Architect*, October, 1913, p 88.

Anon. *Western Architect*, vol 18, no 9, September 1912, pp 93–94, plus 13 plates.

Birrell, James. *Walter Burley Griffin*, University of Queensland Press, Brisbane, 1964.

Bogle, Michael. 'The Cafe Australia', *Australiana*, Sydney, November 1996, pp 92–97.

Brooks, H Allen. 'The Prairie School: the American spirit in midwest residential architecture, 1893–1916', PhD thesis, Northwestern University, 1957.

Brooks, H Allen. 'Steinway Hall: architects and dreams', *Journal of the Society of Architectural Historians*, vol 22, no 3, 1963, pp 171–75.

Brooks, H Allen. 'Frank Lloyd Wright and the Wasmuth Drawings', *The Art Bulletin*, vol 48, June 1966, pp 193–201.

Brooks, H Allen. 'Chicago architecture: its debt to the arts and crafts', *Journal of the Society of Architectural Historians*, vol 30, no 4, 1971, pp 312–17.

Brooks, H Allen. *The Prairie School: Frank Lloyd Wright and his midwest contemporaries*, University of Toronto Press, Toronto, 1972.

Carolan, Jane. *The collegiate furniture of Walter Burley Griffin*, University of Melbourne Museum of Art, 1993.

Duncan, J and Gates, M, eds. *Walter Burley Griffin: a re–view*, Monash University Gallery, Victoria, 1988.

Griffin, Marion Mahony. 'The magic of America', 4 volumes, manuscript held at the New York Historical Society Library and the Burnham Library, Art Institute of Chicago, 1949.

Griffin, M M. 'Democratic architecture – I: its development, its principles and its ideals', *Building*, 12 June 1914, p 101.

Griffin, Walter Burley. 'Planning a capital city complete', *Construction News*, vol 34, no 22, 1912, pp 12–14.

Griffin, W B. 'Planning a federal capital city complete', *Improvement Bulletin*, vol 55, no 25, 6 November 1912, p 16.

[Griffin, W B.] 'Mr. W. B. Griffin's view: architect and social student', *The Salon*, vol 2, September and October 1913, pp 112–13, 183–84.

Griffin, W B. 'Architecture and democracy', *Building*, 11 October 1913, pp 63–64.

Griffin, W B. 'Town planning and its architectural essentials', *Building*, 11 October 1913, p 52.

Griffin, W B. 'Canberra: the architectural and development possibilities of Australia's capital city', *Building*, 12 November 1913, pp 65–66.

Griffin, W B. 'Canberra — II: the Federal city site and its architectural possibilities', *Building*, 12 December 1913, p 68.

Griffin, W B. 'The Canberra plan', paper presented to the Australia and New Zealand Association for the Advancement of Science, Melbourne, 14 August 1914, p 3, unpublished ms, Mitchell Library, Sydney.

Griffin, W B. 'The town plan of Leeton', *The Irrigation Record*, vol 3, nos 4 & 5, 1915, pp 49–50 and 65–66.

Griffin, W B. 'Standards for furnishing', *The Australian Home Builder*, August 1923, pp 34–35.

Griffin, W B. 'The modern architect's field: its limits and discouragements', *Australian Home Builder*, ns, no 6, November 1923, p 38.

Griffin, W B. 'The menace of governments', *Progress*, 1 May 1924, p 3.

Griffin, W B. 'Building for nature', *Advance! Australia*, vol 4, no 3, 1 March 1928, pp 123–27.

Griffin, W B. 'The outdoor arts in Australia', *Advance! Australia*, 1 May 1928, pp 207–11.

Griffin, W B. 'Traditional v. modern contemporary architecture: a discussion', *Architecture*, vol 19, no 12, December 1930, pp 567–68.

Griffin, W B. 'Toward simpler homes', *Architecture*, vol 20, no 8, August 1931, p 171.

Griffin, W B. 'Architecture and the economic impasse', *The Theosophist*, November 1932, pp 186–91.

Griffin, W B. 'Canberra in occupation: recapitulation and projection of the plan', *Canberra Annual*, 1934, p 6.

Griffin, W B. 'Occupational conservation', *Australian Wildlife*, vol 1, no 2, 1935, pp 24–27.

Griffin, W B. 'Architecture in India', unpublished ms, about December 1936.

Griffin, W B. 'Architecture in India', *The Pioneer*, 9 January 1937.

Harrison, P. *Walter Burley Griffin landscape architect*, Freestone, Robert, ed, National Library of Australia, 1995.

Johnson, Donald Leslie. *The architecture of Walter Burley Griffin*, Macmillan, Melbourne, 1977.

Kruty, Paul. 'Walter Burley Griffin and the University of Illinois', *Reflections*, vol 9, 1993.

Kruty, Paul. 'The Gilbert Cooley house, 1925: Walter Burley Griffin's last American building', *Fabrications* (the journal of the Society of Architectural Historians, Australia and New Zealand), vol 6, June 1995, pp 8–23.

Kruty, Paul. 'A new look at the beginnings of the Illinois Architects' Licensing Law', *Illinois Historical Journal*, vol 90, Autumn 1997, pp 154

Kruty, Paul, and Sprague, Paul. *Two American architects in India, Walter B Griffin and Marion M Griffin, 1935–1937*, University of Illinois, School of Architecture, Urbana, 1997.

Maldre, Mati (photographs), and Kruty, Paul (text). *Walter Burley Griffin in America*, University of Illinois Press, Urbana, 1996.

Munchick, Donna Ruff. 'The work of Marion Mahony Griffin: 1894–1913', MA thesis, The Florida State University, School of Visual Arts, December 1974.

Peisch, Mark L. *The Chicago school of architecture: early followers of Sullivan and Wright*, Phaidon, London, 1964.

Pregliasco, Janice. 'The life and work of Marion Mahony Griffin', in *The Prairie School: design vision for the midwest* (issued as *Museum Studies*, vol 21, no 2), The Art Institute of Chicago, Chicago, pp 164–81, 1995.

Price, Nancy. 'Walter Burley Griffin', BArch thesis, University of Sydney, Sydney, 1933.

Proudfoot, Peter. *The secret plan of Canberra*, UNSW Press, Sydney, 1994.

Proudfoot, Peter. 'The symbolism of the crystal in the planning and geometry of the design for Canberra', *Planning Perspectives*, vol 11, no 4, 1996, pp 225–57.

Quinlan Cecil V. 'Walter Burley Griffin: how a great dream came true', *Australian*

National Review, vol 1, no 4, 1937, pp 24–25.

Roe, J. 'The magical world of Marion Mahony Griffin: culture and community in Castlecrag in the interwar years', in Fitzgerald, S, and Wotherspoon, G, eds, *Minorities in cultural diversity in Sydney*, NSW State Library Press, 1995.

Rubbo, Anna. 'Marion and Walter Burley Griffin: a creative partnership', *Architectural Theory Review*, vol 1, no 1, 1996.

Rubbo, Anna. 'The numinous world of Marion Mahony Griffin: architect, artist, writer', *Spirit and place: art in Australia 1861–1966*, Museum of Contemporary Art, Sydney, 1996.

Smith, N K Morris, ed. 'Letters, 1903–1906, by Charles E. White, Jr., from the studio of Frank Lloyd Wright', *Journal of Architectural Education*, vol 25, Fall 1971, pp 104–12.

Van Zanten, David T. 'The early work of Marion Mahony Griffin', *Prairie School Review*, vol 3, Second Quarter, 1966, pp 5–23.

Van Zanten, David T. *Walter Burley Griffin: selected designs*, The Prairie School Press, Palos Park, Illinois, 1970.

Vernon, Christopher. '"Expressing natural conditions with maximum possibility": the American landscape art (1901–c.1912) of Walter Burley Griffin', *Journal of Garden History*, vol 15, no 1, 1995, pp 19–47. Reprinted in *Landscape Australia*, vol 17, nos 2/3, pp 130–37 and 146–52, 214–16.

Vernon, Christopher. 'Wilhelm Miller and the Prairie spirit in landscape gardening', in O'Malley, T, and Treib, M, eds, *Regional garden design in the United States*, Washington DC, Dumbarton Oaks Research Library and Collection, 1995.

Vernon, Christopher. 'Frank Lloyd Wright, Walter Burley Griffin, Jens Jensen and the Jugendstil garden in America', *Die Gartenkunst*, vol 7, no 2, 1995, pp 232–46.

Walker, Meredith, Kabos, Adrienne and Weirick, James. *Building for nature: Walter Burley Griffin and Castlecrag*, The Walter Burley Griffin Society, Incorporated, Castlecrag, 1994.

Watson, Anne. 'Walter Burley Griffin's "other" Canberra legacy', *Australiana*, Sydney, vol 19, no 4, November 1997, pp 99–102, 110.

Weirick, James. 'Walter Burley Griffin, landscape architect: the ideas he brought to Australia', *Landscape Australia*, vol 10, no 3, 1988, pp 241–46, 255–56.

Weirick, James. 'Marion Mahony at M.I.T.', *Transition*, Winter 1988, pp 49–54.

Weirick, James. 'Griffin and Knitlock', *Content*, vol 1, 1995.

Williamson, R K. *American architects and the mechanics of fame*, University of Texas, Austin, 1991.

Wilson, Richard Guy. 'Chicago and the international arts and crafts movement: progressive and conservative tendencies', pp 209–27, in John Zukowsky, ed, *Chicago architecture, 1872–1922: birth of a metropolis*, Prestel–Verlag, Munich, 1987.

Wright, Frank Lloyd. *Ausgeführte Bauten und Entwürfe von Frank Lloyd Wright*, Ernst Wasmuth, Berlin, 1910.

ACKNOWLEDGMENTS

The exhibition that provided the impetus for this book was initiated as a result of the demolition of the Griffins' Pyrmont incinerator, Sydney, in 1992 and the subsequent dispersal of funds by the City of Sydney Council for a travelling exhibition and other Griffin-related projects. Without the generosity of the Council and particularly the support of Council planning staff John McInerney and Peter Romey, neither the exhibition nor this book would have been realised. In the context of the early genesis of the exhibition, to be thanked also are other participants in the 1992 Griffin Incinerator Working Party, including the Walter Burley Griffin Society, Sydney, the National Trust (New South Wales), the Royal Australian Institute of Architects (NSW) and members of the US–Australia Griffin Exchange Program.

The subsequent development of both the exhibition and the book has been substantially assisted by members of the exhibition advisory committee: Griffin scholars, Associate Professor Paul Kruty and Professor Paul Sprague in the United States, Dr Anna Rubbo and Professor James Weirick in Sydney, and Peter Navaretti and Jeffrey Turnbull in Melbourne. Their ideas and advice as well as their essay contributions — and those of other essay authors Christopher Vernon in Fremantle and Dr David Dolan in Perth — have helped make this publication a truly collaborative, scholarly project. Advisory committee member Penelope Amberg formerly at the Australian Embassy, Washington, has also provided invaluable support and advice since the commencement of the project.

Special thanks must go to all the institutions and individuals who have given access to their collections and images and information for publication: in the United States John Zukowsky and Luigi Mumford at the Art Institute of Chicago; David Mickenberg and Amy Winter at the Mary and Leigh Block Museum of Art, Northwestern University, Evanston, Illinois; Janet Parks at the Avery Architectural and Fine Arts Library, Columbia University, New York; and staff at the New-York Historical Society Library. We are particularly indebted to Mati Maldre for unlimited access to his own superb photographs of Griffin projects in the United States and Australia and to Georgia Lloyd and the late Larry Perkins of Chicago, both of whom knew Marion Mahony Griffin.

In Canberra much appreciation is owed to Ian Batterham of the National Archives of Australia and to staff at the National Library of Australia; in Melbourne to Mary Lewis at the State Library of Victoria, David Sampietro, Dianne Betts, Margaret Ferme and particularly to Jane Carolan at Newman College; and in Sydney to Carol Russell at Willoughby City Library, The Archives Authority of New South Wales, Sydney City Archives, Adrienne Kabos and other members of the Walter Burley Griffin Society, Peter Myers and Marie Nicholls.

Many Powerhouse Museum staff have contributed to both the exhibition and the book, but to be singled out for their specific contribution to this publication are our library and photography staff, and particularly Melanie Cariss and assistant curator, Anat Meiri. Diane Tolson, wife of the US Consul-General in Sydney, has provided invaluable support and assistance as a volunteer on the project for several years. Consulting editor Bernadette Foley's comments helped ensure the cohesiveness of the book's essays. **AW**

ABOUT THE AUTHORS

In order of appearance.

Dr Paul Kruty is associate professor at the School of Architecture, University of Illinois at Urbana–Champaign. Professor Kruty studied architectural history at the University of Chicago, the University of Wisconsin–Milwaukee and Princeton University. He has written extensively on Frank Lloyd Wright, Walter Burley Griffin and the architects of the Prairie School, as well as Chicago art and architecture, and such diverse topics as the development of casement–window hardware and America's first architects' licensing law. His book, *Frank Lloyd Wright and Midway Gardens*, was recently published by the University of Illinois Press. Professor Kruty organised 'The Griffins in Context', an international symposium hosted in October 1997 by the University of Illinois.

Dr Paul Sprague is professor emeritus in the Department of Art History at the University of Wisconsin at Milwaukee. His research interests have focused on the evolution of modern architecture in Chicago at the turn of the century, especially on the work of Louis Sullivan, Frank Lloyd Wright and Walter Burley Griffin. His publications include: *The drawings of Louis Sullivan*, 1979; *Frank Lloyd Wright and Madison*, 1990, editor and contributor; and *Two American architects in India*, 1997, contributor. He has written on a range of topics including the origin and evolution of balloon framing in the midwest and the development of crib construction in midwest grain elevators. During the 1970s he was in charge of the architectural and structural surveys in Illinois required by the *Historic Preservation Act of 1966* and since 1974 has consulted in the field through his firm, Historic Preservation Services.

Dr Anna Rubbo is an associate professor in Architecture at the University of Sydney. She has degrees from the University of Melbourne (BArch) and the University of Michigan (DArch). She has written and lectured on Marion Mahony Griffin and is engaged in writing a social and architectural biography of her.

James Weirick is professor of Landscape Architecture at the University of New South Wales, Sydney. His interest in the Griffins, which extends over 30 years, was initiated through his uncle, Colin C Day, who worked as Walter Burley Griffin's last articled pupil and who lived with the Griffins at Castlecrag in the 1930s. He has written and lectured extensively on diverse aspects of the Griffins' work and lives. During the course of his research he has had the privilege of meeting many of their friends and associates, including Ula Baracchi (Maddocks) whose insight into the Griffins was particularly inspirational.

Christopher Vernon is a senior lecturer in Landscape Architecture in the School of Architecture and Fine Arts at the University of Western Australia. He teaches landscape design and the history and theory of landscape architecture.

His current research focuses on the process by which design values have been transferred into and transformed within colonial and post–colonial cultures, and architecture and landscape design as expressions of place and identity. A passion for Griffin's landscape art — particularly as envisaged for Canberra — was a catalyst for his immigration to Australia. He gratefully acknowledges his wife Tanya's unwavering support across two hemispheres, from the North American prairies to the edge of the Antipodes at Fremantle.

Jeffrey John Turnbull, FRAIA, BArch and DipT&RP from the University of Melbourne, MArch at University of California, Berkeley. Jeffrey is now a senior lecturer in Architecture at the University of Melbourne where he teaches architectural design and history and theory of architecture. Since 1994 he has been a PhD candidate studying the architecture of the Griffins' Newman College at University of Melbourne. Since 1988, he has presented papers and lectures on the Griffins at the University of Illinois at Urbana–Champaign, at AIA Chapters in the midwest USA, at the 1996 St Louis Missouri conference of the Society of Architectural Historians, and at the Graham Foundation in Chicago. He and Peter Navaretti are editors of the forthcoming *catalogue raisonné, The Griffins in Australia and India*.

Anne Watson is a curator of decorative arts and design (pre–1945) at the Powerhouse Museum and has an MA in Fine Arts from the University of Sydney. Her area of curatorial specialisation is furniture and architecture, and she has written and lectured widely on many aspects of nineteenth and twentieth–century furniture history and design. She has curated or co–curated a number of exhibitions including *Take a seat, Bush toys and furniture* and the exhibition that this book accompanies, *Beyond architecture: Marion Mahony and Walter Burley Griffin in America, Australia and India*.

Peter Y Navaretti is an architectural historian presently in the position of Heritage Strategy Planner at Royal Melbourne Institute of Technology (RMIT) University, Melbourne. Since compiling a biography, *Melbourne architects: 1900—1940*, in 1971, he has made a study of the work of Walter Burley Griffin and the Prairie School architects in Australia. In 1992, Peter commenced full–time research on the Griffins in Australia and India as a research associate at the University of Melbourne. As well as writing several journal articles on Griffin's architecture in Australia, he is co–author of the forthcoming book, *The Pyrmont incinerator story* and, with Jeffrey Turnbull, is editor of the forthcoming *catalogue raisonné, The Griffins in Australia and India*.

Dr David Dolan is the director of the Research Institute for Cultural Heritage at Curtin University in Western Australia. He was formerly manager of Collection Development and Research at the Powerhouse Museum.

INDEX

Italics denote photos and illustrations.

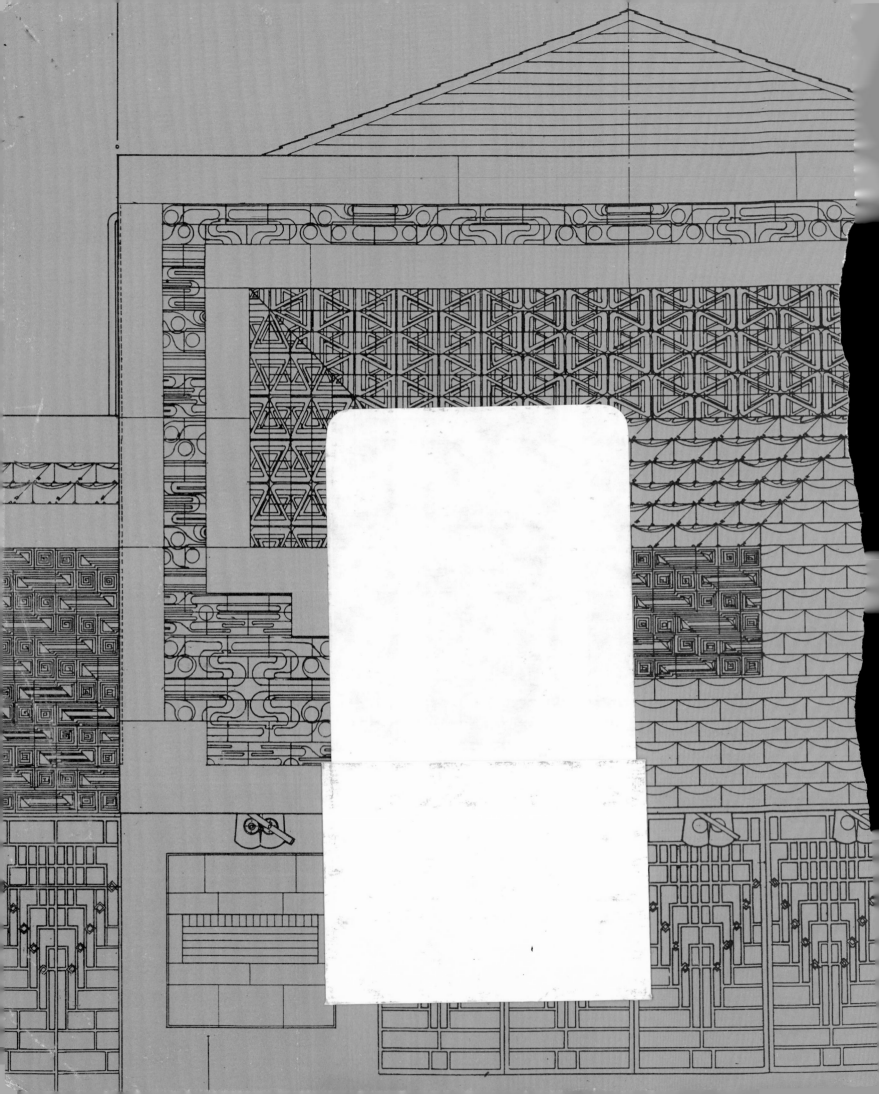